Herbal Medicine for Autoimmune Diseases

Edited by

Cennet Ozay

*Izmir Katip Celebi University, Faculty of Pharmacy,
Department of Basic Pharmaceutical Sciences, Izmir 35620,
Türkiye*

&

Gokhan Zengin

*Department of Biology, Science Faculty, Selcuk University,
Konya 42130, Türkiye*

Herbal Medicine for Autoimmune Diseases

Editors: Cennet Ozay and Gokhan Zengin

ISBN (Online): 978-981-5305-00-5

ISBN (Print): 978-981-5305-01-2

ISBN (Paperback): 978-981-5305-02-9

First published in 2024.

need for a court order if at any point you breach any terms of this License Agreement. In no event will any delay or failure by Bentham Science Publishers in enforcing your compliance with this License Agreement constitute a waiver of any of its rights.

3. You acknowledge that you have read this License Agreement, and agree to be bound by its terms and conditions. To the extent that any other terms and conditions presented on any website of Bentham Science Publishers conflict with, or are inconsistent with, the terms and conditions set out in this License Agreement, you acknowledge that the terms and conditions set out in this License Agreement shall prevail.

Bentham Science Publishers Pte. Ltd.
80 Robinson Road #02-00
Singapore 068898
Singapore
Email: subscriptions@benthamscience.net

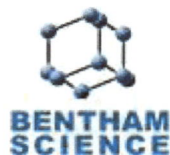

CONTENTS

FOREWORD

Autoimmunity is defined by the presence of self-reactive immune components, while autoimmune diseases result from the combination of autoimmunity and pathology. Both phenomena are significantly increasing worldwide, likely due to changes in our exposure to environmental factors. Significant changes in our diet, exposure to xenobiotics, air quality, infection rates, personal habits, stress levels, and the effects of climate change are all associated with this increase. These factors have significant consequences not only for the individuals and families affected but also for our society and healthcare expenditures. Projections suggest that autoimmune diseases may soon become the most common medical conditions, underscoring the urgency of addressing these complex health challenges.

Autoimmune diseases represent a family of around 100 disorders that share a common pathogenesis, namely an immune-mediated attack on the body's organs. Although immunosuppressive and immunomodulatory drugs represent the fundamental basis for the treatment of autoimmune diseases, there is currently no known radical treatment for these diseases. The use of medicinal plant extracts or secondary plant substances in herbal remedies is currently being investigated as a possible therapeutic approach for autoimmune diseases. Bringing together many studies on autoimmune diseases and herbal remedies in one book titled "Herbal Medicine for Autoimmune Diseases" with great dedication, this will be an excellent resource for researchers studying this topic.

The editors have strived to highlight the potential effectiveness of herbal treatments for autoimmune diseases, while bringing a broad viewpoint from various disciplines, such as pharmacy, medicine, nutrition, and basic sciences. Also, I would like to compliment the authors of all the chapters and acknowledge their efforts in publishing this comprehensive book.

Claudio Ferrante
Pharmaceutical Biology
Department of Pharmacy
Università degli Studi "G. d'Annunzio"
Chieti–Pescara, Italy

PREFACE

Autoimmune diseases are common conditions in which impaired immune activation leads to pathological immune responses directed against either cellular or organ-specific self-antigens. The exact cause of autoimmune diseases is generally unknown, but stress, genetics, and environmental factors have been suggested as possible triggers. However, the connection between these proposed factors and autoimmune diseases is very complex. They are generally undertreated and there is currently no cure for these diseases. Immunosuppressive and immunomodulatory drugs are used in the treatment of autoimmune diseases, but they cannot cure these diseases, only slow down their progression. These medications are also associated with significant adverse effects. Given that the global increase in autoimmune diseases is leading to increased individual and societal suffering as well as higher private and public healthcare costs, the development of appropriate treatments for patients with autoimmune diseases is of great importance.

Therefore, various studies have been carried out to find an effective treatment. Due to their anti-oxidant and anti-inflammatory properties, herbal medicines and their phytochemicals appear to be a promising therapy. Hence, the main purpose of this book is to draw attention to herbal medicines for autoimmune diseases. Data on the therapeutic potential of related medicinal plants for autoimmune diseases can now be accessed from a single source. The book begins with an introductory chapter that serves as a framework for understanding autoimmunity and autoimmune diseases, as well as key principles and components of the immune system. The following chapters of the book, introduce potential medicinal plants and their phytochemicals that can be used in the management of autoimmune diseases such as multiple sclerosis, type 1 diabetes, rheumatoid arthritis, celiac disease, inflammatory bowel disease, Graves' disease, Hashimoto thyroiditis, and systemic lupus erythematosus, which are among the most common autoimmune diseases in the society mentioned with evidence-based data from preclinical and clinical studies. It is known that traditional knowledge about the use of medicinal plants in therapy is an important resource for the discovery of new treatment options and drug targets. One chapter of the book focuses on phyto-nano drug delivery systems that can enhance the efficacy of medicinal plants in the treatment of rheumatoid arthritis. Another chapter provides a comprehensive overview of berry fruits related to autoimmune diseases.

As editors, we would like to express our special thanks to all the contributing authors for making their invaluable chapter contributions in a timely manner, thereby enabling us to publish this book on time. We would also like to express our heartfelt thanks to the team at Bentham Science Publishers for their invaluable help and kind support throughout the editorial process of this book.

Finally, we would like to thank our family members, all the esteemed teachers, friends, colleagues, and students for their constant encouragement, inspiration, and support during the preparation of this book. Together with our contributing authors and publishers, we hope that our efforts will meet the needs of students, academics, researchers, and professionals in the pharmaceutical industry.

Cennet Ozay
Izmir Katip Celebi University, Faculty of Pharmacy
Department of Basic Pharmaceutical Sciences
Izmir 35620, Türkiye

&

Gokhan Zengin
Department of Biology, Science Faculty
Selcuk University, Konya 42130
Türkiye

DEDICATION

We would like to dedicate this book to our beloved fathers, Nurettin and Munir, who passed away in recent years. Our fathers gave us the greatest gift a human being can give another human being: They believed in us. Thanks to them, we could try to touch people's lives through science. Their memories will inspire us every day of our lives.

They will remain forever in our hearts and our prayers.

List of Contributors

Aysun Ozturk	Department of Food Technologies, Ataturk Horticultural Central Research Institution, Yalova 77100, Türkiye
Aybala Temel	Department of Pharmaceutical Microbiology, Faculty of Pharmacy, Izmir Katip Celebi University, Izmir 35620, Türkiye
Abdel Nasser B. Singab	Department of Pharmacognosy, Faculty of Pharmacy, Ain Shams University, Abbassia, Cairo 11566, Egypt Center for Drug Discovery Research and Development, Ain Shams University, Cairo 11566, Egypt
Baran Demir	Department of General Surgery, Faculty of Medicine, Dicle University, Diyarbakır 21280, Türkiye
Betül Rabia Erdoğan	Department of Pharmacology, Faculty of Pharmacy, Izmir Katip Celebi University, Izmir 35620, Türkiye
Cennet Ozay	Izmir Katip Celebi University, Faculty of Pharmacy, Department of Basic Pharmaceutical Sciences, Izmir 35620, Türkiye
Ceylan Dönmez	Department of Pharmacognosy, Faculty of Pharmacy, Selçuk University, Konya, Türkiye
Fatma Ayaz	Department of Pharmacognosy, Faculty of Pharmacy, Selçuk University, Konya, Türkiye
Fatih Gokhan Erbas	Department of Pomiculture, Ataturk Horticultural Central Research Institution, Yalova 77100, Türkiye
Gokhan Zengin	Selcuk University, Faculty of Science, Department of Biology, Konya 42130, Türkiye
Maram M. Aboulwafa	Department of Pharmacognosy, Faculty of Pharmacy, Ain Shams University, Abbassia, Cairo 11566, Egypt
Miray Ilhan	Department of Pharmaceutical Technology, Faculty of Pharmacy, Duzce University, Duzce 81620, Turkiye
Maide Ozturk	Department of Pharmaceutical Technology, Faculty of Pharmacy, Duzce University, Duzce 81620, Turkiye
Mehmet Tolga Kafadar	Department of General Surgery, Faculty of Medicine, Dicle University, Diyarbakır 21280, Türkiye
Nuraniye Eruygur	Department of Pharmacognosy, Faculty of Pharmacy, Selçuk University, Konya, Türkiye
Omayma A. Eldahshan	Department of Pharmacognosy, Faculty of Pharmacy, Ain Shams University, Abbassia, Cairo 11566, Egypt Center for Drug Discovery Research and Development, Ain Shams University, Cairo 11566, Egypt
Shaza H. Aly	Department of Pharmacognosy, Faculty of Pharmacy, Badr University in Cairo (BUC), Cairo 11829, Egypt

Sengul Uysal   Erciyes University Halil Bayraktar Health Services Vocational College, Kayseri 38280, Türkiye
Drug Application and Research Center, Kayseri 38280, Türkiye

Sameh AbouZid   Department of Pharmacognosy, Faculty of Pharmacy, Heliopolis University, Cairo 11785, Egypt

Ünkan Urganci   Department of Food Engineering, Faculty of Engineering, Pamukkale University, Denizli 20160, Türkiye

Yasin Ozdemir   Department of Food Technologies, Ataturk Horticultural Central Research Institution, Yalova 77100, Türkiye

Zinnet Şevval Aksoyalp   Department of Pharmacology, Faculty of Pharmacy, Izmir Katip Celebi University, Izmir 35620, Türkiye

Autoimmune Diseases, Immune System and Herbal Medicine

Cennet Ozay[1,*], Sengul Uysal[2,3] and Gokhan Zengin[4]

[1] *Izmir Katip Celebi University, Faculty of Pharmacy, Department of Basic Pharmaceutical Sciences, Izmir 35620, Türkiye*

[2] *Erciyes University Halil Bayraktar Health Services Vocational College, Kayseri 38280, Türkiye*

[3] *Drug Application and Research Center, Erciyes University, Kayseri 38280, Türkiye*

[4] *Selcuk University, Faculty of Science, Department of Biology, Konya 42130, Türkiye*

Abstract: The immune system is a defense mechanism against infections and illnesses caused by various agents, including bacteria, viruses, and other causative factors. Any disruption in the functioning of the immune system, which is highly organized and precisely regulated, can result in the emergence of immune deficiencies, hypersensitivity reactions, or autoimmune diseases (AIDs). Under certain circumstances, the immune system generates autoantibodies that target their cells, giving rise to AIDs, including multiple sclerosis, type I diabetes, rheumatoid arthritis, inflammatory bowel disease, hashimoto thyroiditis, systemic lupus erythematosus, psoriasis, *etc*. In such cases, the immune system cannot differentiate between foreign substances and the body's own cells. Different factors, such as genetic, epigenetic, and environmental factors, trigger autoimmunity. Currently, autoimmune diseases of various origins are managed using glucocorticoids, non-steroidal anti-inflammatory drugs, immunosuppressive agents, and biological treatments. Nevertheless, a comprehensive cure for these conditions continues to remain beyond our reach. Numerous herbal natural products have been investigated as potential alternative approaches for the management of autoimmune disorders. In this introductory chapter, we summarized the essential concepts of the immune system, the formation, stages, and types of autoimmune diseases, and the role of herbal medicines in the management of AIDs.

Keywords: Autoimmune diseases, Autoimmunity, Herbal medicine, Herbal natural products, Immune system, Natural phytocompounds.

---

* **Corresponding author Cennet Ozay:** Izmir Katip Celebi University, Faculty of Pharmacy, Department of Basic Pharmaceutical Sciences, Izmir 35620, Türkiye; Tel: +90 2323293535, E-mail: cennet.ozay@ikcu.edu.tr

INTRODUCTION

Immunity represents a harmonious equilibrium in which the body possesses effective biological defenses to combat infections, diseases, or unwanted biological intrusions, all while maintaining tolerance to prevent allergies and autoimmune diseases (AIDs). Immune responses result from effective interactions between innate (natural/non-specific) and acquired (adaptive/specific) immune system components. The interaction between phagocytes and micro-organisms in the immune system is a protective pathway, but if inappropriately or improperly organized, it can damage the body and contribute to the development of various long-term inflammatory conditions such as allergies, carcinomas, and AIDs [1].

There are over 80 AIDs known to date, ranging from relatively common to rare conditions. The determination of which AIDs are the most common can vary based on a variety of factors, including patient-reported data, clinical experience, hospital records, and research studies. As of the current information available, some of the more prevalent AIDs include rheumatoid arthritis, multiple sclerosis, type 1 diabetes mellitus, inflammatory bowel disease, hashimoto thyroiditis, Alopecia areata, Graves' disease, celiac disease, systemic lupus erythematosus, and psoriasis, among others. However, the prevalence and ranking of AIDs may change as new research and data emerge [2].

AIDs, arising from the immune system's misalignment targeting the body itself, presents a notable and escalating unmet demand within clinical healthcare. Generally, due to their wide-ranging action rather than being tailored to specific diseases, current treatments are linked to a multitude of side effects. Hence, there is a rising need for the usage of herbal drugs that lead to suppressive effects on the immune system.

The aim of this introductory chapter is (1) to establish a fundamental understanding of the key principles and constituents of the immune system, serving as a framework for comprehending autoimmunity and autoimmune diseases, (2) to provide information about the formation, stages and types of autoimmune diseases, and (3) the role of herbal medicines in the management of autoimmune diseases.

AUTOIMMUNE DISEASES

Autoimmune diseases are a wide range of disorders characterized by chronic inflammation and tissue damage [1, 2]. Autoimmune diseases range from Psoriatic arthritis to Type 1 diabetes mellitus (T1DM), Crohn's disease, Rheumatoid arthritis (RA), Grave's disease (GD), Psoriasis, and Multiple sclerosis (MS). Most of these are incurable, but the symptoms can be managed

[3]. Recently, autoimmune diseases have emerged as a significant health concern with increasing incidence. Autoimmune diseases affect approximately 10% of the population worldwide. These diseases are associated with tremendous economic burden [4, 5]. According to Conrad and Misra [3], autoimmune diseases affect almost one in ten individuals in the UK. In 2019, an estimated 18 million people worldwide were diagnosed with Rheumatoid arthritis [6]. In 2020, the data showed that 2.8 million people were diagnosed with MS worldwide [7]. Crohn's disease has emerged as a global disease and affects over 3.5 million people [8]. There were approximately 8.4 million people worldwide with T1DM in 2021. An estimated number of people with T1DM is expected to reach 13.5-17.4 million by 2040 [9] (Table **1**) (Fig. **1**).

Table 1. Incidence of common autoimmune diseases.

Autoimmune Diseases	*Incidence*	*References*
Psoriatic arthritis (PsA)	0.5-0.8% of the general population.	[10]
Rheumatoid arthritis (RA)	0.5-1% of the global population aged between 25 and 60 years.	[11]
Ankylosing spondylitis (AS)	0.07-0.32% of the general population.	[12]
Multiple sclerosis (MS)	2.8 million people.	[7]
Crohn's disease (CD)	3.5 million people.	[8]
Grave's disease (GD)	1-1.5% of the general population.	[13, 14]
Type 1 diabetes mellitus (T1DM)	8.4 million people.	[15]
Psoriasis	1.5-3% of the general population.	[16]
Scleroderma	30-300 cases per million.	[17]

Causes of Autoimmune Diseases

Autoimmune diseases are multifactorial diseases. The development of AIDs is affected by many factors, including viral infections, genetic predisposition and environmental factors [18, 19]. A large number of autoimmune diseases are more prevalent in women than men [20, 21]. The abnormal activation of chemokine signaling pathways is implicated in the development of several autoimmune diseases including RA and SLE and systemic sclerosis [22]. Tumor necrosis factor-alpha (TNF-α) plays an important role in many AIDs, including RA, MS, PsA, CD, and AS [23].

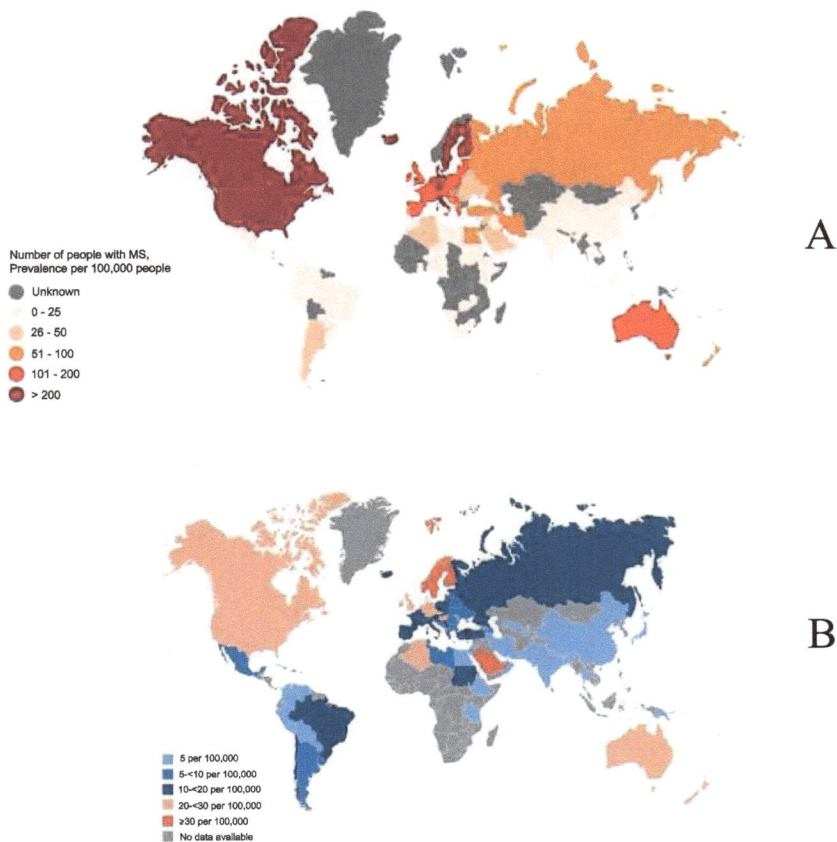

Fig. (1). A: Number of people with MS - prevalence per 100,000 people [7]. B: Map of T1DM in children aged under 15 years [15].

Some Common Factors

Gender

About 78% of people affected by autoimmune diseases are women [24]. Systemic lupus erythematosus (SLE) affects women more commonly than men, with both genetic and hormonal factors. X-chromosome-linked genetic factors have been strongly implicated in the pathogenesis of SLE [25]. MS is more prevalent in women of reproductive years [26]. More than 70% of MS patients are women [27]. Men aged 20-30 years have a higher prevalence of Ankylosing spondylitis (AS) [28]. Graves' disease (GD) is 5-10 times more frequent in women between the ages of 30 and 60 [29].

Genetics

Many genes can contribute to autoimmune diseases. More than 100 genetic loci may confer risk for autoimmune diseases, including SLE and RA [30]. The PTPN22 gene has been demonstrated to be associated with a variety of different autoimmune diseases, including T1DM, RA, and SLE [31]. Rheumatoid arthritis is associated with HLA-DRw4. Furthermore, systemic lupus erythematosus (SLE) has been found to be associated with HLA-DR3 and HLA-B8 [32]. Several studies reported an association between some SNPs in the IFIH1 gene and the risk of various autoimmune diseases, including psoriatic arthritis (PA) and SLE, GD [33]. The NOD2, IL23R and ATG16L1 genes are strongly linked to CD [34, 35]. In T1DM, genetic and familial factors play a significant role in disease susceptibility [36].

External Triggers

In this category, sunlight, diet, stress, drugs, chemicals, viruses, and bacteria can be counted in general. Microorganisms are considered a direct trigger of autoimmune diseases. The pathogenesis of Crohn's disease (CD) is influenced by the gut microbiome [37]. Smoking is a risk factor for the development of RA. This is one example of gene-environment interactions [38]. Furthermore, lifestyle factors including stress, diet, and lack of exercise pose an increased the risk of developing RA [39]. External triggers like smoking, vitamin D, sunlight or infective agents (including Epstein Barr virus) have been implicated in MS pathogenesis [40]. Several viruses have been linked to the development of T1DM, including enteroviruses, such as Coxsackie virus B (CVB), mumps virus, and rotavirus [41]. Obesity has been linked with increased risk of RA, SLE, MS, T1DM [39].

Stages of Autoimmune Diseases

Autoimmune diseases result from the failure of tolerance to self-antigens [42]. Immune tolerance includes central tolerance and peripheral tolerance. Thus, the main problem in the development of autoimmune diseases is the breakdown of some or all of these mechanisms. Currently, autoimmune diseases are triggered by interactions between environmental and genetic factors [43 - 45]. Most autoimmune diseases are long-term diseases. There are three major stage of autoimmune diseases: initiation, propagation, and resolution.

Stage 1 - The Initiation of Autoimmunity

In general, the exact factors responsible for the initiation of autoimmune diseases are not known. Autoimmune diseases are caused by a combination of environmental and genetic factors. Cytokine gene polymorphisms have been linked with a number of autoimmune diseases [46]. The human leukocyte antigen (HLA) is the major genetic factor in autoimmune diseases [47]. IL23R polymorphisms have been determined in ankylosing spondylitis, Crohn's disease, and psoriasis [48].

Stage 2 - The Propagation of Autoimmune Reactions

Propagation phase is defined by tissue damage and progressive inflammation and most patients present with clinical disease in this phase. TNF-α inhibitors play a significant role in the propagation of inflammation in rheumatoid arthritis and psoriatic arthritis. The propagation of autoimmunity can be linked to the progressively growing ratio of effector to regulatory cells [46].

Stage 3 - The Resolution of Autoimmunity

There is generally no care for an autoimmune disease, but the symptoms can be managed by immunosuppression and hormone replacement [49]. The control of autoimmune reactions is probably associated with the induction and activation of regulatory mechanisms. T cells (Tregs) play a significant role in these mechanisms [46].

Types of Autoimmune Diseases

There are 80-100 known autoimmune diseases. Some common autoimmune disorders include Psoriatic arthritis (PsA), Type 1 diabetes mellitus (T1DM), Multiple sclerosis (MS), Crohn's disease (CD), Rheumatoid arthritis (RA), Psoriasis, Graves' disease (GD), Ankylosing spondylitis (AS), Systemic lupus erythematosus (SLE), Celiac disease (CD), Hashimoto thyroiditis (HT) and Inflammatory bowel disease (IBD) [50, 51] (Fig. **2**).

Psoriatic arthritis (PsA) is a chronic inflammatory arthritis and it is characterized as bone proliferation and osteolysis [52, 53]. About 0.5-0.8% of the general population has been infected [10]. The pathogenesis of Psoriatic arthritis is multi-factorial, with demographic, genetic, lifestyle, and clinical [54]. Primarily, psoriatic arthritis is considered to be driven by the IL-23/IL-17 axis and related cytokines [55].

Rheumatoid arthritis (RA) is a chronic autoimmune disease that causes joint inflammation [56]. RA significantly affects their physical function, life quality and emotional state [57]. A total of 18 million people worldwide were living with rheumatoid arthritis in the year 2019 [6]. This disease affects 0.5% to 1% of the global population aged between 25 and 60 years [11]. Rheumatoid arthritis is increasing in the world. The pathogenesis of RA is affected by genetic, immune system and environmental factors (smoking, air pollution, and infections) [58 - 60]. More than 100 have been associated with the RA, and the main influence is associated with HLA-DR (HLA DR1 and HLA DR4) [61]. RA is more common in women than men [62].

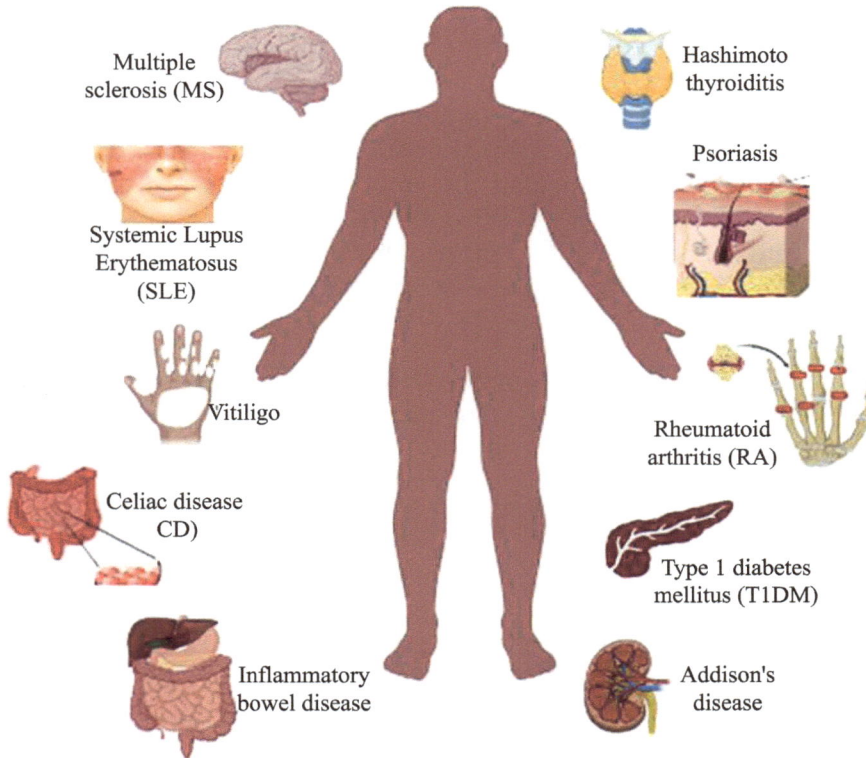

Fig. (2). Some common autoimmune diseases (Drawn in BioRender.com).

Systemic lupus erythematosus (SLE) is a prevalent autoimmune disease related to genetic as well as environmental factors [63]. Women are most affected by Systemic lupus erythematosus [64]. For the past 50 years, the 5-year survival rate of patients with SLE has improved from 50% in the 1950s [65] to 95% in more recent years [66].

Ankylosing spondylitis (AS) is a chronic inflammatory disease [67, 68]. It is characterized by prolonged inflammation of the spine and various joints [69, 70]. The worldwide prevalence of AS ranges from 0.07% to 0.32% [12]. AS occurs more frequently in young adults, most commonly in men aged 20-30 years [28]. AS is strongly linked to human leukocyte antigen (HLA-B27) [71].

Multiple sclerosis (MS) is defined as a chronic inflammatory autoimmune disease of the central nervous system and is associated with gliosis, inflammation, myelin loss, demyelination, and variable degrees of axonal loss [72 - 74]. About 2.8 million people live with MS worldwide [7]. The etiology of MS is not entirely understood. However, genetic and environmental factors (like smoking, vitamin D deficiency, viral infections, sun exposure, gender, and age) may contribute to MS development [75 - 78]. Cytokines are key players during the immunopathogenic process of MS [79].

Crohn's disease (CD) is a chronic inflammatory gastrointestinal disease. This disease is typically characterized by abdominal pain, transmural inflammation, diarrhea, weight loss, and blood in the stool [80, 81]. More than 3.5 million people are affected by Crohn's disease (CD) globally. The prevalence of CD ranged from 3 to 20 cases per 100.000 people [8]. CD is much more common in young people and is a multifactorial disorder caused by genetic, environmental, immunological, and microbial factors [82 - 87].

Graves' disease (GD), the most common cause of hyperthyroidism, is considered a typical autoimmune disease characterized by excessive production of stimulatory antibodies (TSAb) against the TSH receptor [13]. GD is diagnosed in around 1%-1.5% of the global population [13, 14]. Environmental and genetic factors are associated with GD development, such as smoking and stress [14, 88].

Type 1 diabetes mellitus (T1DM) is a chronic autoimmune disorder defined by the destruction of insulin producing β-cells in the pancreas [89]. T1DM in childhood and adolescence is rising and continuously increasing in the world [90]. It is estimated that about 98.200 children under 15 years develop T1DM worldwide in 2019 [15]. T1DM is caused by a combination of environmental, immunological, metabolic, and genetic factors [91].

Psoriasis is a chronic systemic inflammatory skin disorder characterized by vascularization of the skin, erythematous and scaly papules, excessive proliferation of keratinocytes, and plaques [92 - 94]. Psoriasis affects about 1.5-3% of the population globally. This disease occurs equally in women and men [16]. The pathogenesis of psoriasis is complex and still unclear and is determined by a combination of environmental and genetic factors [95].

Systemic sclerosis (SSc), also known as scleroderma, is a complex autoimmune disease characterized by multiple organ involvement, immune system abnormalities, and vasculopathy [96, 97]. Scleroderma predominantly affects women [98]. The prevalence of SSc ranges from 30-300 cases per million individuals [17]. The leading cause of death in scleroderma is pulmonary arterial hypertension (PAH) [99].

Hashimoto's thyroiditis (HT), alternatively referred to as chronic lymphocytic thyroiditis and Hashimoto's disease, is as an autoimmune disorder characterized by the progressive destruction of the thyroid gland. Usually initiating between the ages of 30 and 50, this condition is notably more prevalent in women compared to men [100].

Celiac disease (CD) is an immune reaction to eating gluten, a protein found in wheat, barley and rye, and is sometimes called celiac sprue or gluten-sensitive enteropathy. In celiac disease, the ingestion of gluten begins an immune reaction within the small intestine. As time progresses, this immune response harms the lining of the small intestine, impeding the absorption of certain nutrients (malabsorption). The resultant damage to the intestine frequently gives rise to symptoms like diarrhea, fatigue, weight loss, bloating, and anemia, and it has the potential to give rise to severe complications [101].

Inflammatory bowel disease (IBD) is a group of inflammatory diseases of the colon and small intestine, the most common of which are Crohn's disease and ulcerative colitis. The average incidence of IBD in 2016-2021 was 18 per 100,000 population/year, an increase of 169% compared to 2001-2006 [102].

OVERVIEW OF THE IMMUNE SYSTEM

In principle, the immune system is designed to mount rapid, specific and protective responses against harmful pathogens or their biological products. The mechanisms of immunity operate in a wide range of clinical conditions, ranging from the resolution of infectious diseases, the recognition and rejection of tumors, and the tolerance or rejection of transplanted tissues or organs to autoimmunity and allergy. The immune system consists of two arms, the innate (non-specific) and the adaptive (specific), which are made up of specialized cell types that carry out different effector functions. However, the two arms of the immune system do not operate completely independently. For example, the innate system elicits antigen-specific responses, recruiting cells to the site of infection or injury and delivering antigen to the lymphoid tissue, leading to the activation of adaptive effector cell types [103].

There are two types of adaptive immune response - the primary and the secondary immune response. When a foreign antigen interacts with and activates antigen-specific lymphocytes, a primary immune response is initiated. In general, primary responses are quite effective in resolving infection in combination with innate mechanisms. Immunological memory, which protects against secondary challenges, is also initiated by this first antigenic encounter. Immunological memory is the basis of vaccine strategies and leads to rapid, highly specific clearance of the infectious agent by high-affinity antibody molecules [103].

Innate Immune System

The innate immune system consists of a variety of different mechanisms that perform different functions in host defense. These include, but are not limited to: (i) the phagocytic system; (ii) the acute phase response and complement; (iii) natural killer (NK) cells; and (iv) dendritic cells (DCs) [104]. Speed is a distinguishing feature of the innate immune system, as it swiftly initiates a protective inflammatory response within minutes of encountering a pathogen. Additionally, innate immunity holds a pivotal role in triggering the subsequent adaptive immune response. The innate immune system is emerging as a critical regulator of human inflammatory diseases, although it is critical for host defense against infectious challenges. In fact, the innate immune system is involved in the development of asthma, atopy and several autoimmune diseases, including inflammatory bowel disease, type 1 diabetes and systemic lupus erythematosus [105].

Cells of both haematopoietic and non-haematopoietic origin provide innate immune protection. Mast cells, macrophages, neutrophils, eosinophils, dendritic cells, NK cells and NK T cells are haematopoietic cells involved in the innate immune response. To complement these cellular defensive mechanisms, innate immunity also has a humoral component, including well-characterized components such as complement proteins, C-reactive protein, LPS binding protein, and other collectins, pentraxins, and antimicrobial peptides, including defensins [105].

Adaptive Immune System

In adaptive (acquired/specific) immunity, white blood cells called lymphocytes (B cells and T cells) come across an invader, learn how to attack it, and remember the specific invader so that they can attack it even more efficiently the next time they encounter it. The establishment of acquired immunity requires a period of time following the initial encounter with a novel invader, as lymphocytes need to undergo adaptation to effectively respond to it. But after that, the response is quick. B and T cells work together to kill the invaders. To recognize invaders, T cells need to be helped by cells called antigen-presenting cells, including dendritic cells. These cells ingest an invader and break it into fragments [106].

The adaptive immune system, so called because it is shaped by exposure to antigens, is made up of T and B lymphocytes. Unlike the innate immune system, which relies on a restricted set of pathogen receptors, the adaptive immune system boasts an exceptionally wide-ranging and randomly generated collection of receptors [107]. The advantage of this diversity of receptors is that the adaptive immune system is able to recognize virtually any antigen, but there is a price to pay for this diversity. Firstly, there is the AIDs risk. Receptors designed to recognize self-proteins, such as insulin and myelin, emerge through the stochastic mechanism of gene rearrangement, responsible for producing the receptors expressed by T and B cells. As a result, sophisticated tolerance mechanisms have evolved for the elimination or regulation of self-reactive cells. Secondly, after initial exposure to a pathogen, there is a delay in the generation of a protective adaptive immune response [106].

Cytokines: The Language of Immunity

Cytokines, small soluble proteins, emerge in reaction to antigens, serving as molecular messengers that govern the orchestration of both the innate and adaptive immune systems. These proteins are generated by nearly all cells participating in innate and adaptive immunity, but especially by T- helper (Th) lymphocytes. Activation of cytokine-producing cells triggers their synthesis and secretion of cytokines. The cytokines are then able to bind to specific cytokine receptors on other cells of the immune system and influence their activity in some way [108].

Cytokines display pleiotropy, redundancy, and multifunctionality. Pleiotropy signifies that a given cytokine can influence numerous cell types rather than just one. Redundancy pertains to multiple cytokines having the capability to perform the same role. Multifunctionality denotes that a single cytokine is capable of overseeing various functions [109]. Certain cytokines exhibit antagonistic behavior, where one cytokine triggers a specific defensive action while another cytokine inhibits that same action. On the other hand, some cytokines display synergy, where the combined effect of two different cytokines surpasses the impact of each individual cytokine. Cytokines can be categorized into three functional groups: (i) Cytokines that govern innate immune reactions, (ii) cytokines that regulate adaptive immune reactions, and (iii) cytokines that induce hematopoiesis [110].

Cytokines assume vital roles in the context of innate immunity against various categories of microorganisms. They are discharged during infections caused by pyogenic (pus-forming) extracellular bacteria. These encompass TNF-α, IL-1, IL-10, IL-12, IL-6, IL-18, interferons, as well as chemokines. In addition, the cytokines required for the development and activity of the adaptive immune system are IL-2, IL-4, IL-5, TGFβ, IL-10 and IFN-γ [111].

Immune System and Autoimmune Diseases

Autoimmune disease is regulated by a combination of host genes and environmental factors. Both of these components can enhance vulnerability to autoimmunity by influencing the general responsiveness and characteristics of immune system cells. They also control which antigens, and therefore which organs, are targeted by the immune system. The specificity of antigens and target organs is influenced by factors such as antigen presentation and recognition, antigen expression, and the condition and response of the targeted organs [112].

The immune system is a delicate and active process that balances antimicrobial effector functions with adequate mechanisms for the resolution of inflammation and prevention of self-damage. Certainly, when immune responses become dysregulated, and the equilibrium among these mechanisms is disrupted, it can result in tissue damage, inflammation, and the emergence of autoimmune conditions. The term 'autoimmunity' encompasses a diverse array of conditions where the immune system generates or fails to eliminate antibodies and immune cells that exhibit reactivity against self-antigens (also referred to as autoantigens). This process leads to harm inflicted upon targeted tissues and the development of distinct diseases. The path leading to autoimmunity is intricate and multifaceted and involves numerous presumed stages that entail intricate interactions among diverse immune and stromal cells. This process is affected by external exposures, genetic and epigenetic elements, and unpredictable stochastic incidents that are not yet fully comprehended [113, 114].

The treatment of autoimmune diseases can be seen as a jigsaw puzzle in progress. Current treatments for autoimmune diseases include physiotherapy, non-steroidal anti-inflammatory drugs (NSAIDs), disease-modifying anti-inflammatory drugs (DMARDs), corticosteroids, anti-cytokine therapies, biological inhibitors of T-cell function, inhibition of intracellular signaling pathways, regulatory T cells, B-cell anergy and depletion, stem cell transplantation [115].

Although there is no permanent cure for AIDs, standard treatments aim to reduce the signs and symptoms of the disease and limit the autoimmune processes. The development of more effective medicines to treat and prevent these diseases is therefore urgently needed.

HERBAL MEDICINE WITH THE POTENTIAL ROLE IN THE MANAGEMENT OF AUTOIMMUNE DISEASES

Typical and widely used therapeutic approaches for AIDs encompass the use of analgesics, NSAIDs, and glucocorticoids. In recent years, however, therapeutic immunosuppression and biological agents have also been demonstrated to be beneficial in the treatment of AIDs [116]. Indeed, even as these treatments can alleviate the inflammatory symptoms or slow down disease progression, a complete and definitive cure for AIDs continues to be out of reach. Dietary and herbal natural products are also widely studied as potential strategies for treating AIDs [117, 118].

Herbal medicines and the metabolites extracted from them have a rich historical background in the treatment of immune system disorders. The theory and application of herbal medicines have demonstrated that many of them exhibit immune-regulating properties and are commonly employed to address immune-related ailments [119]. Most of the active constituents of herbal medicines are being investigated for their immunosuppressive properties. These medicinal plants are useful in several immune-mediated diseases, such as autoimmune diseases. Various plants, such as *Curcuma longa, Artemisia annua, Camellia sinensis, Andrographis paniculata, Salvia miltiorrhiza, and Tripterygium wilfordii, etc.* exert their suppressive effects on the immune system [120].

Artemisia annua has been widely used in traditional Chinese medicine to treat autoimmune diseases such as systemic lupus erythematosus and rheumatoid arthritis. In a study evaluating the immunosuppressive effect of ethanol extract of *A. annua* on specific antibodies and cellular responses of mice against ovalbumin, a single dose of 0.25, 0.5 and 1.0 mg of the extract significantly reduced the ovalbumin-specific serum lgG, lgG1 and lgG2b antibody levels and suppressed the splenocyte proliferation [121]. Green tea, derived from the dried leaves of *Camellia sinensis*, is employed in the management of autoimmune arthritis. This is attributed to the anti-inflammatory properties of the polyphenolic compound catechin found in green tea [122]. A study has identified *Cornus officinalis* and *Paeonia lactiflora* as potential therapeutic candidates for treating Rheumatoid arthritis. This is based on their main active compounds, ursolic acid and paeoniflorin, which have been shown to decrease synovial hyperplasia and inflammatory infiltration of joint tissues while promoting synovial apoptosis in a rat model of collagen-induced arthritis [123].

Withania somnifera is extensively utilized in the treatment of Rheumatoid arthritis and Psoriasis. This plant contains various chemical constituents, including alkaloids (such as isopelletierine and anaferine), steroidal lactones (including withanolides and withaferins), saponins (like sitoindoside VII and VIII), and withanolides. These phytochemicals are responsible for exerting immunosuppressive effects by modulating the activity of B and T cells in hyperimmune states [124]. Quercetin is a natural flavonoid found in many fruits, herbs and vegetables. It has been shown to have a wide range of beneficial effects and biological activities, including anti-inflammatory, antioxidant and neuroprotective properties. In several recent studies, quercetin has been reported to attenuate multiple sclerosis, rheumatoid arthritis, systemic lupus erythematosus, and inflammatory bowel disease in human or animal models [125]. As a result, numerous medicinal plants have been used for the treatment of diverse autoimmune disorders. Substantial research has been conducted to elucidate how the constituents of these plants function as immunosuppressive agents. Therefore, their pharmacological properties provide a strong foundation for further confirmatory studies and the potential expansion of their applications in various immunosuppressive therapies.

CONCLUDING REMARKS

Autoimmune diseases represent a global health concern, with increasing rates of morbidity. They are marked by the malfunction and dysregulation of the immune system. The development and pathogenesis of autoimmune diseases involve multiple associations and interacting factors. Many potent conventionally used drugs are available for these diseases, but severe adverse effects besides a high cost accompany their prolonged use. Therefore, there is an unmet need for effective but less expensive medications for AIDs.

Natural plant products belonging to the traditional systems of medicine offer a vast and promising resource in this regard. Several ongoing scientific studies are investigating the use of natural plant products to develop drugs for the treatment of autoimmune diseases. The herbal medicines due to their antioxidant and anti-inflammatory properties have an important role in the management of AIDs. Nonetheless, the scientific evidence for herbal medicines' effects on diseases linked to immune responses and inflammatory processes remains limited. The evidence regarding their clinical effectiveness and safety is even scarcer, often hindered by inadequate characterization/description of the substances being studied.

REFERENCES

[1]   Cao F, Hu LQ, Yao SR, *et al.* P2X7 receptor: A potential therapeutic target for autoimmune diseases. Autoimmun Rev 2019; 18(8): 767-77.
        [http://dx.doi.org/10.1016/j.autrev.2019.06.009] [PMID: 31181327]

[2]   Wigerblad G, Kaplan MJ. Neutrophil extracellular traps in systemic autoimmune and autoinflammatory diseases. Nat Rev Immunol 2023; 23(5): 274-88.
        [http://dx.doi.org/10.1038/s41577-022-00787-0] [PMID: 36257987]

[3]   Conrad N, Misra S, Verbakel JY, *et al.* Incidence, prevalence, and co-occurrence of autoimmune disorders over time and by age, sex, and socioeconomic status: a population-based cohort study of 22 million individuals in the UK. Lancet 2023; 401(10391): 1878-90.
        [http://dx.doi.org/10.1016/S0140-6736(23)00457-9] [PMID: 37156255]

[4]   Ghobadinezhad F, Ebrahimi N, Mozaffari F, *et al.* The emerging role of regulatory cell-based therapy in autoimmune disease. Front Immunol 2022; 13: 1075813.
        [http://dx.doi.org/10.3389/fimmu.2022.1075813] [PMID: 36591309]

[5]   American Autoimmune Related Disease Association. Available from: https://autoimmune.org

[6]   Vos T, Lim SS, Abbafati C, *et al.* Global burden of 369 diseases and injuries in 204 countries and

territories, 1990–2019: a systematic analysis for the Global Burden of Disease Study 2019. Lancet 2020; 396(10258): 1204-22.
[http://dx.doi.org/10.1016/S0140-6736(20)30925-9] [PMID: 33069326]

[7]   Atlas of MS 2020.https://www.atlasofms.org/map/global/epidemiology/number-of-people-with-ms

[8]   Ng SC, Bernstein CN, Vatn MH, *et al.* Geographical variability and environmental risk factors in inflammatory bowel disease. Gut 2013; 62(4): 630-49.
[http://dx.doi.org/10.1136/gutjnl-2012-303661] [PMID: 23335431]

[9]   Gregory GA, Robinson TIG, Linklater SE, *et al.* Global incidence, prevalence, and mortality of type 1 diabetes in 2021 with projection to 2040: a modelling study. Lancet Diabetes Endocrinol 2022; 10(10): 741-60.
[http://dx.doi.org/10.1016/S2213-8587(22)00218-2] [PMID: 36113507]

[10]   Alinaghi F, Calov M, Kristensen LE, *et al.* Prevalence of psoriatic arthritis in patients with psoriasis: A systematic review and meta-analysis of observational and clinical studies. J Am Acad Dermatol 2019; 80(1): 251-265.e19.
[http://dx.doi.org/10.1016/j.jaad.2018.06.027] [PMID: 29928910]

[11]   Alivernini S, Tolusso B, Petricca L, Ferraccioli G, Gremese E. Rheumatoid Arthritis. In: Perricone C, Shoenfeld Y, Eds. Mosaic of Autoimmunity. 2019; pp. 501-26.
[http://dx.doi.org/10.1016/B978-0-12-814307-0.00046-3]

[12]   Zhang X, Sun Z, Zhou A, *et al.* Association Between Infections and Risk of Ankylosing Spondylitis: A Systematic Review and Meta-Analysis. Front Immunol 2021; 12: 768741.
[http://dx.doi.org/10.3389/fimmu.2021.768741] [PMID: 34745144]

[13]   Kahaly GJ. Management of Graves Thyroidal and Extrathyroidal Disease: An Update. J Clin Endocrinol Metab 2020; 105(12): 3704-20.
[http://dx.doi.org/10.1210/clinem/dgaa646] [PMID: 32929476]

[14]   Ehlers M, Schott M, Allelein S. Graves rsquo disease in clinical perspective. Front Biosci 2019; 24(1): 35-47.
[http://dx.doi.org/10.2741/4708] [PMID: 30468646]

[15]   Patterson CC, Karuranga S, Salpea P, Saeedi P, Dahlquist G, Solttimtimesz G, *et al.* Worldwide estimates of incidence, prevalence and mortality of type 1 diabetes in children and adolescents: Results from the International Diabetes Federation Diabetes Atlas. 9th ed. Diabetes Research and Clinical Practice 2019; p. 157.

[16]   Zhou X, Chen Y, Cui L, Shi Y, Guo C. Advances in the pathogenesis of psoriasis: from keratinocyte perspective. Cell Death Dis 2022; 13(1): 81.
[http://dx.doi.org/10.1038/s41419-022-04523-3] [PMID: 35075118]

[17]   van de Zande SC, Abdulle AE, Al-Adwi Y, *et al.* Self-Reported Systemic Sclerosis-Related Symptoms Are More Prevalent in Subjects with Raynaud's Phenomenon in the Lifelines Population: Focus on Pulmonary Complications. Diagnostics (Basel) 2023; 13(13): 2160.
[http://dx.doi.org/10.3390/diagnostics13132160] [PMID: 37443554]

[18]   Fujinami RS, von Herrath MG, Christen U, Whitton JL. Molecular mimicry, bystander activation, or viral persistence: infections and autoimmune disease. Clin Microbiol Rev 2006; 19(1): 80-94.
[http://dx.doi.org/10.1128/CMR.19.1.80-94.2006] [PMID: 16418524]

[19]   Incorvaia E, Sicouri L, Petersen-Mahrt SK, Schmitz KM. Hormones and AID: Balancing immunity and autoimmunity. Autoimmunity 2013; 46(2): 128-37.
[http://dx.doi.org/10.3109/08916934.2012.748752] [PMID: 23181348]

[20]   Angum F, Khan T, Kaler J, Siddiqui L, Hussain A. The Prevalence of Autoimmune Disorders in Women: A Narrative Review. Cureus Journal of Medical Science 2020; 12(5).
[http://dx.doi.org/10.7759/cureus.8094]

[21]   Desai MK, Brinton RD. Autoimmune Disease in Women: Endocrine Transition and Risk Across the

Lifespan. Front Endocrinol (Lausanne) 2019; 10: 265.
[http://dx.doi.org/10.3389/fendo.2019.00265] [PMID: 31110493]

[22]   Miyabe Y, Lian J, Miyabe C, Luster AD. Chemokines in rheumatic diseases: pathogenic role and therapeutic implications. Nat Rev Rheumatol 2019; 15(12): 731-46.
[http://dx.doi.org/10.1038/s41584-019-0323-6] [PMID: 31705045]

[23]   Jang D, Lee AH, Shin HY, *et al.* The role of tumor necrosis factor alpha (TNF-α) in autoimmune disease and current TNF-α inhibitors in therapeutics. Int J Mol Sci 2021; 22(5): 2719.
[http://dx.doi.org/10.3390/ijms22052719] [PMID: 33800290]

[24]   Fairweather D, Frisancho-Kiss S, Rose NR. Sex differences in autoimmune disease from a pathological perspective. Am J Pathol 2008; 173(3): 600-9.
[http://dx.doi.org/10.2353/ajpath.2008.071008] [PMID: 18688037]

[25]   Jiwrajka N, Toothacre NE, Beethem ZT, *et al.* Impaired dynamic X-chromosome inactivation maintenance in T cells is a feature of spontaneous murine SLE that is exacerbated in female-biased models. J Autoimmun 2023; 139: 103084.
[http://dx.doi.org/10.1016/j.jaut.2023.103084] [PMID: 37399593]

[26]   Portaccio E, Bellinvia A, Fonderico M, *et al.* Progression is independent of relapse activity in early multiple sclerosis: a real-life cohort study. Brain 2022; 145(8): 2796-805.
[http://dx.doi.org/10.1093/brain/awac111] [PMID: 35325059]

[27]   Walkiewicz D, Adamczyk B, Maluchnik M, *et al.* The Rate of Hospitalization of Pregnant Women with Multiple Sclerosis in Poland. J Clin Med 2022; 11(19): 5615.
[http://dx.doi.org/10.3390/jcm11195615] [PMID: 36233482]

[28]   Saraux A, Guillemin F, Guggenbuhl P, *et al.* Prevalence of spondyloarthropathies in France: 2001. Ann Rheum Dis 2005; 64(10): 1431-5.
[http://dx.doi.org/10.1136/ard.2004.029207] [PMID: 15817661]

[29]   Subekti I, Pramono LA. Current Diagnosis and Management of Graves' Disease. Acta Med Indones 2018; 50(2): 177-82.
[PMID: 29950539]

[30]   Pisetsky DS. Pathogenesis of autoimmune disease. Nat Rev Nephrol 2023; 19(8): 509-24.
[http://dx.doi.org/10.1038/s41581-023-00720-1] [PMID: 37165096]

[31]   Stanford SM, Mustelin TM, Bottini N, Eds. Lymphoid tyrosine phosphatase and autoimmunity: human genetics rediscovers tyrosine phosphatases Seminars in immunopathology. Springer 2010.

[32]   Kaur G, Mohindra K, Singla S. Autoimmunity—Basics and link with periodontal disease. Autoimmun Rev 2017; 16(1): 64-71.
[http://dx.doi.org/10.1016/j.autrev.2016.09.013] [PMID: 27664383]

[33]   Xiao Z, Luo S, Zhou Y, *et al.* Association of the rs1990760, rs3747517, and rs10930046 polymorphisms in the *IFIH1* gene with susceptibility to autoimmune diseases: a meta-analysis. Front Immunol 2023; 14: 1051247.
[http://dx.doi.org/10.3389/fimmu.2023.1051247] [PMID: 37426657]

[34]   Tsianos EV, Katsanos KH, Tsianos VE. Role of genetics in the diagnosis and prognosis of Crohn's disease. World J Gastroenterol 2011; 17(48): 5246-59.
[http://dx.doi.org/10.3748/wjg.v17.i48.5246] [PMID: 22219593]

[35]   Danese S, Fiorino G, Fernandes C, Peyrin-Biroulet L. Catching the therapeutic window of opportunity in early Crohn's disease. Curr Drug Targets 2014; 15(11): 1056-63.
[http://dx.doi.org/10.2174/1389450115666140908125738] [PMID: 25198784]

[36]   Redondo MJ, Jeffrey J, Fain PR, Eisenbarth GS, Orban T. Concordance for islet autoimmunity among monozygotic twins. N Engl J Med 2008; 359(26): 2849-50.
[http://dx.doi.org/10.1056/NEJMc0805398] [PMID: 19109586]

[37]   Gao X, Sun R, Jiao N, *et al.* Integrative multi-omics deciphers the spatial characteristics of host-gut microbiota interactions in Crohn's disease. Cell Rep Med 2023; 4(6): 101050.
[http://dx.doi.org/10.1016/j.xcrm.2023.101050]

[38]   Klareskog L, Stolt P, Lundberg K, *et al.* A new model for an etiology of rheumatoid arthritis: Smoking may trigger HLA–DR (shared epitope)–restricted immune reactions to autoantigens modified by citrullination. Arthritis Rheum 2006; 54(1): 38-46.
[http://dx.doi.org/10.1002/art.21575] [PMID: 16385494]

[39]   Frazzei G, van Vollenhoven RF, de Jong BA, Siegelaar SE, van Schaardenburg D. Preclinical Autoimmune Disease: a Comparison of Rheumatoid Arthritis, Systemic Lupus Erythematosus, Multiple Sclerosis and Type 1 Diabetes. Front Immunol 2022; 13: 899372.
[http://dx.doi.org/10.3389/fimmu.2022.899372] [PMID: 35844538]

[40]   Ortiz GG, Torres-Mendoza BMG, Ramírez-Jirano J, *et al.* Genetic Basis of Inflammatory Demyelinating Diseases of the Central Nervous System: Multiple Sclerosis and Neuromyelitis Optica Spectrum. Genes (Basel) 2023; 14(7): 1319.
[http://dx.doi.org/10.3390/genes14071319] [PMID: 37510224]

[41]   Limanaqi F, Vicentini C, Saulle I, Clerici M, Biasin M. The role of endoplasmic reticulum aminopeptidases in type 1 diabetes mellitus. Life Sci 2023; 323: 121701.
[http://dx.doi.org/10.1016/j.lfs.2023.121701] [PMID: 37059356]

[42]   Ahmad S, Al-Hatamleh MAI, Mohamud R. Targeting immunosuppressor cells with nanoparticles in autoimmunity: How far have we come to? Cell Immunol 2021; 368: 104412.
[http://dx.doi.org/10.1016/j.cellimm.2021.104412] [PMID: 34340162]

[43]   Anaya JM, Ramirez-Santana C, Alzate MA, Molano-Gonzalez N, Rojas-Villarraga A. The Autoimmune ecology. Front Immunol 2016; 7: 139.
[http://dx.doi.org/10.3389/fimmu.2016.00139] [PMID: 27199979]

[44]   Bogdanos DP, Smyk DS, Rigopoulou EI, *et al.* Twin studies in autoimmune disease: Genetics, gender and environment. J Autoimmun 2012; 38(2-3): J156-69.
[http://dx.doi.org/10.1016/j.jaut.2011.11.003] [PMID: 22177232]

[45]   Ellis JA, Kemp AS, Ponsonby AL. Gene–environment interaction in autoimmune disease. Expert Rev Mol Med 2014; 16: e4.
[http://dx.doi.org/10.1017/erm.2014.5] [PMID: 24602341]

[46]   Rosenblum MD, Remedios KA, Abbas AK. Mechanisms of human autoimmunity. J Clin Invest 2015; 125(6): 2228-33.
[http://dx.doi.org/10.1172/JCI78088] [PMID: 25893595]

[47]   Goris A, Liston A. The immunogenetic architecture of autoimmune disease. Cold Spring Harb Perspect Biol 2012; 4(3): a007260.
[http://dx.doi.org/10.1101/cshperspect.a007260] [PMID: 22383754]

[48]   Vandenbroeck K. Cytokine gene polymorphisms and human autoimmune disease in the era of genome-wide association studies. J Interferon Cytokine Res 2012; 32(4): 139-51.
[http://dx.doi.org/10.1089/jir.2011.0103] [PMID: 22191464]

[49]   Hundt JE, Hoffmann MH, Amber KT, Ludwig RJ. Editorial: Autoimmune pre-disease. Front Immunol 2023; 14: 1159396.
[http://dx.doi.org/10.3389/fimmu.2023.1159396] [PMID: 36865538]

[50]   Mané-Damas M, Hoffmann C, Zong S, *et al.* Autoimmunity in psychotic disorders. Where we stand, challenges and opportunities. Autoimmun Rev 2019; 18(9): 102348.
[http://dx.doi.org/10.1016/j.autrev.2019.102348] [PMID: 31323365]

[51]   Rengasamy KRR, Khan H, Gowrishankar S, *et al.* The role of flavonoids in autoimmune diseases: Therapeutic updates. Pharmacol Ther 2019; 194: 107-31.
[http://dx.doi.org/10.1016/j.pharmthera.2018.09.009] [PMID: 30268770]

[52]   Belasco J, Wei N. Psoriatic arthritis: what is happening at the joint? Rheumatol Ther 2019; 6(3): 305-15.
[http://dx.doi.org/10.1007/s40744-019-0159-1] [PMID: 31102105]

[53]   Merola JF, Espinoza LR, Fleischmann R. Distinguishing rheumatoid arthritis from psoriatic arthritis. RMD Open 2018; 4(2): e000656.
[http://dx.doi.org/10.1136/rmdopen-2018-000656] [PMID: 30167326]

[54]   Zabotti A, De Lucia O, Sakellariou G, *et al.* Predictors, Risk Factors, and Incidence Rates of Psoriatic Arthritis Development in Psoriasis Patients: A Systematic Literature Review and Meta-Analysis. Rheumatol Ther 2021; 8(4): 1519-34.
[http://dx.doi.org/10.1007/s40744-021-00378-w] [PMID: 34596875]

[55]   Fragoulis GE, Siebert S, McInnes IB. Therapeutic Targeting of IL-17 and IL-23 Cytokines in Immune-Mediated Diseases.
[http://dx.doi.org/10.1146/annurev-med-051914-021944]

[56]   Gibofsky A. Epidemiology, pathophysiology, and diagnosis of rheumatoid arthritis: A Synopsis. Am J Manag Care 2014; 20(7) (Suppl.): S128-35.
[PMID: 25180621]

[57]   Malm K, Bergman S, Andersson MLE, Bremander A, Larsson I. Quality of life in patients with established rheumatoid arthritis: A phenomenographic study. SAGE Open Med 2017; 5
[http://dx.doi.org/10.1177/2050312117713647] [PMID: 28611920]

[58]   Nemtsova MV, Zaletaev DV, Bure IV, *et al.* Epigenetic Changes in the Pathogenesis of Rheumatoid Arthritis. Front Genet 2019; 10: 570.
[http://dx.doi.org/10.3389/fgene.2019.00570] [PMID: 31258550]

[59]   Giannini D, Antonucci M, Petrelli F, Bilia S, Alunno A, Puxeddu I. One year in review 2020: pathogenesis of rheumatoid arthritis. Clin Exp Rheumatol 2020; 38(3): 387-97.
[http://dx.doi.org/10.55563/clinexprheumatol/3uj1ng] [PMID: 32324123]

[60]   Radu AF, Bungau SG. Management of Rheumatoid Arthritis: An Overview. Cells 2021; 10(11): 2857.
[http://dx.doi.org/10.3390/cells10112857] [PMID: 34831081]

[61]   Raychaudhuri S, Thomson BP, Remmers EF, *et al.* Genetic variants at CD28, PRDM1 and CD2/CD58 are associated with rheumatoid arthritis risk. Nat Genet 2009; 41(12): 1313-8.
[http://dx.doi.org/10.1038/ng.479] [PMID: 19898481]

[62]   Wu F, Gao J, Kang J, *et al.* B Cells in Rheumatoid Arthritis:Pathogenic Mechanisms and Treatment Prospects. Front Immunol 2021; 12: 750753.
[http://dx.doi.org/10.3389/fimmu.2021.750753] [PMID: 34650569]

[63]   Fava A, Petri M. Systemic lupus erythematosus: Diagnosis and clinical management. J Autoimmun 2019; 96: 1-13.
[http://dx.doi.org/10.1016/j.jaut.2018.11.001] [PMID: 30448290]

[64]   Bentham J, Morris DL, Cunninghame Graham DS, *et al.* Genetic association analyses implicate aberrant regulation of innate and adaptive immunity genes in the pathogenesis of systemic lupus erythematosus. Nat Genet 2015; 47(12): 1457-64.
[http://dx.doi.org/10.1038/ng.3434] [PMID: 26502338]

[65]   Merrell M, Shulman LE. Determination of prognosis in chronic disease, illustrated by systemic lupus erythematosus. J Chronic Dis 1955; 1(1): 12-32.
[http://dx.doi.org/10.1016/0021-9681(55)90018-7] [PMID: 13233308]

[66]   Borchers AT, Keen CL, Shoenfeld Y, Gershwin ME. Surviving the butterfly and the wolf: mortality trends in systemic lupus erythematosus. Autoimmun Rev 2004; 3(6): 423-53.
[http://dx.doi.org/10.1016/j.autrev.2004.04.002] [PMID: 15351310]

[67]   Sieper J, Poddubnyy D. Axial spondyloarthritis. Lancet 2017; 390(10089): 73-84.

[http://dx.doi.org/10.1016/S0140-6736(16)31591-4] [PMID: 28110981]

[68]   Ritchlin CT, Colbert RA, Gladman DD. Psoriatic Arthritis. N Engl J Med 2017; 376(10): 957-70.
[http://dx.doi.org/10.1056/NEJMra1505557] [PMID: 28273019]

[69]   Garcia-Montoya L, Gul H, Emery P. Recent advances in ankylosing spondylitis: understanding the disease and management. F1000 Res 2018; 7: 1512.
[http://dx.doi.org/10.12688/f1000research.14956.1] [PMID: 30345001]

[70]   Houzou P, Koffi-Tessio VE, Oniankitan S, *et al.* Clinical profile of ankylosing spondylitis patients in Togo. Egypt Rheumatol 2022; 44(1): 1-4.
[http://dx.doi.org/10.1016/j.ejr.2021.07.002]

[71]   Picozzi M, Weber M, Frey R, Baumberger H.

[72]   TaŞKapilioĞLu Ö. TaŞKapilioĞLu Ö. Recent advances in the treatment for multiple sclerosis; current new drugs specific for multiple sclerosis. Noro Psikiyatri Arsivi 2018; 55 (Suppl. 1): S15-20.
[PMID: 30692849]

[73]   Sipe JC. Cladribine for multiple sclerosis: review and current status. Expert Rev Neurother 2005; 5(6): 721-7.
[http://dx.doi.org/10.1586/14737175.5.6.721] [PMID: 16274330]

[74]   Carson DA, Wasson DB, Taetle R, Yu A. Specific toxicity of 2-chlorodeoxyadenosine toward resting and proliferating human lymphocytes. Blood 1983; 62(4): 737-43.
[http://dx.doi.org/10.1182/blood.V62.4.737.737] [PMID: 6136305]

[75]   Olsson T. Interactions between genetic, lifestyle/environmental risk factors for multiple sclerosis. Mult Scler J 2022; 28(3) (Suppl.): 4.

[76]   Ramagopalan SV, Dobson R, Meier UC, Giovannoni G. Multiple sclerosis: risk factors, prodromes, and potential causal pathways. Lancet Neurol 2010; 9(7): 727-39.
[http://dx.doi.org/10.1016/S1474-4422(10)70094-6] [PMID: 20610348]

[77]   Afshar B, Khalifehzadeh-Esfahani Z, Seyfizadeh N, Rezaei Danbaran G, Hemmatzadeh M, Mohammadi H. The role of immune regulatory molecules in multiple sclerosis. J Neuroimmunol 2019; 337: 577061.
[http://dx.doi.org/10.1016/j.jneuroim.2019.577061] [PMID: 31520791]

[78]   Compston A, Coles A. Multiple sclerosis. Lancet (Lond, Engl) 2008; 372: 1502-17.

[79]   Egwuagu CE, Larkin J III. Therapeutic targeting of STAT pathways in CNS autoimmune diseases. JAK-STAT 2013; 2(1): e24134.
[http://dx.doi.org/10.4161/jkst.24134] [PMID: 24058800]

[80]   Dulai PS, Singh S, Vande Casteele N, *et al.* Should we divide Crohn's disease into ileum-dominant and isolated colonic diseases? Clin Gastroenterol Hepatol 2019; 17(13): 2634-43.
[http://dx.doi.org/10.1016/j.cgh.2019.04.040] [PMID: 31009791]

[81]   Roda G, Chien Ng S, Kotze PG, *et al.* Crohn's disease. Nat Rev Dis Primers 2020; 6(1): 22.
[http://dx.doi.org/10.1038/s41572-020-0156-2] [PMID: 32242028]

[82]   Rustgi SD, Kayal M, Shah SC. Sex-based differences in inflammatory bowel diseases: a review. Therap Adv Gastroenterol 2020; 13
[http://dx.doi.org/10.1177/1756284820915043] [PMID: 32523620]

[83]   Lungaro L, Costanzini A, Manza F, *et al.* Impact of Female Gender in Inflammatory Bowel Diseases: A Narrative Review. J Pers Med 2023; 13(2): 165.
[http://dx.doi.org/10.3390/jpm13020165] [PMID: 36836400]

[84]   Severs M, Spekhorst LM, Mangen MJJ, *et al.* Sex-Related Differences in Patients With Inflammatory Bowel Disease: Results of 2 Prospective Cohort Studies. Inflamm Bowel Dis 2018; 24(6): 1298-306.
[http://dx.doi.org/10.1093/ibd/izy004] [PMID: 29688413]

[85]   Romberg-Camps M, Dagnelie P, Kester A, Hesselink-Van De Kruijs M, Cilissen M, Engels L, *et al.* Influence of phenotype at diagnosis and of other potential prognostic factors on the course of inflammatory bowel disease. Official journal of the American College of Gastroenterology. ACG 2009; 104(2): 371-83.
[http://dx.doi.org/10.1038/ajg.2008.38]

[86]   Peyrin-Biroulet L, Harmsen SW, Tremaine WJ, Zinsmeister AR, Sandborn WJ, Loftus EV Jr. Surgery in a population-based cohort of Crohn's disease from Olmsted County, Minnesota (1970-2004). Am J Gastroenterol 2012; 107(11): 1693-701.
[http://dx.doi.org/10.1038/ajg.2012.298] [PMID: 22945286]

[87]   Shah SC, Khalili H, Gower-Rousseau C, Olen O, Benchimol EI, Lynge E, *et al.* Sex-based differences in incidence of inflammatory bowel diseases—pooled analysis of population-based studies from western countries. Gastroenterology 2018; 155(4): 1079-83.

[88]   Effraimidis G, Wiersinga WM. MECHANISMS IN ENDOCRINOLOGY: Autoimmune thyroid disease: old and new players. Eur J Endocrinol 2014; 170(6): R241-52.
[http://dx.doi.org/10.1530/EJE-14-0047] [PMID: 24609834]

[89]   DiMeglio LA, Evans-Molina C, Oram RA. Type 1 diabetes. Lancet 2018; 391(10138): 2449-62.
[http://dx.doi.org/10.1016/S0140-6736(18)31320-5] [PMID: 29916386]

[90]   Ziegler R, Neu A. Diabetes in childhood and adolescence: A guideline-based approach to diagnosis, treatment, and follow-up. Dtsch Arztebl Int 2018; 115(9): 146-56.
[PMID: 29563012]

[91]   Cerna M. Epigenetic Regulation in Etiology of Type 1 Diabetes Mellitus. Int J Mol Sci 2019; 21(1): 36.
[http://dx.doi.org/10.3390/ijms21010036] [PMID: 31861649]

[92]   Lima EA, Lima MA. Reviewing concepts in the immunopathogenesis of psoriasis. An Bras Dermatol 2011; 86(6): 1151-8.
[http://dx.doi.org/10.1590/S0365-05962011000600014] [PMID: 22281904]

[93]   Frischknecht L, Vecellio M, Selmi C. The role of epigenetics and immunological imbalance in the etiopathogenesis of psoriasis and psoriatic arthritis. Ther Adv Musculoskelet Dis 2019; 11: 1759720X1988650.
[http://dx.doi.org/10.1177/1759720X19886505] [PMID: 31723358]

[94]   Azuaga AB, Ramírez J, Cañete JD. Psoriatic Arthritis: Pathogenesis and Targeted Therapies. Int J Mol Sci 2023; 24(5): 4901.
[http://dx.doi.org/10.3390/ijms24054901] [PMID: 36902329]

[95]   Lowes MA, Suarez-Farinas M, Krueger JG. Immunology of Psoriasis.
[http://dx.doi.org/10.1146/annurev-immunol-032713-120225]

[96]   Bruni C, Ross L. Cardiac involvement in systemic sclerosis: Getting to the heart of the matter. Best Pract Res Clin Rheumatol 2021; 35(3): 101668.
[http://dx.doi.org/10.1016/j.berh.2021.101668] [PMID: 33736950]

[97]   Truchetet ME, Brembilla NC, Chizzolini C. Current Concepts on the Pathogenesis of Systemic Sclerosis. Clin Rev Allergy Immunol 2021; 64(3): 262-83.
[http://dx.doi.org/10.1007/s12016-021-08889-8] [PMID: 34487318]

[98]   Cutolo M, Soldano S, Smith V. Pathophysiology of systemic sclerosis: current understanding and new insights. Expert Rev Clin Immunol 2019; 15(7): 753-64.
[http://dx.doi.org/10.1080/1744666X.2019.1614915] [PMID: 31046487]

[99]   Tyndall AJ, Bannert B, Vonk M, *et al.* Causes and risk factors for death in systemic sclerosis: a study from the EULAR Scleroderma Trials and Research (EUSTAR) database. Ann Rheum Dis 2010; 69(10): 1809-15.
[http://dx.doi.org/10.1136/ard.2009.114264] [PMID: 20551155]

[100] Ragusa F, Fallahi P, Elia G, *et al.* Hashimotos' thyroiditis: Epidemiology, pathogenesis, clinic and therapy. Best Pract Res Clin Endocrinol Metab 2019; 33(6): 101367.
[http://dx.doi.org/10.1016/j.beem.2019.101367] [PMID: 31812326]

[101] Iversen R, Sollid LM. The Immunobiology and Pathogenesis of Celiac Disease. Annu Rev Pathol 2023; 18(1): 47-70.
[http://dx.doi.org/10.1146/annurev-pathmechdis-031521-032634] [PMID: 36067801]

[102] Caviglia GP, Garrone A, Bertolino C, *et al.* Epidemiology of Inflammatory Bowel Diseases: A Population Study in a Healthcare District of North-West Italy. J Clin Med 2023; 12(2): 641.
[http://dx.doi.org/10.3390/jcm12020641] [PMID: 36675570]

[103] Medina KL. Overview of the immune system Handbook of clinical neurology 133. Elsevier 2016; pp. 61-76.

[104] Yatim KM, Lakkis FG. A brief journey through the immune system. Clin J Am Soc Nephrol 2015; 10(7): 1274-81.
[http://dx.doi.org/10.2215/CJN.10031014] [PMID: 25845377]

[105] Turvey SE. Broide DHJJoA, Immunology C. Innate Immun 2010; 125(2): S24-32.

[106] Gray KJ, Gibbs JE. Adaptive immunity, chronic inflammation and the clock. Semin Immunopathol 2022; 44(2): 209-24.
[http://dx.doi.org/10.1007/s00281-022-00919-7] [PMID: 35233691]

[107] Chaplin DDJJoa, immunology c. Overview of the immune response. 2010; 125(2): S3-S23.

[108] Gulati K, Guhathakurta S, Joshi J, Rai N, Ray AJMI. Cytokines and their role in health and disease: a brief overview. 2016; 4(2): 00121.

[109] Ramani T, Auletta CS, Weinstock D, *et al.* Cytokines. Int J Toxicol 2015; 34(4): 355-65.
[http://dx.doi.org/10.1177/1091581815584918] [PMID: 26015504]

[110] Dinarello CAJEjoi. Historical insights into cytokines. 2007; 37(S1): S34-S45.

[111] Abraha RJAVAS. Review on the role and biology of cytokines in adaptive and innate immune system. 2020; 2: 2.

[112] Marrack P, Kappler J, Kotzin BLJNm. Autoimmune disease: why and where it occurs. 2001; 7(8): 899-905.

[113] Firestein GS, McInnes IB. Immunopathogenesis of Rheumatoid Arthritis. Immunity 2017; 46(2): 183-96.
[http://dx.doi.org/10.1016/j.immuni.2017.02.006] [PMID: 28228278]

[114] Ma L, Roach T, Morel L. Immunometabolic alterations in lupus: where do they come from and where do we go from there? Curr Opin Immunol 2022; 78: 102245.
[http://dx.doi.org/10.1016/j.coi.2022.102245] [PMID: 36122544]

[115] Rosato E, Pisarri S, Salsano F. Current strategies for the treatment of autoimmune diseases. J Biol Regul Homeost Agents 2010; 24(3): 251-9.
[PMID: 20846473]

[116] Alexander T, Bondanza A, Muraro P, Greco R, Saccardi R, Daikeler T, *et al.* SCT for severe autoimmune diseases: consensus guidelines of the European Society for Blood and Marrow Transplantation for immune monitoring and biobanking. 2015; 50(2): 173-80.
[http://dx.doi.org/10.1038/bmt.2014.251]

[117] Javadi B, Sahebkar A. Natural products with anti-inflammatory and immunomodulatory activities against autoimmune myocarditis. Pharmacol Res 2017; 124: 34-42.
[http://dx.doi.org/10.1016/j.phrs.2017.07.022] [PMID: 28757189]

[118] Busto R, Serna J, Perianes-Cachero A, *et al.* Ellagic acid protects from myelin-associated sphingolipid loss in experimental autoimmune encephalomyelitis. Biochim Biophys Acta Mol Cell Biol Lipids

2018; 1863(9): 958-67.
[http://dx.doi.org/10.1016/j.bbalip.2018.05.009] [PMID: 29793057]

[119] Divya M, Vijayakumar S. Traditional South Indian Herbal Plants for a Strong Immune System Traditional Herbal Therapy for the Human Immune System. CRC Press 2021; pp. 245-54.
[http://dx.doi.org/10.1201/9781003137955-9]

[120] Sahoo B, Banik BJICR. Medicinal plants: Source for immunosuppressive agents. 2018; 2: 106.

[121] Zhang Y, Sun H. Immunosuppressive effect of ethanol extract of *Artemisia annua* on specific antibody and cellular responses of mice against ovalbumin. Immunopharmacol Immunotoxicol 2009; 31(4): 625-30.
[http://dx.doi.org/10.3109/08923970902932954] [PMID: 19874232]

[122] Lorenzo JM, Munekata PESJAPJoTB. Phenolic compounds of green tea: Health benefits and technological application in food. 2016; 6(8): 709-19.

[123] Huang L, Hu S, Shao M, Wu X, Zhang J, Cao G. Combined Cornus Officinalis and Paeonia Lactiflora Pall Therapy Alleviates Rheumatoid Arthritis by Regulating Synovial Apoptosis *via* AMPK-Mediated Mitochondrial Fission. Front Pharmacol 2021; 12: 639009.
[http://dx.doi.org/10.3389/fphar.2021.639009] [PMID: 33897428]

[124] Vetvicka V, Vetvickova JJNAjoms. Immune enhancing effects of WB365, a novel combination of Ashwagandha (Withania somnifera) and Maitake (Grifola frondosa) extracts. 2011; 3(7): 320.

[125] Shen P, Lin W, Deng X, *et al.* Potential Implications of Quercetin in Autoimmune Diseases. Front Immunol 2021; 12: 689044.
[http://dx.doi.org/10.3389/fimmu.2021.689044] [PMID: 34248976]

CHAPTER 2

Role of Herbalism in Systemic Lupus Erythematosus Treatment

Maram M. Aboulwafa[1], Shaza H. Aly[2], Sameh AbouZid[3], Omayma A. Eldahshan[1,4,*] and Abdel Nasser B. Singab[1,4,*]**

[1] *Department of Pharmacognosy, Faculty of Pharmacy, Ain Shams University, Abbassia, Cairo 11566, Egypt*

[2] *Department of Pharmacognosy, Faculty of Pharmacy, Badr University in Cairo (BUC), Cairo 11829, Egypt*

[3] *Department of Pharmacognosy, Faculty of Pharmacy, Heliopolis University, Cairo 11785, Egypt*

[4] *Center for Drug Discovery Research and Development, Ain Shams University, Cairo 11566, Egypt*

Abstract: The well-known inflammatory and autoimmune condition known as systemic lupus erythematosus (SLE) causes symptoms in the kidneys, the skin, the brain, and the heart. It can also cause complications that affect several organs. The diversity in organ involvement and heterogeneous conditions of patients led to the complicated management of SLE. Increasingly, there is evidence highlighting the importance of phytochemicals in both dietary and non-dietary contexts in the management of SLE without side effects.

Herein, we discuss the role of different plant extracts with their metabolites and their modes of action against SLE updated to 2023, in addition to the incorporation of herbal formulas in the management of the SLE. The present work is an overview of different plant extracts and their secondary metabolites with significant anti-inflammatory, antioxidant, and immunomodulation in SLE. The current chapter focuses on the various targets, mechanisms, and pathways of natural products that manage SLE. Based on the current work, it can be inferred that natural products show potential as effective agents in the medical care of SLE.

Keywords: Autoimmune, Anti-inflammatory, Diet, Herbalism, Immunomodulation, Mode of action, Natural compounds, Plant extract, Systemic lupus erythematosus, Treatment.

***Corresponding authors Omayma Eldahshan and Abdel Nasser B. Singab:** Department of Pharmacognosy, Faculty of Pharmacy, Ain Shams University, Abbassia, Cairo 11566, Egypt & Center for Drug Discovery Research and Development, Ain Shams University, Cairo 11566, Egypt; Tel: +20 0224051120; E-mails: oeldahshan@pharma.asu.edu.eg, dean@pharma.asu.edu.eg

INTRODUCTION

Systemic lupus erythematosus (SLE) exemplifies a typical autoimmune-related multisystemic condition [1]. SLE is a persistent and recurrent autoimmune disorder characterized by inflammation that impacts various organs, such as the skin, joints, blood, and kidneys. The involvement of macrophages in the pathogenesis of this condition has been deemed significant [2]. Numerous immunological abnormalities and excessive inflammatory responses that affect numerous organs throughout the body are features of SLE [3, 4]. Manifestations vastly differ across patients, SLE can manifest with a range of symptoms, such as malar, discoid, and photosensitive skin rashes, arthralgias, and arthritis, constitutional symptoms like pain and fatigue, psychiatric disturbances, and potentially extensive internal organ disease involving renal, pulmonary, cardiac, neurologic, and/or gastrointestinal systems. Additionally, SLE is characterized by the production of autoantibodies, which can be detected by the presence of an antinuclear antibody (ANA) (Fig. **1**). Systemic lupus erythematosus is reported to have an incidence ranging from 0.3 to 31.5 instances per 100,000 people annually, and its adjusted prevalence is predicted to be close to or greater than 50 to 100 cases per 100,000 people [5].

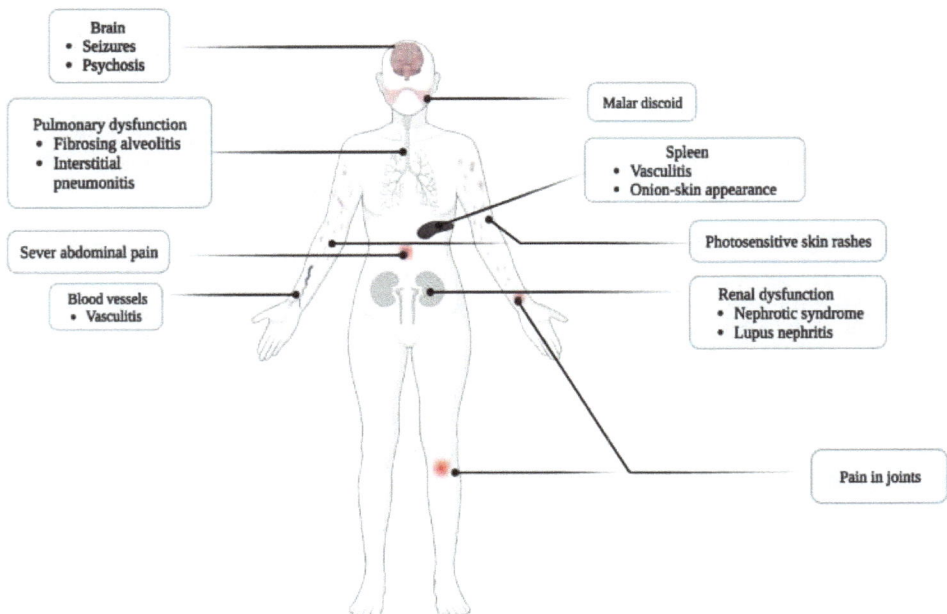

Fig. (1). Manifestations of systemic lupus erythematosus (SLE).

Treatment for SLE as a whole necessitates a comprehensive, interdisciplinary strategy that goes well beyond treating immunological dysfunction and takes into account the patient's distinct and particular demands. For dermatologic indications, strategies might range from conservative treatments like acetaminophen and non-steroidal anti-inflammatory medicines to alleviate joint pain, and the use of topical steroid creams and cautious sunscreen to more targeted immunologic therapy with varying degrees of immunosuppressive potential. Complementary and alternative medicine (CAM) is frequently used in conjunction with conventional treatment. Patients with active SLE, who often have a diminished quality of life and significant unmet needs, commonly turn to CAM as an additional approach to managing their condition [6]. CAM usage is linked to worse health status in Yucatan, Mexico individuals with SLE [7].

Increasingly, there is evidence highlighting the importance of herbalism as well as its secondary metabolites in the management of different conditions of inflammation, oxidative stress, and apoptosis [8 - 12]. Also, the presence of variable secondary metabolites belong to different classes, including volatile oils, alkaloids, flavonoids, terpenoids, and fatty acids [13 - 16] that regulate abnormal responses in the innate and adaptive immune systems, kidneys, intestines, bone system (including chondrocytes, osteoclasts, joints, and paw tissues). This suggests that plant metabolites could be a potential target for managing SLE without adverse effects [17]. Many reports have documented the utilization of diverse plant species in the management of SLE; most of them belong to families namely, Celastraceae, Lamiaceae, Apiaceae, Ranunculaceae, Oleaceae, Theaceae, Simaroubaceae, Achariaceae, Campanulaceae, Urticaceae, Oxalidaceae, Clusiaceae, Hypericaceae, Schisandraceae, Menispermaceae, Orobanchaceae, Rubiaceae, Paeoniaceae, Rutaceae, Dioscoreaceae, Alismataceae, Cornaceae, Rosaceae, Alismataceae, Lauraceae, Nelumbonaceae, Linaceae, Solanaceae, Polygonaceae, Equisetaceae and others. Fungi are also involved such as fungi from Ganodermataceae, Ophiocordycipitaceae and Polyporaceae families [18 - 20].

This aim of this chapter is to assemble and analyse the prospective applications of herbalism, including plant extracts and isolated bioactive compounds, in managing SLE. The focus is on exploring the efficacy and mechanisms of action of these natural remedies, as well as discussing the role of isolated bioactive compounds in combating the disease. It is hoped that this chapter will inspire further research by scientists towards the development of potent medications for the therapy of SLE.

PLANT EXTRACTS WITH POTENTIAL ROLE IN THE MANAGEMENT OF SLE

Among the most common plant species historically used to treat a variety of inflammatory and autoimmune conditions such as SLE is *Tripterygium wilfordii,* a native Asian plant known as Thundergod vine (Celastraceae) [21], which is a Chinese herbal medicine that has a role in urinary protein reduction with a slight reduction in the severity of lymphadenopathy and arthritis, as well as the extension of mice survival at a dose of 20 mg/kg, three times a week [22]. The roots are well known for their immunosuppressive glycosides [23, 24] that have immunosuppression and anti-inflammatory effects, but with a potential to induce hepatotoxicity with long-term use, which is linked to the control of the signaling pathway for interleukin-17 (IL-17) and T helper 17 (Th17) cell differentiation where their effectiveness in the treatment of SLE is based on the same mechanisms [25]. It is important to be cautious about the prolonged use of *T. wilfordii* in women with SLE, as it may lead to a reduction in their bone mineral density levels [26].

In China, in addition to *T. wilfordii,* the roots of the *Glycyrrhizaglabra* (Fabaceae) are also used [27]. Where the extract from the roots of *G.glabra* could prevent the abnormal development of immune complexes linked to SLE [28, 29].

Artemisia annua (Sweet wormwood) (Asteraceae) has been widely used to treat SLE as well. It also contains a lot of vitamins and amino acids, and its function in the immunological and pro-inflammatory pathways is apparent through its immunosuppression and anti-inflammatory activities [19, 30]. Another preliminary trial found that *Artemisia apiacea* (Sweet Annie) (Asteraceae) was successful in treating SLE through its immunosuppressive properties [23, 31].

The roots of *Sophora flavescens* (Fabaceae) at a dose of 5.8 mg/mouse daily decrease glomerular capillaries, serum anti-dsDNA antibodies, and proteinuria, and IFN-γ expression in splenocyte culture and corrects Th1/Th2 imbalances. Also, it demonstrated a substantial improvement in renal glomerular damage [32].

The ethanolic extract of *Nelumbo nucifera* (Nelumbonaceae) has the potential to function as an immunomodulatory agent for treating SLE, it inhibited the growth of cells and the generation of cytokines in human peripheral blood mononuclear cells, which were activated by phytohemagglutinin, a mitogen that specifically targets T lymphocytes [33].

In vitro experiments have shown that *Atractylodes ovata* (Asteraceae)and *Ligustrum lucidum* (Oleaceae) can enhance the impaired production of IL-2 in SLE patients. *Angelica sinensis*, known as female ginseng (Apiaceae), has been observed to enhance the impaired production of IL-2 in SLE patients *in vitro* and extend the lifespan of female mice. Also, *Codonopsis pilosula* (Campanulaceae) exhibits the same activity *via* inhibiting anti-ds DNA production [34].

Bupleurum smithii var. parvifolium (Apiaceae) is known to have advantageous effects on inflammatory conditions, and the crude polysaccharides derived from its roots have been shown to have potent immunomodulatory properties in murine peritoneal macrophages. These effects were achieved by enhancing phagocytic activity while also restraining the production of pro-inflammatory mediators that are associated with the lupus [35].

Centella asiatica (Apiaceae) has been used by Ayurveda, Chinese, and Sri Lankan Traditional Medicines to treat lupus [36]. In 1956, the healing properties of *Centella* extract were studied, which showed a tendency to promote quicker healing of wounds and a positive effect on the overall healing process. However, in 1965, the local application of *Centella* extract in powder form for the treatment of lupus erythematosus was found to cause signs of intolerance [37].

Tinospora cordifolia (Menispermaceae) is an Ayurveda treatment for SLE. For patients with vasculitis, this particular treatment has been successfully used without any complications or relapses for over a year, and it has been effective in saving limbs [1].

Eurycoma longifolia (Simaroubaceae) can suppress key cellular pathways in endothelial cells that inhibit angiogenesis, it has been suggested that this substance could be utilized as a treatment for SLE, which is a pathophysiological condition that is believed to be dependent on angiogenesis [38].

Tripterygium hypoglaucum Hutch (Celastraceae), is the plant source of Kunming Shanhaitang, a traditional Chinese medicine that was initially documented in the Compendium of Materia Medica and is extensively employed in the management of several autoimmune disorders, including SLE. The therapeutic properties of *T. hypoglaucum* are largely attributed to its unique compound composition, with terpenoids and alkaloids being the essential active components. Two of these components namely triptolide and celastrol have demonstrated strong immunosuppressive and anti-inflammatory activities [39].

Withania somnifera (Solanaceae), known as ashwagandha, root powder has a prophylactic effect against SLE. In a mouse model of lupus, it has been demonstrated to suppress multiple indicators of inflammation, including pro-inflammatory cytokines like IL-6 and tumor necrosis factor (TNF)-α, as well as nitric oxide and reactive oxygen species (ROS) in both serum and ascitic fluid [40].

The agglutinin of *Urtica dioica* (Urticaceae), known as common nettle alters the production of autoantibodies and does not cause evident clinical signs of lupus and nephritis in mice [41]. Flavonoids found in the leaves and lectin present in the roots have been reported to possess immune-stimulating properties that could be a valuable therapeutic option for managing systemic lupus [42].

Regarding lupus nephritis, a severe SLE manifestation with a negative prognostic effect [43], *Linum usitatissimum* (Linaceae), rich in inflammation-modulating omega-3 essential fatty acids and phytoestrogen lignans makes it advantageous for individuals with lupus nephritis, as it serves as a renoprotective agent [23, 44]. *Averrhoa carambola* (Oxalidaceae) fruit juice and *Plantago major* (Plantaginaceae) decoction can be used generally for the treatment of lupus nephritis in Singapore [45].

Regarding cutaneous lupus erythematosus, green tea; *Camellia sinensis* (Theaceae) functions as an immune-modulating agent derived from food [46]. Studies indicate that Epigallocatechin gallate (EGCG) can boost the number of regulatory T cells, which have a vital role in immune function by regulating cytokine production and controlling cutaneous lupus erythematosus [47]. *Illicium verum* Hook. f. (Schisandraceae) extract directly impacts the treatment of IFN-γ-dependent elements *via* influencing keratinocyte-T cell interactions [48].

Olea europaea (Oleaceae) produces olive oil that possesses anti-inflammatory, immunomodulatory, and antioxidant characteristics, making it a potentially effective remedy for inflammatory and ROS-related disorders [49].

PLANTS' SECONDARY METABOLITES WITH POTENTIAL ROLE IN THE MANAGEMENT OF SLE

Plant-derived secondary metabolites offer a range of biological functions and therapeutic benefits, and are often studied for their potential therapeutic applications including alkaloids, flavonoids, terpenoids, and polyphenols [50 - 55]. Several compounds derived from plant species have potential activity against the management of SLE [56, 57].

Isogarcinol [1], a polyisoprenylated benzophenone, is derived from *Garcinia mangostana* (Clusiaceae) and exhibits a substantial immunosuppressive effect on SLE. Significant reductions in proteinuria, correction of abnormal serum biochemical indicators, following oral treatment of 60 mg/kg, lower kidney histopathology scores and lower serum antibody levels were observed. By regulating the irregular activation of CD4 T cells responsible for inflammation, it was able to lower the expression of inflammatory genes and cytokines in the kidneys and peritoneal macrophages, resulting in reduced proteinuria and decreased levels of serum antibodies [58].

Astiblin [2], a flavonoid isolated from *Hypericum perforatum* (Hypericaceae), was observed to delay disease development when administered orally as a preventative measure before or after beginning of the disease in lupus prone MRL/*lpr* mice. Treatment with astiblin resulted in reduced levels of circulating anti-nuclear antibodies, as well as several serum cytokines IFN-g, IL-17A, IL-1b, TNF-a, and IL-6, and a prominent reduction in the number of functional activated T and B cells [59].

Oridonin [3], a terpenoid isolated from *Isodon serra* (Lamiaceae), regulates B-cell activating factor. It slows down B-cell maturation and differentiation, which improves the symptoms of SLE in MRL/*lpr* mice [60].

Dihydroartemisinin [4], a sesquiterpene lactone and the primary active artemisinin metabolite, which is obtained from the *Artemisia annua* has the potential to be therapeutically useful in the treatment of SLE by suppressing lupus-induced cell activation in mice. This is achieved by reducing Toll-like receptor 4-mediated inflammatory signaling through the inhibition of its expression and interferon (IFN) regulatory factor activation in spleen cells of mice [3]. Artemisinin and Arteether, a potent semisynthetic analog of dihydroartemisinin, have a selective immunosuppressive activity [61].

Celastrol [5], a highly potent bioactive triterpenoid extracted from *Tripterygium wilfordii*, is recognized for its potential therapeutic benefits in treating autoimmune disorders such as SLE. It functions by regulating the activity of several signaling proteins, including IL-10, TNF, and matrix metalloprotein 9, which control pathways related to mitogen-activated protein kinase, TNF, and apoptosis. Celastrol is anticipated to influence networks primarily associated with cytokine activity, cytokine receptor binding, receptor-ligand activity, receptor regulator activity, and cofactor binding [62]. Celastrol has shown promise as a potential treatment for autoimmune diseases that are dependent on the interferon (IFN) response. This is because it targets the activation of interferon regulatory factor 3 (IRF3), resulting in the downregulation of IFN response that can be induced by cytosolic nucleic acids in both *in vitro* and *in vivo* studies. In mouse models, celastrol has been observed to reduce the development of autoantibodies and excessive T-cell activation [63].

Another diterpenoid from *T. wilfordii* is triptolide [6], which has a role in the management of the treatment of SLE through the migration of Tc and Th cells to Tcl and Tc2 to keep the relative state of equilibrium, maintaining the integrity of Tc and Th cells at a distinct level, influencing inflammatory response and immunological response [64]. Both *in vivo* and *in vitro*, triptolide might activate regulatory T cells (T_{reg}) [65].

(S)-Armepavine [7] the major isolated compound from the seeds of *Nelumbo nucifera*, was observed to hinder the development of lymphadenopathy and increase the lifespan of MRL/MpJ-*lpr/lpr* mice. This outcome seems to be accomplished by reducing splenocyte proliferation, inhibiting the expression of genes related to interleukin-2 (IL-2), interleukin-4, interleukin-10, and interferon-γ (IFN-γ), lowering urinary protein and anti-double stranded DNA autoantibody synthesis, immunological complex accumulation in glomeruli, and hypercellularity; hence a mitigating impact on SLE symptoms [33].

Total glucosides of Paeony (TGP), extracted from Paeony root, is one of the traditional Chinese medicines. Studies have demonstrated that it possesses anti-inflammatory and immuno-regulatory properties, and can be therapeutically beneficial in SLE through the downregulation of Foxp3 promoter methylation levels that alter DNA methylation status in T cell subset to improve SLE. They could also induce regulatory T cell (Treg) differentiation in lupus CD4+ T cells [66].

Paeoniflorin [8], a nitrogen glycoside isolated from the roots of *Paeonia lactiflora* (Paeoniaceae) has immunosuppressive and anti-inflammatory properties by inhibiting the IL-1 receptor-associated kinase1- nuclear factor kappa-B (IRAK1-NNF-κB) pathway in peritoneal mouse macrophages [67].

Aconitine [9], an alkaloid and the main active constituent of *Aconitum lamarckii* (Ranunculaceae), decreases elevated blood leukocyte counts, reduces the serum level of anti-double-stranded DNA (anti-dsDNA) antibody, ameliorates renal histopathologic damage, reduces IgG deposit in glomerular, decreases the levels prostaglandin E2, IL-17a and IL-6 in murine model of SLE and hence inhibits the progression of disease and ameliorates the pathologic lesion of SLE [68].

Icariin [10], a prenylated flavonol glycoside, the main bioactive component isolated from Chinese medicine *Epimedium alpinum* (Berberidaceae), alleviates murine lupus nephritis *via* inhibiting NF-κB activation and NLRP3 inflammasome activation [69]. Icaritin, obtained from *Epimedium alpinum* L. (Berberidaceae) at a dose of 2 mg/kg daily inhibits CD4 (+) T cell overactivity, promotes forkhead box P3 (FoxP3)-IL17a balance and promotes the inhibition of Treg cell in both human SLE peripheral blood mononuclear cells (PBMC) and mice. It has immunosuppressive action by lowering Th1/Th2 cytokines and inhibiting the activation of T cells [70].

Apigenin [11], 4',5,7-trihydroxyflavone can be found abundantly in various dietary plants, including parsley, thyme, peppermint, olives, and chamomile, and is considered a natural inhibitor of cyclooxygenase-2 (COX-2) and NF-κB derived from dietary plants. It is capable of suppressing inflammation in lupus. It suppresses autoantigen-presenting and stimulatory antigen-presenting cell capabilities that are required for the activation and growth of autoreactive Th1 and Th17 cells, as well as B cells, in lupus [71].

Kaempferol [12], is an anti-inflammatory polyphenol antioxidant that has been found in several plant species and is frequently used in conventional medicine to treat and prevent inflammatory illnesses like SLE. Kaempferol exerts its anti-inflammatory action *via* increasing FOXP3 expression level in Treg cells and hence enhancing their suppressive function [72].

Curcumin [13], the active ingredient of *Curcuma longa* (Zingiberaceae) [19], has the potential to be used in SLE treatment. It acts primarily against hyperproliferative cells through modulating Th17/Treg balance specifically on CD4+ T cells of SLE patients [73]. Curcumin exerts a protective effect, which may be *via* its interaction with Treg cells, against lupus nephritis in mice. Curcumin can decrease the proteinuria level and serum levels of IgG1, IgG2a, and anti-dsDNA IgG antibodies, along with reducing IgG immune complex deposition in the glomeruli and hence decreasing renal inflammation [43]. It intensely decreases spleen size as well as decreased serum anti-dsDNA levels-induced NLR Family Pyrin Domain Containing 3 (NLRP3) inflammasome activation in podocytes of lupus-prone mice, which is a key player in lupus nephritis [74]. It inhibits the expression and activation of the signaling protein, proline-rich tyrosine kinase 2 (PYK2), in peripheral blood mononuclear cells *in vitro* and in lupus nephritis patients, it inhibits the production of the costimulatory molecules CD40L and CTLA-4 along with PBMC proliferation [75].

Resveratrol [14], represents a prominent bioactive component of stilbene phytoalexins, which was initially extracted from the roots of an oriental medicinal plant *Polygonum cuspidatum* (Polygonaceae) [76]. It has mitigating effects in lupus mice *via* attenuating proteinuria, immunoglobulin deposition in kidney and glomerulonephritis as well as IgG1 and IgG2a in the serum. Additionally, resveratrol reduces CD4 IFN+ Th1 cells and the Th1/Th2 cell ratio, and inhibits *in vitro* antibody formation, and B cell proliferation. It also suppresses CD69 and CD71 activity on CD4+ T cells and also decreases CD4+ T cell proliferation [77]. It can inhibit pro-inflammatory mediators *via* enhancing FcγRIIB gene transcription and hence FcγRIIB expression in B cells, which results in selectively depleted plasma cells in both spleen and bone marrow, leading to a decrease in serum autoantibody titers, leading to the improvement of lupus nephritis and prolonged survival. Resveratrol is considered here as an anti-inflammatory agent [78], in addition to its beneficial role in reducing lipid deposition and atherosclerosis in SLE patients as well [79].

Piperine [15] is an alkaloid that led to reductions in proteinuria and creatinine in the urine of lupus mice. Combining 25 mg/kg body weight of resveratrol with 2.5 mg/kg body weight of piperine resulted in additional decreases in IFN-α, IL-6, TNF-α expression, and oxidative stress in lupus mice [80].

Quercetin [16], derived from *Fagopyrum tataricum* (Polygonaceae), is a potent immunomodulator as in mice with SLE-like symptoms, it can lower the levels of serum antibodies, CD4+ T cell activation, and the expression of T-bet, GATA-3, and certain cytokines [19, 81].

Salvianolic acid A [17], obtained from the roots of *Salvia miltiorrhiza* (Lamiaceae), reduces kidney damage in mice with SLE *via* the suppression of phosphorylation of IkappaB kinases, IkappaB, and NFκB [82].

Cryptotanshinone [18], a prominent quinoid diterpene found in the dried roots of Salvia miltiorrhiza, has the potential to serve as a novel therapeutic agent for SLE. It inhibits STAT3 activation in double-negative T cells, which hence postpones the onset of lupus nephritis and ameliorates SLE progression [83].

Arctigenin [19], is a bioactive component found in the seeds of *Arctium lappa* (Asteraceae) and could be a promising therapeutic target for SLE treatment. Studies have revealed that it functions as a negative regulator of inflammatory responses by controlling the IFN-I-mediated differentiation of germinal center B cells and the pathogenesis of SLE [84].

Andrographolide [20], an abundant component of the plant Andrographis, inhibits NF-κB activity [85].

Linear Furanocoumarins, also referred to as psoralens, are a subclass of phenolic compounds in the coumarins group that exhibit an exclusive behavior when exposed to UVA light, making the use of these molecules possible in extracorporeal photopheresis or combination therapy with psoralen and UVA radiation for the treatment of various autoimmune disorders, including SLE [86].

H1-A, an isolated, pure molecule that is a kind of ergosterol, is helpful in SLE because it can reduce lymph node hyperplasia and the formation of anti-ds-DNA antibodies *in vitro*, which helps to extend mice's life. It is also beneficial in lupus nephritis because it slows the evolution of proteinuria by reducing the growth of glomerular mesangial cells [87].

Traditional medicine is considered an alternative treatment option for SLE, which can be achieved by using herbal remedies or fungi. *Ganoderma tsugae* (Ganodermataceae), a fungus [88], reduces anti-dsDNA autoantibody formation, and cellular infiltration of internal organs [23], decreases the impact of proteinuria, and improves mice's chances of survival [89]. Fungi, *Ophiocordyceps sinensis* [formerly known as *Cordyceps sinensis*] (Ophiocordycipitaceae) can improve defective IL-2 production in patients with SLE *in vitro* and prolong the life span of female mice *via* inhibiting anti-ds DNA production [34]. In Mauritius, *Polygonum aviculare* (Polygonaceae) seeds are used traditionally for lupus [20].

Cordyceps sinensis could reduce lymphadenectasis and enhance renal function [90]. Cordyceps protein could improve lupus nephritis as in mice, it prevents the formation of proteinuria and renal inflammatory infiltration, which diminishes renal fibrosis. In mice, it modifies the STAT3/mTOR/NF-κB signaling pathway and significantly reduces the levels of IL-6 and IL-1β [91].

The structures of secondary metabolites with the potential role in SLE management are shown in Fig. (**2**).

HERBAL FORMULAS WITH POTENTIAL ROLE IN THE MANAGEMENT OF SLE

Several herbal formulas are effective in treating SLE. *Rehmannia glutinosa* (Orobanchaceae), *Artemisia annua*, *Hedyotis diffusa* (Rubiaceae), *Paeonia veitchii* (Paeoniaceae), *Centella asiatica*, *Paeonia suffruticosa* (Paeoniaceae), *Citrus medica* (Rutaceae), *Cimicifuga foetida* (Ranunculaceae) and *Glycyrrhiza uralensis* (Fabaceae) are utilised in China to create a recognized, efficient hospital prescription for the treatment of SLE, which is named 'Jieduquyuziyin'. It may inhibit the activation of peritoneal macrophages in lupus mice [92] and the inflammatory activity of their bone marrow-derived macrophages [93]. It affects macrophage activation and pro-inflammatory response *via* the inhibition of the NOTCH1/NF-κB pathway [94]. In the hepatocytes of mice, it could dramatically decrease the expression of glucocorticoid-induced gluconeogenesis [94]. It increases prednisone efficacy in SLE and lupus nephritis treatment *via* increasing nuclear factor erythroid 2-related factor 2 expression, hence reducing the kidneys' degree of stress caused by oxidation [95]. It prevents the development of aortic plaque, promotes lipid metabolism, and boosts the expression of genes that control cholesterol efflux and prevent the creation of foam cells in macrophages [96].

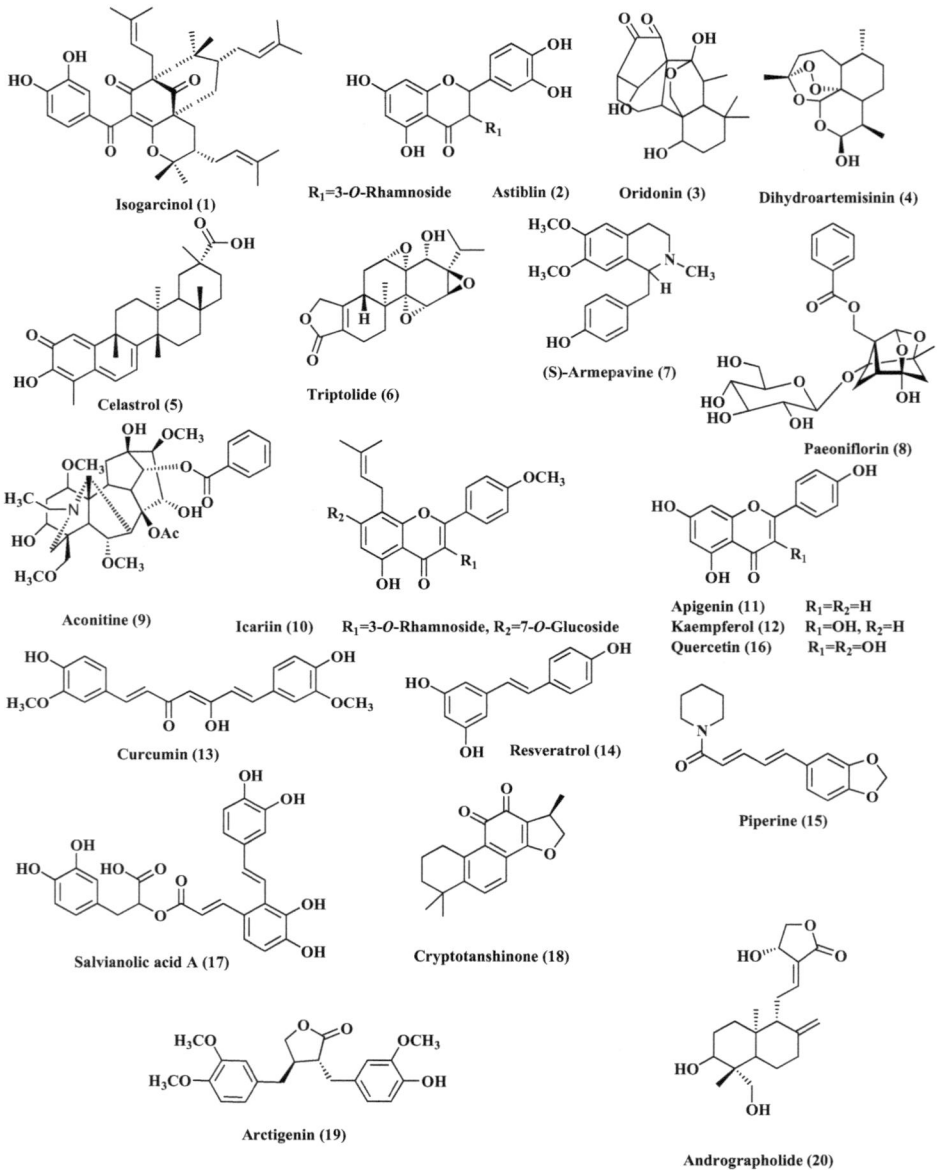

Fig. (2). The chemical structure of secondary metabolites with a potential role in SLE management.

Another formula known as Jiedu-Quyu-Ziyin Fang (JQZF) consists of Chinese medicinal herbs *Rehmannia glutinosa*, *Artemisia annua*, *Hedyotis diffusa*, *Paeonia anomala* (Paeoniaceae), *Centella asiatica*, *Citrus medica*, *Actaea cimicifuga* (Ranunculaceae), *Glycyrrhiza uralensis* and Coix lacryma-jobi (Poaceae) have been shown to be beneficial in the treatment of SLE by preventing lymphocyte proliferation and survival when given in a dry form. The formula JQZF has the ability to activate blood and remove stasis while also cooling blood and eliminating toxins [97].

The prepared root of *Rehmannia glutinosa*, rhizome of *Dioscorea opposite* (Dioscoreaceae), sclerotia of fungus *Poria cocos* (Polyporaceae), root bark of *Paeonia suffruticosa*, rhizome of *Alisma plantago-aquatica* (Alismataceae), processed fruit of *Cornus officinalis* (Cornaceae), root of *Salvia miltiorrhiza* and root of *Panax Notoginseng* (Araliaceae) are used to formulate "Dan-Chi-Liu-Wei" combination, which has an effect on decreasing SLE activity [98].

Oral administration of Ba-Wei-Di-Huang-Wan, traditional Chinese medicine which is composed of *Rehmannia glutinosa* root, *Cornus officinalis* fruit, *Dioscorea batatas* (Dioscoreaceae) rhizome, *Alisma orientale* (sometimes listed as a subspecies of *Alisma plantago-aquatica*) [99] (Alismataceae) rhizome, hoelen (Poria cocos), root bark of *Paeonia suffruticosa*, *Cinnamomum cassia* (Lauraceae) bark and *Aconitum carmichaelii* (Ranunculaceae) tuber [100], improves IL-4 production in mice while inhibiting IFN production and IL-12 mRNA expression.

Hachimi-jio-gan, another name for (ba-wei-di-huang-wan), historical Japanese herbal remedy [101, 102], that reduces proteinuria and immune complex deposition in the kidney can be used to treat lupus [89].

Another herbal powder San-Miao-San, "four marvels" consisting of *Atractylodes macrocephala* (Asteraceae), *Phellodendron chinensis* (Rutaceae), *Achyranthes bidentata* (Amaranthaceae) and *Coix lacryma-jobi* (Poaceae) extract along with fungi *Ganoderma lucidum* (Ganodermataceae) has been found to reduce anti-dsDNA antibodies concentrations, induce Treg and Breg formation, reduce IL-21, IL-10, and IL-17A and increase IL-2 and IL-12p70 in the serum. This traditional medicine is used in cutaneous lupus erythematosus [19, 103].

Foeniculum vulgare (Apiacae), the dried woody septum inside the walnut *Juglans regia* (Juglandaceae) fruit hull/kernel, dried leaves of *Epimediium brevicornu* (Berberidaceae), *Zanthoxylum bungeanum* (Rutaceae), Aconitum root, *Cyathula officinalis* (Amaranthaceae), *Allium sativum* bulb (Amaryllidaceae) and *Piper wallichii* (Piperaceae) are used to formulate a prescription and Chinese patent medicine for the relief from various infections and itching caused by lupus erythematosus [104].

The root of *Astragalus membranaceus* (Fabaceae), *Rehmannia glutinosa*, *Cornus officinalis* fruit, *Paeonia lactiflora*, root bark of *Paeonia suffruticosa*, and Hedyotidis diffuse are used to formulate "Zi Shen Qing", which is a safe and effective Chinese herbal medication to reduce SLE disease and reduce the dosage of corticosteroids in people with mild to moderate SLE [105].

Bupleurum falcatum (Apiaceae), *Pinellia ternate* (Araceae0, *Scutellaria baicalensis* (Lamiaceae), *Panax ginseng* (Araliaceae, *Glycyrrhiza uralensis*, *Ziziphus jujuba* (Rhamnaceae), *Zingiber officinale* (Zingiberaceae), *Atractylodes lancea* (Asteraceae), *Polyporus umbellatus* (lyporaceae), *Alisma orientale*, Hoelen (*Wolfiporia cocos*) [106] and *Cinnamomum cassia* are used to formulate "Sairei-to" [107]. It is a Japanese herbal formula which decreases the titers of anti-DNA antibodies, the quantity of IgG deposited at the dermo-epidermal interface, and lymphoproliferation [107].

Gentiana rigescens (Gentianaceae), *Scutellaria baicalensis*, *Gardenia jasminoides* (Rubiaceae), *Alisma orientale*, *Clematis montana* (Ranunculaceae), *Plantago asiatica* (Plantaginaceae), *Angelica sinensis*, *Rehmannia glutinosa*, *Bupleurum chinense* (Apiaceae) and *Glycyrrhizae uralensis* are used to formulate a Chinese herbal medicine "Longdan Xiegan Tang" [108], which is useful in reducing distress in SLE as it decreases oxidative stress linked to the development of the illness in animals [108].

Kan Jang (a combination of extracts from the plants *Andrographis paniculata* (Acanthaceae) and *Eleutherococcus senticosus* (Araliaceae) and *Andrographis* has been widely used in Asia as a folk treatment to treat inflammatory diseases [85], and is possibly beneficial for treating SLE by deregulating the IFN signalling pathway [109].

IM253, a new formulation of herbal extract originating from *Rosa canina* (Rosaceae), *Tanacetum vulgare* (Asteraceae), and *Urtica dioica*, which has been enriched with selenium, reduces IL-17 cytokine expression, which is increased in SLE, considerably [110].

Herbal shampoo and a combination of extracts from plants namely, leaf extract of *Urtica urens* and root extract of *Urtica dioica* (Urticaceae), flower extract *of Matricaria chamomilla* (Asteraceae), aerial part extract of *Achillea millefolium* (Asteraceae), *Ceratonia siliqua* (Fabaceae) fruit extract and *Equisetum arvense* (Equisetaceae) leaf extract can be used in the management of Telogen effluvium a temporary hair loss condition [111] that represents the overall SLE disease activity throughout time [112].

It is vital to improve the patient's nutritional status, which may be done with the help of tonics, healthy food, bracing air, cod liver oil, and the thoughtful application of stimulants. Mercury and iodides must be banned [113]. By providing enough potential macronutrients and micronutrients to control the overall disease activity, a low-calorie, low-protein diet with high levels of fiber, polyunsaturated fatty acids, vitamins, minerals, and polyphenols controls the immunological and inflammatory activities of SLE [18]. Calorie restriction improves survival in murine lupus models by delaying the onset of the disease, eliminating the abnormal increase in IL-12, IFN-γ, IgA, and IgG2 productions, abolishing the decline in CD8+ T lymphocytes, and delaying the development of kidney disease and age-related immune dysfunction and complications [89].

In lupus animal models, the quantity and quality of dietary fat change immune responses and influence the severity of illness. It has been discovered that reducing the severity of autoimmune illnesses may be accomplished by increasing the daily consumption of dietary omega-3 polyunsaturated fatty acids like fish oil and linseed oil. A diet low in essential fatty acids (linoleic and linolenic acid) can lower arachidonic acid, which in turn lowers the formation of pro-inflammatory eicosanoids, prostaglandins, and leukotriene metabolites, suppresses the creation of autoantibodies, and lessens the severity of nephritis [89].

Retinoids are already used to treat dermatologic illnesses. Retinoic acids, the oxidised version of vitamin A, play significant regulatory functions in cellular proliferation and differentiation [89]. Th17 and Treg are out of balance in vitamin A deficiency, which worsens the course of SLE [114]. Given that the T lymphocyte and macrophage contain considerable amounts of vitamin D and its receptor, vitamin D plays a crucial role in immunomodulation. According to a survey, vitamin D needs enough calcium to stop the onset of SLE, but bone health and metabolism should also be taken into account. For SLE patients seeking protection against oxidative stress, optimal vitamin E intake is advised. Unless there is an increase in oxidative stress, very high vitamin E consumption should be avoided [89].

SLE mostly affects females throughout their reproductive years, however amenorrhea is frequently linked to it [115]. Studies have shown how oestrogen contributes to the development of SLE and speeds up the illness. Due to their structural resemblance to 17β-estradiol, phytoestrogens, a varied range of naturally occurring plant chemicals, seem to bind to estrogen receptors more preferentially (immunosuppressive impact) than estrogen receptors (immuno-stimulatory role). One of the most prevalent phytoestrogens, isoflavone also has anti-inflammatory properties that are advantageous for chronic renal illness. It has been discovered that soy germ isoflavone prevents from immune complex deposition and renal inflammation. Selective oestrogen receptor modulators have demonstrated favorable effects on the severity of the illness in lupus mice and exert an anti-inflammatory impact. Examples include *Medicago sativa* (Fabaceae) (alfalfa) sprout extracted in ethyl acetate and indole-3-carbinol (in Cruciferous vegetables) [89]. Although, the non-protein amino acid L-canavanine in alfalfa may exacerbate the disease severity in patients with SLE [116]. Phytoestrogens such as coumestrol may be valuable in treating lupus [23].

Tar and lead solutions are advantageous in treating lupus erythematosus. Similarly, internal administration of arsenic may be utilized with considerable benefits. There are various techniques available to prevent ulceration. One such method involves using caustics such as chloride of zinc or acid nitrate of mercury to dress the affected area. This can result in complete healing of the patch with just a single application, and the sores tend to granulate well and heal quickly. Another method involves using actual cautery, which is highly effective but may cause slow healing of burns despite causing less pain. The erosion treatment is another option that causes less pain and leads to rapid and complete healing of the sore. This treatment can be employed during the early stages of ulceration [113].

Traditional Chinese Medicine diagnostic expert system, designed using the latent class model and disease pattern coding system (B-code), can perform well in identifying the disease patterns of SLE and may be clinically useful for Traditional Chinese Medicine physicians who have identified different SLE patterns [117]. By using B-code with nonlinear canonical correlation analysis, pattern differentiation and principle of treatment for SLE can be assessed using clinical datasets [118].

CONCLUDING REMARKS

In this book chapter, various extracts and isolated compounds were examined for their potential in managing SLE. Earlier studies have identified numerous plant extracts from the Fabaceae, Asteraceae, Apiaceae, and Linaceae families that exhibit impressive anti-inflammatory and immunosuppressive effects, which play a crucial role in controlling SLE symptoms. Furthermore, we investigated bioactive compounds that have been identified and isolated from various parts of plants belonging to flavonoids, alkaloids, and terpenoids. Additionally, we examined the role of several herbal formulas, primarily in Chinese traditional medicine, and their constituents' effects on managing SLE. Based on our findings, we can conclude that plant extracts, isolated compounds, and herbal formulas hold promise as potential candidates for developing new drugs aimed at managing SLE symptoms. However, in order to conduct a comprehensive examination of the efficacy, bioavailability, safety profile, and clinical trial results of the isolated compounds and diverse extracts as agents derived from plants, further research is necessary.

REFERENCES

[1]   Gururaja D, Hegde V. Ayurvedic management of systemic lupus erythematosus overlap vasculitis. J Ayurveda Integr Med 2019; 10(4): 294-8. Available from: https://www.sciencedirect.com/science/article/pii/S0975947617304333
[http://dx.doi.org/10.1016/j.jaim.2018.08.007] [PMID: 31421962]

[2]   Katsiari CG, Liossis SNC, Sfikakis PP. The pathophysiologic role of monocytes and macrophages in systemic lupus erythematosus: a reappraisal. Semin Arthritis Rheum 2010; 39(6): 491-503. Available from: https://www.sciencedirect.com/science/article/pii/S0049017208002011
[http://dx.doi.org/10.1016/j.semarthrit.2008.11.002] [PMID: 19147182]

[3]   Huang X, Xie Z, Liu F, *et al.* Dihydroartemisinin inhibits activation of the Toll-like receptor 4 signaling pathway and production of type I interferon in spleen cells from lupus-prone MRL/lpr mice. Int Immunopharmacol 2014; 22(1): 266-72. Available from: https://www.sciencedirect.com/science/article/pii/S1567576914002562
[http://dx.doi.org/10.1016/j.intimp.2014.07.001] [PMID: 25027631]

[4]   Yu H, Nagafuchi Y, Fujio K. Clinical and immunological biomarkers for systemic lupus erythematosus. Biomolecules 2021; 11(7): 928.
[http://dx.doi.org/10.3390/biom11070928] [PMID: 34206696]

[5]   Gergianaki I, Fanouriakis A, Repa A, *et al.* Epidemiology and burden of systemic lupus erythematosus in a Southern European population: data from the community-based lupus registry of Crete, Greece. Ann Rheum Dis 2017; 76(12): 1992-2000.
[http://dx.doi.org/10.1136/annrheumdis-2017-211206] [PMID: 28780511]

[6]   Haija AJ, Schulz SW. The role and effect of complementary and alternative medicine in systemic lupus erythematosus. Rheum Dis Clin North Am 2011; 37(1): 47-62. Available from: https://www.sciencedirect.com/science/article/pii/S0889857X10000980
[http://dx.doi.org/10.1016/j.rdc.2010.11.005] [PMID: 21220085]

[7]   Alvarez-Nemegyei J, Bautista-Botello A. Complementary or alternative therapy use and health status in systemic lupus erythematosus. Lupus 2009; 18(2): 159-63.
[http://dx.doi.org/10.1177/0961203308095946] [PMID: 19151118]

[8]   Saber FR, Aly SH, Khallaf MA, El-Nashar HAS, Fahmy NM, El-Shazly M, *et al.* Hyphaene thebaica (Areceaeae) as a Promising Functional Food: Extraction, Analytical Techniques, Bioactivity, Food, and Industrial Applications. Food Anal Methods 2022; 1-21.

[9]   Aly SH, El-Hassab MA, Elhady SS, Gad HA. Comparative Metabolic Study of *Tamarindus indica* L.'s Various Organs Based on GC/MS Analysis, *In Silico* and *In Vitro* Anti-Inflammatory and Wound Healing Activities. Plants 2022; 12(1): 87.
[http://dx.doi.org/10.3390/plants12010087] [PMID: 36616217]

[10]   Aly SH, Eldahshan OA, Al-Rashood ST, *et al.* Chemical Constituents, Antioxidant, and Enzyme Inhibitory Activities Supported by *In-Silico* Study of *n*-Hexane Extract and Essential Oil of Guava Leaves. Molecules 2022; 27(24): 8979.
[http://dx.doi.org/10.3390/molecules27248979] [PMID: 36558111]

[11]   El-Nashar HAS, Aly SH, Ahmadi A, El-Shazly M. The Impact of Polyphenolics in the Management of Breast Cancer: Mechanistic Aspects and Recent Patents. Recent Patents Anticancer Drug Discov 2022; 17(4): 358-79.
[http://dx.doi.org/10.2174/1574892816666211213090623] [PMID: 34961465]

[12]   Elebeedy D, Ghanem A, Aly SH, *et al.* Synergistic antiviral activity of Lactobacillus acidophilus and Glycyrrhiza glabra against Herpes Simplex-1 Virus (HSV-1) and Vesicular Stomatitis Virus (VSV): experimental and In Silico insights. BMC Microbiol 2023; 23(1): 173. Available from: https://bmcmicrobiol.biomedcentral.com/articles/10.1186/s12866-023-02911-z
[http://dx.doi.org/10.1186/s12866-023-02911-z] [PMID: 37391715]

[13] Hussiny , Elissawy A, Eldahshan O, Elshanawany M, Singab AN. Phytochemical investigation using GC/MS analysis and evaluation of antimicrobial and cytotoxic activities of the lipoidal matter of leaves of Sophora secundiflora and Sophora tomentosa. Archives of Pharmaceutical Sciences Ain Shams University 2020; 4(2): 207-14.
[http://dx.doi.org/10.21608/aps.2020.38371.1039]

[14] Aly SH, Kandil NH, Hemdan RM, *et al.* GC/MS Profiling of the Essential Oil and Lipophilic Extract of *Moricandia sinaica* Boiss. and Evaluation of Their Cytotoxic and Antioxidant Activities. Molecules 2023; 28(5): 2193.
[http://dx.doi.org/10.3390/molecules28052193] [PMID: 36903440]

[15] Aly SH, Elissawy AM, Mahmoud AMA, *et al.* Synergistic Effect of *Sophora japonica* and *Glycyrrhiza glabra* Flavonoid-Rich Fractions on Wound Healing: *In Vivo* and Molecular Docking Studies. Molecules 2023; 28(7): 2994.
[http://dx.doi.org/10.3390/molecules28072994] [PMID: 37049756]

[16] Aly SH, Elissawy AM, Salah D, *et al.* Phytochemical Investigation of Three *Cystoseira* Species and Their Larvicidal Activity Supported with In Silico Studies. Mar Drugs 2023; 21(2): 117.
[http://dx.doi.org/10.3390/md21020117] [PMID: 36827158]

[17] Cao F, Cheng MH, Hu LQ, *et al.* Natural products action on pathogenic cues in autoimmunity: Efficacy in systemic lupus erythematosus and rheumatoid arthritis as compared to classical treatments. Pharmacol Res 2020; 160: 105054. Available from: https://www.sciencedirect.com/science/article/pii/S1043661820313621
[http://dx.doi.org/10.1016/j.phrs.2020.105054] [PMID: 32645358]

[18] Islam MA, Khandker SS, Kotyla PJ, Hassan R. Immunomodulatory effects of diet and nutrients in systemic lupus erythematosus (SLE): a systematic review. Front Immunol 2020; 11: 1477.
[http://dx.doi.org/10.3389/fimmu.2020.01477] [PMID: 32793202]

[19] Lubov JE, Jamison AS, Baltich Nelson B, Amudzi AA, Haas KN, Richmond JM. Medicinal plant extracts and natural compounds for the treatment of cutaneous lupus erythematosus: a systematic review. Front Pharmacol 2022; 13: 802624.
[http://dx.doi.org/10.3389/fphar.2022.802624] [PMID: 35431950]

[20] Suroowan S, Pynee KB, Mahomoodally MF. A comprehensive review of ethnopharmacologically important medicinal plant species from Mauritius. S Afr J Bot 2019; 122: 189-213. Available from: https://www.sciencedirect.com/science/article/pii/S0254629918311116
[http://dx.doi.org/10.1016/j.sajb.2019.03.024]

[21] Zhuang XM, Liu PX, Zhang YJ, *et al.* Simultaneous determination of triptolide and its prodrug MC002 in dog blood by LC–MS/MS and its application in pharmacokinetic studies. J Ethnopharmacol 2013; 150(1): 131-7. Available from: https://www.sciencedirect.com/science/article/pii/S0378874113005722
[http://dx.doi.org/10.1016/j.jep.2013.08.018] [PMID: 23994469]

[22] Zhang XY, Tsuchiya N, Dohi M, *et al.* Prolonged survival of MRL-lpr/lpr mice treated with Tripterygium Wilfordii Hook-F. Clin Immunol Immunopathol 1992; 62(1): 66-71. Available from: https://www.sciencedirect.com/science/article/pii/009012299290023H
[http://dx.doi.org/10.1016/0090-1229(92)90023-H] [PMID: 1728981]

[23] Yarnell E, Abascal K. Lupus erythematosus and herbal medicine. Altern Complement Ther 2008; 14(1): 9-12.
[http://dx.doi.org/10.1089/act.2008.14105]

[24] Ye X, Zhao H, Liu J, Lu B, Shao J, Wang J. 1530/EJE-20-0857). Eur J Endocrinol 2021; 184(2): X1.
[http://dx.doi.org/10.1530/EJE-20-0857z] [PMID: 33539318]

[25] Chen Y, Wang YF, Song SS, Zhu J, Wu LL, Li XY. Potential shared therapeutic and hepatotoxic mechanisms of Tripterygium wilfordii polyglycosides treating three kinds of autoimmune skin diseases by regulating IL-17 signaling pathway and Th17 cell differentiation. J Ethnopharmacol 2022;

296: 115496. Available from: https://www.sciencedirect.com/science/article/pii/S0378874122005359 [http://dx.doi.org/10.1016/j.jep.2022.115496] [PMID: 35750104]

[26]   Huang L, Feng S, Wang H. Decreased bone mineral density in female patients with systemic lupus erythematosus after long-term administration of Tripterygium Wilfordii Hook. F. Chin Med J (Engl) 2000; 113(2): 159-61.
[PMID: 11775543]

[27]   Chang C. Unmet needs in the treatment of autoimmunity: From aspirin to stem cells. Autoimmun Rev 2014; 13(4-5): 331-46. Available from: https://www.sciencedirect.com/science/article/pii/ S1568997214000640
[http://dx.doi.org/10.1016/j.autrev.2014.01.052] [PMID: 24462645]

[28]   Hasan MK, Ara I, Mondal MSA, Kabir Y. Phytochemistry, pharmacological activity, and potential health benefits of *Glycyrrhiza glabra*. Heliyon 2021; 7(6): e07240.
[http://dx.doi.org/10.1016/j.heliyon.2021.e07240] [PMID: 34189299]

[29]   Damle M. Glycyrrhiza glabra (Liquorice)-a potent medicinal herb. Int J Herb Med 2014; 2(2): 132-6.

[30]   Das S. Artemisia annua (Qinghao): a pharmacological review. Int J Pharm Sci Res 2012; 3(12): 4573-7.

[31]   Zhuang GK. [Clinical study on the treatment of lupus erythematosus with Artemisia apiacea Hce]. Zhonghua Yi Xue Za Zhi 1982; 62(6): 365-7.
[PMID: 6812928]

[32]   Ko E, Lee Y, Park N, *et al.* Sophorae radix reduces autoimmune response in NZB/w F1 systemic lupus erythematosus mouse model. Lupus 2007; 16(5): 335-41.
[http://dx.doi.org/10.1177/0961203307078228] [PMID: 17576735]

[33]   Liu CP, Tsai WJ, Shen CC, *et al.* Inhibition of (S)-armepavine from Nelumbo nucifera on autoimmune disease of MRL/MpJ-lpr/lpr mice. Eur J Pharmacol 2006; 531(1-3): 270-9. Available from: https://www.sciencedirect.com/science/article/pii/S0014299905012781
[http://dx.doi.org/10.1016/j.ejphar.2005.11.062] [PMID: 16413531]

[34]   Chen J-R, Yen J-H, Lin C-C, Tsai W-J, Liu W-J, Tsai J-J, *et al.* The effects of Chinese herbs on improving survival and inhibiting anti-ds DNA antibody production in lupus mice. Am J Chin Med 1993; 21(03n04): 257-62.
[http://dx.doi.org/10.1142/S0192415X93000303]

[35]   Cheng XQ, Li H, Yue XL, *et al.* Macrophage immunomodulatory activity of the polysaccharides from the roots of Bupleurum smithii var. parvifolium. J Ethnopharmacol 2010; 130(2): 363-8. Available from: https://www.sciencedirect.com/science/article/pii/S0378874110003259
[http://dx.doi.org/10.1016/j.jep.2010.05.019] [PMID: 20546871]

[36]   Okselni T, Septama AW, Pamungkas RA, Rahmi EP, Efdi M, Koketsu M. A systematic review and meta-analysis extraction techniques to reach the optimum asiaticoside content from the edible plant of Centella asiatica. S Afr J Bot 2023; 155: 261-73. Available from: https://www.sciencedirect. com/science/article/pii/S0254629923000807
[http://dx.doi.org/10.1016/j.sajb.2023.02.019]

[37]   Brinkhaus B, Lindner M, Schuppan D, Hahn EG. Chemical, pharmacological and clinical profile of the East Asian medical plant Centella aslatica. Phytomedicine 2000; 7(5): 427-48. Available from: https://www.sciencedirect.com/science/article/pii/S0944711300800653
[http://dx.doi.org/10.1016/S0944-7113(00)80065-3] [PMID: 11081995]

[38]   Al-Salahi OSA, Kit-Lam C, Majid AMSA, *et al.* Anti-angiogenic quassinoid-rich fraction from Eurycoma longifolia modulates endothelial cell function. Microvasc Res 2013; 90: 30-9. Available from: https://www.sciencedirect.com/science/article/pii/S002628621300109X
[http://dx.doi.org/10.1016/j.mvr.2013.07.007] [PMID: 23899415]

[39]   Wei J, Chen L, Gao S, Wang J, Wang Y, Zhang Z, *et al.* 2022. Available from:

https://www.sciencedirect.com/science/article/pii/S2667142522000550

[40]   Minhas U, Minz R, Bhatnagar A. Prophylactic effect of *Withania somnifera* on inflammation in a non-autoimmune prone murine model of lupus. Drug Discov Ther 2011; 5(4): 195-201.
        [http://dx.doi.org/10.5582/ddt.2011.v5.4.195] [PMID: 22466301]

[41]   Musette P, Galelli A, Chabre H, *et al. Urtica dioica* agglutinin, a Vβ8.3-specific superantigen, prevents the development of the systemic lupus erythematosus-like pathology of MRL *lpr* / *lpr mice.* Eur J Immunol 1996; 26(8): 1707-11.
        [http://dx.doi.org/10.1002/eji.1830260807] [PMID: 8765010]

[42]   Sharma S, Singh D, Gurung YB, Shrestha SP, Pantha C. Immunomodulatory effect of Stinging nettle (*Urtica dioica)* and Aloe vera (*Aloe barbadensis)* in broiler chickens. Vet Anim Sci 2018; 6: 56-63.
        Available from: https://www.sciencedirect.com/science/article/pii/S2451943X18300887
        [http://dx.doi.org/10.1016/j.vas.2018.07.002] [PMID: 32734053]

[43]   Lee H, Kim H, Lee G, Chung HS, Bae H. Curcumin attenuates lupus nephritis upon interaction with regulatory T cells in New Zealand Black/White mice. Br J Nutr 2013; 110(1): 69-76.
        [http://dx.doi.org/10.1017/S0007114512004734] [PMID: 23181951]

[44]   Clark WF, Kortas C, Heidenheim AP, Garland J, Spanner E, Parbtani A. Flaxseed in lupus nephritis: a two-year nonplacebo-controlled crossover study. J Am Coll Nutr 2001; 20(2) (Suppl.): 143-8.
        [http://dx.doi.org/10.1080/07315724.2001.10719026] [PMID: 11349937]

[45]   Siew YY, Zareisedehizadeh S, Seetoh WG, Neo SY, Tan CH, Koh HL. Ethnobotanical survey of usage of fresh medicinal plants in Singapore. J Ethnopharmacol 2014; 155(3): 1450-66. Available from: https://www.sciencedirect.com/science/article/pii/S0378874114005431
        [http://dx.doi.org/10.1016/j.jep.2014.07.024] [PMID: 25058874]

[46]   Aboulwafa MM, Youssef FS, Gad HA, Altyar AE, Al-Azizi MM, Ashour ML. A comprehensive insight on the health benefits and phytoconstituents of Camellia sinensis and recent approaches for its quality control. Antioxidants 2019; 8(10): 455.
        [http://dx.doi.org/10.3390/antiox8100455] [PMID: 31590466]

[47]   Aparicio-Soto M, Sánchez-Hidalgo M, Alarcón-de-la-Lastra C. An update on diet and nutritional factors in systemic lupus erythematosus management. Nutr Res Rev 2017; 30(1): 118-37.
        [http://dx.doi.org/10.1017/S0954422417000026] [PMID: 28294088]

[48]   Sung YY, Kim HK. Illicium verum extract suppresses IFN-γ-induced ICAM-1 expression *via* blockade of JAK/STAT pathway in HaCaT human keratinocytes. J Ethnopharmacol 2013; 149(3): 626-32.
        [http://dx.doi.org/10.1016/j.jep.2013.07.013] [PMID: 23872327]

[49]   De Cicco P, Maisto M, Tenore GC, Ianaro A. Olive leaf extract, from Olea europaea L., reduces palmitate-induced inflammation *via* regulation of murine macrophages polarization. Nutrients 2020; 12(12): 3663.
        [http://dx.doi.org/10.3390/nu12123663] [PMID: 33260769]

[50]   El-Nashar HAS, Eldehna WM, Al-Rashood ST, Alharbi A, Eskandrani RO, Aly SH. GC/MS analysis of essential oil and enzyme inhibitory activities of Syzygium cumini (Pamposia) grown in Egypt: chemical characterization and molecular docking studies. Molecules 2021; 26(22): 6984.
        [http://dx.doi.org/10.3390/molecules26226984] [PMID: 34834076]

[51]   Aly SH, Elissawy AM, Fayez AM, Eldahshan OA, Elshanawany MA, Singab ANB. Neuroprotective effects of *Sophora secundiflora, Sophora tomentosa* leaves and formononetin on scopolamine-induced dementia. Nat Prod Res 2021; 35(24): 5848-52.
        [http://dx.doi.org/10.1080/14786419.2020.1795853] [PMID: 32696670]

[52]   Ads EN, Hassan SI, Rajendrasozhan S, Hetta MH, Aly SH, Ali MA. Isolation, structure elucidation and antimicrobial evaluation of natural pentacyclic triterpenoids and phytochemical investigation of different fractions of Ziziphus spina-christi (L.) stem bark using LCHRMS analysis. Molecules 2022; 27(6): 1805.

[http://dx.doi.org/10.3390/molecules27061805] [PMID: 35335169]

[53]   Aly SH, Elissawy AM, Allam AE, *et al.* New quinolizidine alkaloid and insecticidal activity of *Sophora secundiflora* and *Sophora tomentosa* against *Culex pipiens* (Diptera: Culicidae). Nat Prod Res 2022; 36(11): 2722-34.
[http://dx.doi.org/10.1080/14786419.2021.1919108] [PMID: 33974474]

[54]   Elgindi MR, Singab AE-NB, Aly SH, Mahmoud II. Phytochemical investigation and antioxidant activity of Hyophorbe verschaffeltii (Arecaceae). J Pharmacogn Phytochem 2016; 5(2): 39-46.

[55]   Aly SH, Elgindi MR, Singab AENB, Mahmoud II. Hyophorbe verschaffeltii DNA profiling, chemical composition of the lipophilic fraction, antimicrobial, anti-inflammatory and cytotoxic activities. Res J Pharm Biol Chem Sci 2016; 7(2): 120-30.

[56]   Balkrishna A, Thakur P, Singh S, Chandra Dev SN, Varshney A. Mechanistic paradigms of natural plant metabolites as remedial candidates for systemic lupus erythromatosus. Cells 2020; 9(4): 1049.
[http://dx.doi.org/10.3390/cells9041049] [PMID: 32331431]

[57]   Asenso J, Yang XD, Yu J, Zhou P, Wang C, Wei W. Plant-based anti-inflammatory agents: Progress from Africa and China. Clin Anti-Inflamm Anti-Allergy Drugs 2016; 2(1): 52-66.
[http://dx.doi.org/10.2174/2212703802999151230113431]

[58]   Li W, Li H, Zhang M, *et al.* Isogarcinol Extracted from *Garcinia mangostana* L. Ameliorates Systemic Lupus Erythematosus-like Disease in a Murine Model. J Agric Food Chem 2015; 63(38): 8452-9.
[http://dx.doi.org/10.1021/acs.jafc.5b03425] [PMID: 26330173]

[59]   Guo L, Liu W, Lu T, *et al.* Decrease of functional activated T and B cells and treatment of glomerulonephitis in lupus-prone mice using a natural flavonoid astilbin. PLoS One 2015; 10(4): e0124002.
[http://dx.doi.org/10.1371/journal.pone.0124002] [PMID: 25867237]

[60]   Zhou L, Sun L, Wu H, *et al.* Oridonin ameliorates lupus-like symptoms of MRLlpr/lpr mice by inhibition of B-cell activating factor (BAFF). Eur J Pharmacol 2013; 715(1-3): 230-7.
[http://dx.doi.org/10.1016/j.ejphar.2013.05.016] [PMID: 23712004]

[61]   Tawfik AF, Bishop SJ, Ayalp A, El-Feraly FS. Effects of artemisinin, dihydroartemisinin and arteether on immune responses of normal mice. Int J Immunopharmacol 1990; 12(4): 385-9. Available from: https://www.sciencedirect.com/science/article/pii/019205619090019J
[http://dx.doi.org/10.1016/0192-0561(90)90019-J] [PMID: 2202689]

[62]   Xinqiang S, Yu Z, Ningning Y, Erqin D, Lei W, Hongtao D. Molecular mechanism of celastrol in the treatment of systemic lupus erythematosus based on network pharmacology and molecular docking technology. Life Sci 2020; 240: 117063. Available from: https://www.sciencedirect.com/science/article/pii/S0024320519309907
[http://dx.doi.org/10.1016/j.lfs.2019.117063] [PMID: 31734262]

[63]   Liu Y, Xiao N, Du H, *et al.* Celastrol ameliorates autoimmune disorders in Trex1-deficient mice. Biochem Pharmacol 2020; 178: 114090. Available from: https://www.sciencedirect.com/science/article/pii/S0006295220303269
[http://dx.doi.org/10.1016/j.bcp.2020.114090] [PMID: 32565148]

[64]   Liu Y-F, He H-Q, Ding Y-L, Wu S-Y, Chen D-S, e CL. [Effects of Triptolide on Tc and Th Cell Excursion in Peripheral Blood of Nude Mice with Systemic Lupus Erythematosus BALB/c-un]. Zhongguo Shi Yan Xue Ye Xue Za Zhi 2019; 27(5): 1691-5.
[PMID: 31607333]

[65]   Zhao X, Tang X, Yan Q, *et al.* Triptolide ameliorates lupus *via* the induction of miR-125a-5p mediating Treg upregulation. Int Immunopharmacol 2019; 71: 14-21. Available from: https://www.sciencedirect.com/science/article/pii/S1567576918313341
[http://dx.doi.org/10.1016/j.intimp.2019.02.047] [PMID: 30861393]

[66]   Zhao M, Liang G, Tang M, *et al.* Total glucosides of paeony induces regulatory CD4+CD25+ T cells by increasing Foxp3 demethylation in lupus CD4+ T cells. Clin Immunol 2012; 143(2): 180-7.
[http://dx.doi.org/10.1016/j.clim.2012.02.002] [PMID: 22406048]

[67]   Ji L, Hou X, Liu W, *et al.* Paeoniflorin inhibits activation of the IRAK1-NF-κB signaling pathway in peritoneal macrophages from lupus-prone MRL/lpr mice. Microb Pathog 2018; 124: 223-9.
[http://dx.doi.org/10.1016/j.micpath.2018.08.051] [PMID: 30149133]

[68]   Li X, Gu L, Yang L, Zhang D, Shen J. Aconitine: A potential novel treatment for systemic lupus erythematosus. J Pharmacol Sci 2017; 133(3): 115-21.
[http://dx.doi.org/10.1016/j.jphs.2017.01.007] [PMID: 28302448]

[69]   Su B, Ye H, You X, Ni H, Chen X, Li L. Icariin alleviates murine lupus nephritis *via* inhibiting NF-κB activation pathway and NLRP3 inflammasome. Life Sci 2018; 208: 26-32. Available from: https://www.sciencedirect.com/science/article/pii/S0024320518303850
[http://dx.doi.org/10.1016/j.lfs.2018.07.009] [PMID: 30146016]

[70]   Liao J, Liu Y, Wu H, *et al.* The role of icaritin in regulating Foxp3/IL17a balance in systemic lupus erythematosus and its effects on the treatment of MRL/lpr mice. Clin Immunol 2016; 162: 74-83.
[http://dx.doi.org/10.1016/j.clim.2015.11.006] [PMID: 26604013]

[71]   Kang HK, Ecklund D, Liu M, Datta SK. Apigenin, a non-mutagenic dietary flavonoid, suppresses lupus by inhibiting autoantigen presentation for expansion of autoreactive Th1 and Th17 cells. Arthritis Res Ther 2009; 11(2): R59.
[http://dx.doi.org/10.1186/ar2682] [PMID: 19405952]

[72]   Lin F, Luo X, Tsun A, Li Z, Li D, Li B. Kaempferol enhances the suppressive function of Treg cells by inhibiting FOXP3 phosphorylation. Int Immunopharmacol 2015; 28(2): 859-65. Available from: https://www.sciencedirect.com/science/article/pii/S1567576915001460
[http://dx.doi.org/10.1016/j.intimp.2015.03.044] [PMID: 25870037]

[73]   Handono K, Pratama MZ, Endharti AT, Kalim H. Treatment of low doses curcumin could modulate Th17/Treg balance specifically on CD4+ T cell cultures of systemic lupus erythematosus patients. Cent Eur J Immunol 2015; 4(4): 461-9.
[http://dx.doi.org/10.5114/ceji.2015.56970] [PMID: 26862311]

[74]   Zhao J, Wang J, Zhou M, Li M, Li M, Tan H. Curcumin attenuates murine lupus *via* inhibiting NLRP3 inflammasome. Int Immunopharmacol 2019; 69: 213-6. Available from: https://www.sciencedirect.com/science/article/pii/S1567576918313286
[http://dx.doi.org/10.1016/j.intimp.2019.01.046] [PMID: 30738291]

[75]   Wang M, Zhou G, Lv J, Zeng P, Guo C, Wang Q. Curcumin modulation of the activation of PYK2 in peripheral blood mononuclear cells from patients with lupus nephritis. Reumatologia/Rheumatology 2017; 55(6): 269-75.
[http://dx.doi.org/10.5114/reum.2017.72623]

[76]   Pervaiz S. Resveratrol: from grapevines to mammalian biology. FASEB J 2003; 17(14): 1975-85.
[http://dx.doi.org/10.1096/fj.03-0168rev] [PMID: 14597667]

[77]   Wang ZL, Luo XF, Li MT, *et al.* Resveratrol possesses protective effects in a pristane-induced lupus mouse model. PLoS One 2014; 9(12): e114792.
[http://dx.doi.org/10.1371/journal.pone.0114792] [PMID: 25501752]

[78]   Jhou JP, Chen SJ, Huang HY, Lin WW, Huang DY, Tzeng SJ. Upregulation of FcγRIIB by resveratrol *via* NF-κB activation reduces B-cell numbers and ameliorates lupus. Exp Mol Med 2017; 49(9): e381-1.
[http://dx.doi.org/10.1038/emm.2017.144] [PMID: 28960214]

[79]   Voloshyna I, Teboul I, Littlefield MJ, *et al.* Resveratrol counters systemic lupus erythematosus-associated atherogenicity by normalizing cholesterol efflux. Exp Biol Med (Maywood) 2016; 241(14): 1611-9.

[http://dx.doi.org/10.1177/1535370216647181] [PMID: 27190277]

[80]   Pannu N, Bhatnagar A. Prophylactic effect of resveratrol and piperine on pristane-induced murine model of lupus-like disease. Inflammopharmacology 2020; 28(3): 719-35.
[http://dx.doi.org/10.1007/s10787-020-00717-3] [PMID: 32415428]

[81]   Li Y, Yao J, Han C, *et al.* Quercetin, inflammation and immunity. Nutrients 2016; 8(3): 167.
[http://dx.doi.org/10.3390/nu8030167] [PMID: 26999194]

[82]   Lin Y, Yan Y, Zhang H, *et al.* Salvianolic acid A alleviates renal injury in systemic lupus erythematosus induced by pristane in BALB/c mice. Acta Pharm Sin B 2017; 7(2): 159-66. Available from: https://www.sciencedirect.com/science/article/pii/S2211383516300879
[http://dx.doi.org/10.1016/j.apsb.2016.07.001] [PMID: 28303221]

[83]   Du Y, Du L, He Z, Zhou J, Wen C, Zhang Y. Cryptotanshinone ameliorates the pathogenesis of systemic lupus erythematosus by blocking T cell proliferation. Int Immunopharmacol 2019; 74: 105677. Available from: https://www.sciencedirect.com/science/article/pii/S1567576919306848
[http://dx.doi.org/10.1016/j.intimp.2019.105677] [PMID: 31177018]

[84]   Zhang X, Zou M, Liang Y, *et al.* Arctigenin inhibits abnormal germinal center reactions and attenuates murine lupus by inhibiting IFN-I pathway. Eur J Pharmacol 2022; 919: 174808. Available from: https://www.sciencedirect.com/science/article/pii/S0014299922000693
[http://dx.doi.org/10.1016/j.ejphar.2022.174808] [PMID: 35151645]

[85]   Xia YF, Ye BQ, Li YD, *et al.* Andrographolide attenuates inflammation by inhibition of NF-κ B activation through covalent modification of reduced cysteine 62 of p50. J Immunol 2004; 173(6): 4207-17.
[http://dx.doi.org/10.4049/jimmunol.173.6.4207] [PMID: 15356172]

[86]   Del Río JA, Díaz L, García-Bernal D, Blanquer M, Ortuño A, Correal E, *et al.* 2014. Available from: https://www.sciencedirect.com/science/article/pii/B9780444634306000059

[87]   Yang LY, Chen A, Kuo YC, Lin CY. Efficacy of a pure compound H1-A extracted from Cordyceps sinensis on autoimmune disease of MRL lpr/lpr mice. J Lab Clin Med 1999; 134(5): 492-500. Available from: https://www.sciencedirect.com/science/article/pii/S0022214399901713
[http://dx.doi.org/10.1016/S0022-2143(99)90171-3] [PMID: 10560943]

[88]   Lai N-S, Lin R-H, Lai R-S, Kun U-C, Leu S-C. Prevention of autoantibody formation and prolonged survival in New Zealand Black/New Zealand White F1 mice with an ancient Chinese herb, Ganoderma tsugae. Lupus 2001; 10(7): 461-5.
[http://dx.doi.org/10.1191/096120301678416006] [PMID: 11480842]

[89]   Hsieh CC, Lin BF. Dietary factors regulate cytokines in murine models of systemic lupus erythematosus. Autoimmun Rev 2011; 11(1): 22-7. Available from: https://www.sciencedirect.com/science/article/pii/S1568997211001510
[http://dx.doi.org/10.1016/j.autrev.2011.06.009] [PMID: 21763466]

[90]   Fu T, Lin J. [Effect of Cordyceps sinensis on inhibiting systemic lupus erythematosus in MRL 1pr/1pr mice (correction of rats)]. Zhong Yao Cai 2001; 24(9): 658-9.
[PMID: 11799778]

[91]   He L, Niu S, Yang C, *et al.* Cordyceps proteins alleviate lupus nephritis through modulation of the STAT3/mTOR/NF-κB signaling pathway. J Ethnopharmacol 2023; 309: 116284. Available from: https://www.sciencedirect.com/science/article/pii/S0378874123001526
[http://dx.doi.org/10.1016/j.jep.2023.116284] [PMID: 36828195]

[92]   Ji L, Hou X, Deng X, Fan X, Zhuang A, Zhang X, *et al.* Jieduquyuziyin prescription-treated rat serum suppresses activation of peritoneal macrophages in MRL/Lpr lupus mice by inhibiting IRAK1 signaling pathway. Evidence-based Complement Altern Med 2019.
[http://dx.doi.org/10.1155/2019/2357217]

[93]   Ji L, Fan X, Hou X, *et al.* Jieduquyuziyin prescription suppresses inflammatory activity of MRL/lpr

mice and their bone marrow-derived macrophages *via* inhibiting expression of IRAK1-NF-κb signaling pathway. Front Pharmacol 2020; 11: 1049.
[http://dx.doi.org/10.3389/fphar.2020.01049] [PMID: 32760274]

[94] Ji L, Wu S, Fu D, *et al.* Jieduquyuziyin Prescription alleviates hepatic gluconeogenesis *via* PI3K/Akt/PGC-1α pathway in glucocorticoid-induced MRL/lpr mice. J Ethnopharmacol 2022; 284: 114815. Available from: https://www.sciencedirect.com/science/article/pii/S037887412101045X
[http://dx.doi.org/10.1016/j.jep.2021.114815] [PMID: 34763039]

[95] Du L, Feng Y, Wang C, *et al.* Jieduquyuziyin prescription promotes the efficacy of prednisone *via* upregulating Nrf2 in MRL/lpr kidneys. J Ethnopharmacol 2022; 298: 115643. Available from: https://www.sciencedirect.com/science/article/pii/S0378874122006821
[http://dx.doi.org/10.1016/j.jep.2022.115643] [PMID: 36031105]

[96] He Y, Tian W, Zhang M, *et al.* Jieduquyuziyin prescription alleviates SLE complicated by atherosclerosis *via* promoting cholesterol efflux and suppressing TLR9/MyD88 activation. J Ethnopharmacol 2023; 309: 116283. Available from: https://www.sciencedirect.com/science/article/pii/S0378874123001514
[http://dx.doi.org/10.1016/j.jep.2023.116283] [PMID: 36898449]

[97] Gao Y, Zhou J, Huang Y, *et al.* Jiedu-Quyu-Ziyin Fang (JQZF) inhibits the proliferation and activation of B cells in MRL/lpr mice *via* modulating the AKT/mTOR/c-Myc signaling pathway. J Ethnopharmacol 2023; 315: 116625. Available from: https://www.sciencedirect.com/science/article/pii/S0378874123004932
[http://dx.doi.org/10.1016/j.jep.2023.116625] [PMID: 37236380]

[98] Liao YN, Liu CS, Tsai TR, *et al.* Preliminary study of a traditional Chinese medicine formula in systemic lupus erythematosus patients to taper steroid dose and prevent disease flare-up. Kaohsiung J Med Sci 2011; 27(7): 251-7. Available from: https://www.sciencedirect.com/science/article/pii/S1607551X11000751
[http://dx.doi.org/10.1016/j.kjms.2011.03.001] [PMID: 21757141]

[99] Hendricks AJ. A Revision of the Genus Alisma (Dill.) L. Am Midl Nat 1957; 58(2): 470-93.
[http://dx.doi.org/10.2307/2422629]

[100] Isobe H, Yamamoto K, Cyong J-C. Components of Hachimi-jio-gan (Ba-Wei-Di-Huang-Wan) and changes in blood flow in the human central retinal artery. J Tradit Med (Toyama) 2002; 19(3): 105-13.

[101] Furuya Y, Kawakita T, Nomoto K. Immunomodulating effect of a traditional Japanese medicine, Hachimi-jio-gan (Ba-Wei-Di-Huang-Wan), on Th1 predominance in autoimmune MRL/MP-lpr/lpr mice. Int Immunopharmacol 2001; 1(3): 551-9. Available from: https://www.sciencedirect.com/science/article/pii/S1567576900000242
[http://dx.doi.org/10.1016/S1567-5769(00)00024-2] [PMID: 11367538]

[102] Isobe H, Yamamoto K, Cyong JC. Effects of hachimi-jio-gan (ba-wei-di-huang-wan) on blood flow in the human central retinal artery. Am J Chin Med 2003; 31(3): 425-35.
[http://dx.doi.org/10.1142/S0192415X03001181] [PMID: 12943173]

[103] Cai Z, Wong CK, Dong J, *et al.* Anti-inflammatory activities of Ganoderma lucidum (Lingzhi) and San-Miao-San supplements in MRL/lpr mice for the treatment of systemic lupus erythematosus. Chin Med 2016; 11(1): 23.
[http://dx.doi.org/10.1186/s13020-016-0093-x] [PMID: 27134645]

[104] Wang J, Wang H, Yu J, *et al.* Traditional uses, chemical composition, and pharmacological effects of diaphragma juglandis fructus: A review. J Ethnopharmacol 2023; 312: 116440. Available from: https://www.sciencedirect.com/science/article/pii/S0378874123003082
[http://dx.doi.org/10.1016/j.jep.2023.116440] [PMID: 37023838]

[105] Zhong LLD, Bian ZX, Gu JH, Zhou X, Tian Y, Mao JC, *et al.* 2013.
[http://dx.doi.org/10.1155/2013/327245]

[106] Matsushima H, Hishikawa H, Miki H, *et al.* Cinnamomi Cortex and Scutellariae Radix in the Japanese

herbal medicine Kampo saireito inhibit expression of INOS through different mechanisms in hepatocytes. Tradit Kampo Med 2020; 7(1): 38-47.
[http://dx.doi.org/10.1002/tkm2.1241]

[107]   Kanauchi H, Imamura S, Takigawa M, Furukawa F. Evaluation of the Japanese-Chinese herbal medicine, kampo, for the treatment of lupus dermatoses in autoimmune prone MRL/Mp-lpr/lpr mice. J Dermatol 1994; 21(12): 935-9.
[http://dx.doi.org/10.1111/j.1346-8138.1994.tb03315.x] [PMID: 7868765]

[108]   Lee T-Y, Chang H-H. Longdan Xiegan Tang has immunomodulatory effects on CD4+CD25+ T cells and attenuates pathological signs in MRL/lpr mice. Int J Mol Med 2010; 25(5): 677-85.
[PMID: 20372809]

[109]   Panossian A, Seo EJ, Wikman G, Efferth T. Synergy assessment of fixed combinations of Herba Andrographidis and Radix Eleutherococci extracts by transcriptome-wide microarray profiling. Phytomedicine 2015; 22(11): 981-92. Available from: https://www.sciencedirect.com/science/article/pii/S0944711315002408
[http://dx.doi.org/10.1016/j.phymed.2015.08.004] [PMID: 26407940]

[110]   Esmaeilzadeh E, Soleimani M, Khorram Khorshid HR. Protective effects of Herbal Compound (IM253) on the inflammatory responses and oxidative stress in a mouse model of multiple sclerosis. Mult Scler Relat Disord 2022; 67: 104076. Available from: https://www.sciencedirect.com/science/article/pii/S2211034822005843
[http://dx.doi.org/10.1016/j.msard.2022.104076] [PMID: 35961059]

[111]   Chien Yin GO, Siong-See JL, Wang ECE. Telogen Effluvium – a review of the science and current obstacles. J Dermatol Sci 2021; 101(3): 156-63. Available from: https://www.sciencedirect.com/science/article/pii/S0923181121000086
[http://dx.doi.org/10.1016/j.jdermsci.2021.01.007] [PMID: 33541773]

[112]   Udompanich S, Chanprapaph K, Suchonwanit P. Hair and scalp changes in cutaneous and systemic lupus erythematosus. Am J Clin Dermatol 2018; 19(5): 679-94.
[http://dx.doi.org/10.1007/s40257-018-0363-8] [PMID: 29948959]

[113]   Hutchinson J. On lupus & its treatment. BMJ 1880; 1(1009): 650-2.
[http://dx.doi.org/10.1136/bmj.1.1009.650] [PMID: 20749473]

[114]   Fettouh DS, Saif DS, El Gazzar SF, Sonbol AA. Study the relationship between vitamin A deficiency, T helper 17, regulatory T cells, and disease activity in patients with systemic lupus erythematosus. Egypt Rheumatol Rehabil 2019; 46(4): 244-50.
[http://dx.doi.org/10.4103/err.err_5_19]

[115]   Erill S. Corticotrophins and corticosteroids. In: Dukes MNG, Aronson JK, Eds. Side Effects of Drugs Annual. Elsevier 1992; pp. 447-56. Available from: https://www.sciencedirect.com/science/article/pii/S0378608005805215

[116]   Akaogi J, Barker T, Kuroda Y, *et al.* Role of non-protein amino acid l-canavanine in autoimmunity. Autoimmun Rev 2006; 5(6): 429-35.
[http://dx.doi.org/10.1016/j.autrev.2005.12.004] [PMID: 16890899]

[117]   Wu WH, Liu JY, Chang HH. Latent class model based diagnostic system utilizing traditional Chinese medicine for patients with systemic lupus erythematosus. Expert Syst Appl 2011; 38(1): 281-7. Available from: https://www.sciencedirect.com/science/article/pii/S0957417410005622
[http://dx.doi.org/10.1016/j.eswa.2010.06.058]

[118]   Liu CY, Wu WH, Huang TP, Lee TY, Chang HH. A novel model for exploring the correlation between patterns and prescriptions in clinical practice of traditional Chinese medicine for systemic lupus erythematosus. Complement Ther Med 2014; 22(3): 481-8. Available from: https://www.sciencedirect.com/science/article/pii/S0965229914000375
[http://dx.doi.org/10.1016/j.ctim.2014.03.006] [PMID: 24906588]

CHAPTER 3

Type 1 Diabetes Mellitus and Herbal Medicines

Zinnet Şevval Aksoyalp[1,*] and **Betül Rabia Erdoğan**[1]

¹ Department of Pharmacology, Faculty of Pharmacy, Izmir Katip Celebi University, Izmir 35620, Türkiye

Abstract: The global incidence of type 1 diabetes mellitus (T1DM) is rising substantially and T1DM remains a marked economic burden despite advances in the diagnosis, prevention, and treatment of complications. T1DM, often associated with autoimmune disease, is characterized by insulin deficiency and insufficiency due to beta cell destruction. The primary treatment for T1DM is insulin therapy, limited by the risk of hypoglycemia and weight gain. Other treatments for T1DM are teplizumab and donislecel, which have recently received FDA approval. Beyond these treatment options, T1DM patients are interested in non-pharmacological interventions and are willing to use herbal products. Therefore, we reviewed the effects of herbal medicines used for T1DM, including fenugreek, ficus extracts, cinnamon, berberine, silymarin, silibinin, curcumin, resveratrol, catechins, ginseng, olive leaf, allicin, thymoquinone, and mangiferin to understand their level of evidence and associated effects, and their potential for use as antidiabetic agents in the clinic. As a result of our research, the majority of the studies were conducted on diabetic animal models. There are limited clinical studies investigating herbal medicines in T1DM. Studies show that the abovementioned herbal medicines are beneficial in T1DM by lowering glucose levels, increasing insulin levels, and exerting anti-oxidant, anti-inflammatory, and pancreas islet β-cell protective mechanisms. However, these studies are insufficient to recommend the use of existing herbs in treating T1DM on a clinical level.

Keywords: Alloxan, Autoimmune diabetes, Insulin-mimetics, Insulin-dependent diabetes mellitus, Streptozotocin, Type 1 diabetes mellitus.

INTRODUCTION

Diabetes mellitus is a severe and chronic disease characterized by insufficient insulin production or utilization, resulting in elevated levels of circulating blood glucose [1]. Prolonged insulin deficiency and sustained hyperglycemia can lead to serious complications such as retinopathy, nephropathy, neuropathy, and cardiovascular disease. The prevalence of diabetes mellitus is escalating as a

* **Corresponding author Zinnet Şevval Aksoyalp:** Department of Pharmacology, Faculty of Pharmacy, Izmir Katip Celebi University, Izmir 35620, Türkiye; Tel: +90(232)3293535; Fax: +90(232)3860888; E-mail: zinnetsevval.aksoyalp@ikcu.edu.tr

Cennet Ozay & Gokhan Zengin (Eds.)

global health challenge, with the number of people affected increasing every year. According to the 10th edition of the International Diabetes Federation (IDF) Diabetes Atlas, the global prevalence of diabetes is estimated to reach 537 million people in 2021, a number that is projected to increase to 783 million by 2045 [2]. The Atlas suggests that diabetes affects men and women equally, with a higher prevalence observed in people aged 75-79 years. The economic burden of diabetes-related conditions is estimated to have reached $966 billion in 2021, with a projected increase to $1,054 billion by 2045 [2].

Diabetes mellitus is classified into four subgroups: Type 1 diabetes mellitus (T1DM), type 2 diabetes mellitus (T2DM), specific types of diabetes, and gestational diabetes mellitus [3]. T1DM is characterized by insulin deficiency and insufficiency, resulting from β-cell destruction, often associated with autoimmune disease. Conversely, T2DM is often non-autoimmune and characterized by reduced insulin secretion and insulin resistance [3]. Contrary to the misconception that T1DM only affects children, T1DM can also occur in adulthood [4]. T2DM is not age restricted but is more prevalent in adults over the age of 40. T2DM is associated with overweight conditions, insulin resistance, and relative insulin insufficiency. Patients with T2DM are managed with lifestyle interventions and glucose-lowering medications [5]. The primary treatment for T1DM is insulin therapy with continuous blood glucose monitoring. Nonetheless, the risk of hypoglycemia and weight gain are limitations of insulin therapy. In recent years, the FDA has approved a monoclonal antibody called teplizumab [6] and a cellular therapy called donislecel for treating patients with T1DM [7]. In addition to these therapeutic options, there is a growing trend among patients with T1DM to explore non-pharmacological interventions. Alongside regular physical activity and a healthy diet, patients are also willing to use herbal products.

This chapter aims to evaluate the effects of herbs and herbal metabolites on the pathophysiology and symptoms of T1DM through preclinical and clinical studies. The herbs and herbal metabolites most frequently studied for their effects on T1DM, including fenugreek, ficus extracts, cinnamon, berberine, silymarin, silibinin, curcumin, resveratrol, catechins, ginseng, olive leaf, allicin thymoquinone, and mangiferin are reviewed comprehensively in this chapter.

TYPE 1 DIABETES MELLITUS

Epidemiology

T1DM affects all age cohorts; however, data on the epidemiology of T1DM in adults are limited [8]. The incidence of diabetes among children and adolescents is increasing, with projections from the 10th IDF Atlas indicating an estimated number of over 1.2 million affected children and adolescents by 2021 [9].

Given the lack of comprehensive global epidemiological data on the prevalence and incidence of T1DM, a meta-analysis of 193 studies was conducted [10]. The global incidence of T1DM is estimated to be 15 per 100,000 individuals, while its prevalence is 9.5% [10]. In 2017, a study estimated the number of global incidences as 234,710 and prevalence as 9,004,610 for T1DM cases in all age groups [11]. High-income countries contributed to 49% of the global incidence of T1DM and 52% of its prevalence [11]. Furthermore, a study conducted in 2018 revealed that individuals aged 31-60 years accounted for 42% of T1DM cases, representing 4% of all diabetes patients diagnosed after the age of 30 [5].

Diagnosis

The diagnosis of diabetes is established through several criteria, as outlined in the "Standards of Care in Diabetes" published by the American Diabetes Association in 2023 [3]. These include a fasting blood glucose (FBG) concentration of ≥ 126 mg/dL, an oral glucose tolerance test at blood glucose concentration of ≥ 200 mg/dL, or a hemoglobin A1c (HbA1c) level of $\geq 6.5\%$. In addition, many patients are diagnosed based on a random blood glucose concentration of ≥ 200 mg/dL, accompanied by classic symptoms such as dysglycemia, polyuria, polydipsia, and weight loss [12]. T1DM is diagnosed by hyperglycemia, ketosis, rapid weight loss, short-term symptoms, an early onset, lower body mass index, and autoimmune disease history.

Most cases of diabetes among young individuals are attributed to T1DM, which is easily diagnosed. In people over 30, however, T1DM can be challenging to distinguish from T2DM [5]. Measurement of circulating C-peptide levels, indicating endogenous insulin secretion and detection of autoantibodies against islet antigens can help differentiate T1DM from T2DM. However, it is noteworthy that these biomarkers are not routinely tested.

Clinical Manifestations

Patients diagnosed with T1DM progress through three distinct stages [13]. In the first stage, patients have two or more islet autoantibodies. Subsequently, in the second stage, patients develop glucose intolerance and dysglycemia. Ultimately, the third and final stage is characterized by the manifestation of clinical symptoms characteristic of the disease (Fig. **1**). The clinical presentation of both T1DM and T2DM is remarkably similar, with patients presenting with symptoms including polyuria, polydipsia, fatigue, dehydration, vision impairment, susceptibility to infections, and weight loss [14]. In the context of T1DM, these symptoms tend to be more severe and occur more rapidly, although the progression of immune-mediated damage is slow [14]. A critical complication associated with T1DM is diabetic ketoacidosis, a potentially life-threatening condition [15]. Individuals with T1DM may experience symptoms such as nausea, vomiting, abdominal pain, dehydration, shortness of breath, and coma, all of which indicate diabetic ketoacidosis.

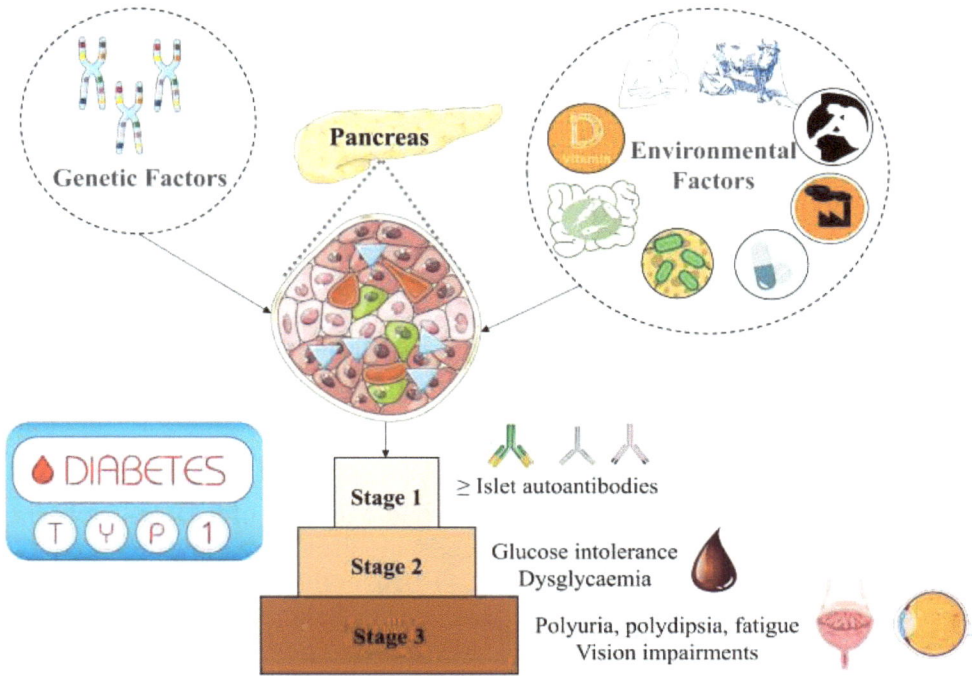

Fig. (1). The contributing factors and the stages of T1DM. T1DM is strongly associated with genetic factors, but environmental factors are also thought to play an important role, including early life dietary patterns, vitamin D levels, gut microbiota composition, infections, medications, pollutants, and psychological stress. T1DM is divided into three stages. In the first stage, patients have two or more islet autoantibodies. In the second stage, patients develop glucose intolerance and dysglycemia. In the third stage, clinical symptoms specific to the disease appear. The figure has been prepared using the Servier Medical Art and Pixabay website (https://smart.servier.com/; https://pixabay.com/tr/).

Pathogenesis

T1DM is a complex autoimmune disease with multiple factors contributing to its intricate pathophysiology. Autoimmune processes and pancreatic β-cell dysfunction are recognized hallmarks of T1DM, but the exact etiology and pathology of T1DM remain unclear [16]. The development of T1DM has been proposed to encompass three pivotal conditions [17]. First, T-cell activation of the immune system against pancreatic β-cell antigens is required. Second, there has to be a strong proinflammatory response. Third, the autoimmune response has to become uncontrolled. Thus, this response becomes chronic and leads to β-cell destruction [17].

Genetic and environmental factors affect the development of T1DM [16]. Genetically, T1DM is strongly associated with human leukocyte antigen (HLA)-DR and HLA-DQ complexes, which present antigens to T lymphocytes [18]. In the non-HLA region, many T1DM-associated loci contain insulin gene polymorphisms [12]. Nevertheless, genetic factors are not entirely responsible for T1DM. Environmental factors such as early life dietary patterns (breastfeeding and cow's milk), vitamin D levels, gut microbiota composition, infections, medications (pentamidine and antibiotics), pollutants, and psychological stress are thought to play an important role [19] (Fig. 1).

T1DM is closely associated with the immune system, and patients with T1DM have circulating islet cell antibodies. Predominant autoantibodies identified in the serum include insulin autoantibodies (IAA), glutamic acid decarboxylase antibody (GADA), insulinoma-associated-2 autoantibodies (IA-2A), and zinc transporter 8 (ZnT8A) antibody [20]. β-cell autoantibodies are often detectable prior to clinical manifestations [12], and a correlation has been established between the rapid progression of T1DM and the presence of multiple islet autoantibodies in children [21].

Multiple immune players are involved in the pathogenesis of T1DM, including T cells, B cells, neutrophils, natural killer cells, macrophages and dendritic cells [17]. T helper 1 (TH1) and T helper 2 (TH2) cells orchestrate cellular and humoral immunity, respectively. They function in balance to maintain immune homeostasis. Disruption of this balance leads to inflammation, prompting insulitis and diabetes. Insulitis, characterized by inflammation resulting from immune cell infiltration into the pancreatic islets, sheds light on the immune-mediated destruction of β-cells. Predominantly, CD4+ and CD8+ T cells mediate this destruction [22], with a notable emphasis on cytotoxic CD8+ T cells in the pathogenesis of T1DM [23]. Cytokines released by immune cells are involved in the destruction of β-cells. Proinflammatory cytokines, including interleukin-2 (IL-2), IL-1β, IL-6, IL-12, interferon-gamma (IFN-γ) and tumor necrosis factor-alpha (TNF-α) released by TH1 cells, exert cytotoxic effects on pancreatic β-cells [24]. IFN-γ, IL-17, TNF-α, and IL-6 induced nuclear factor kappa B (NF-κB) activation contributes to β-cell destruction and dysfunction [25]. These proinflammatory cytokines activate cytotoxic macrophages and cytotoxic T cells and lead to β-cell loss. Conversely, TH2 cells secrete anti-inflammatory cytokines, such as IL-4 and IL-10, which attenuate the inflammation and destruction of pancreatic β-cells [24] (Fig. 2).

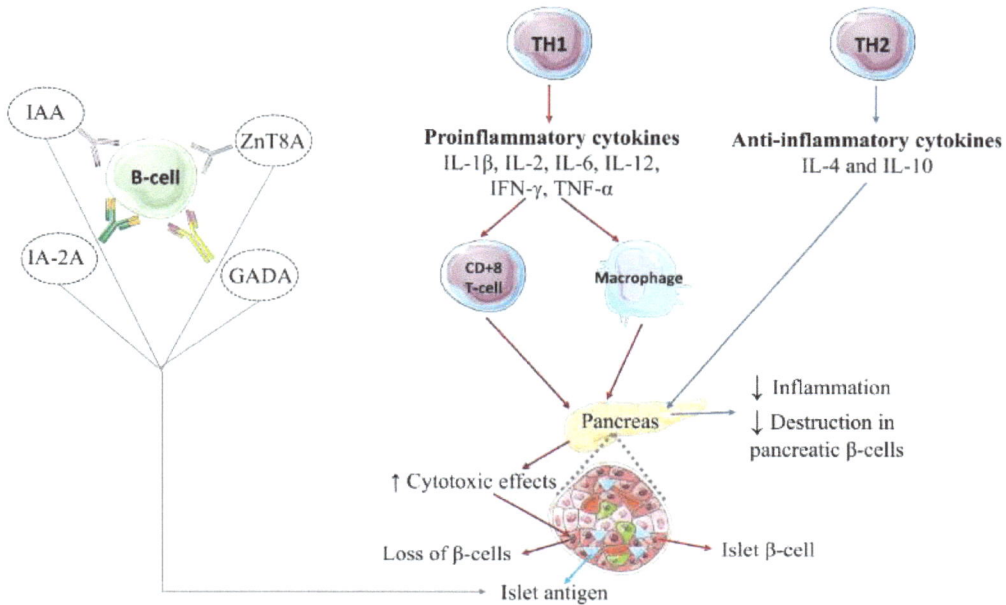

Fig. (2). The immune system and type 1 diabetes pathogenesis. TH1 activation is responsible for the release of proinflammatory cytokines, while TH2 activation mediates the release of anti-inflammatory cytokines. These proinflammatory cytokines activate cytotoxic macrophages and cytotoxic CD+8 T cells and lead to the loss of β-cells. Anti-inflammatory cytokines decrease the pancreatic β-cells destruction. Autoantibodies released by B cells are also involved in the pathology of T1DM by binding to antigens in pancreatic beta cells. The figure has been prepared using the Servier Medical Art and Pixabay website (https://smart.servier.com/; https://pixabay.com/tr/). *Abbreviations: IAA: Insulin autoantibodies, GADA: Glutamic acid decarboxylase antibody, IA-2A: Insulinoma-associated-2 autoantibodies, IFN-γ: Interferon-gamma, IL: Interleukin, TH: T helper, TNF-α: Tumor necrosis factor-alpha, ZnT8A: Zinc transporter 8 antibody.*

PHARMACOLOGICAL MANAGEMENT OF TYPE 1 DIABETES MELLITUS

The pharmacological management of T1DM represents a significant advance since the discovery of insulin. The breakthrough discovery by Frederick Banting and colleagues in 1922 led to the isolation of insulin, and T1DM became a manageable condition [26]. The activation of multiple pathways may explain the multifaceted effects of insulin. Insulin hormone is present in the form of preproinsulin and proinsulin. Glucose enters the pancreas through the glucose transporter (GLUT)-2 located in β-cells and stimulates the pancreas. Subsequently, proinsulin cleavage produces equal amounts of insulin and C-peptide, which are released into the circulation [27]. Circulating insulin binds to its membrane receptor on the target cells, and phosphorylation of the receptor leads to tyrosine kinase activation. Notably, insulin receptor substrates (IRS) 1 and 2 are phosphorylated, triggering downstream signaling [28]. Insulin affects the function of almost every tissue in the body and is responsible for energy storage in the liver, muscles, and adipose tissues. Insulin stimulates the entry of glucose into skeletal muscle and adipose tissue *via* GLUT-4, which is in the cell membranes.

Insulin preparations are designed to mimic physiological insulin secretion and have evolved from purified animal insulins to genetically engineered human insulins and insulin analogs [29]. Many different types of insulin have been developed with different onset and duration of action, including rapid, short, intermediate, and long-acting and premixed [29]. Insulin lispro, glulisine, and aspart are rapid-acting insulins. Human neutral protamine Hagedorn (NPH) insulin is an intermediate-acting insulin. Insulin glargine and degludec are long-acting insulins. Long-acting basal insulin and rapid-acting bolus insulin injections allow patients to achieve tight blood glucose control. The adverse effects of insulin are hypoglycemia and weight gain. A state of normoglycemia without hypoglycemia or weight increase remains an unmet treatment goal for patients with T1DM [29]. According to the "Standards of Care in Diabetes" by the American Diabetes Association, the glycemic targets are FBG 80-130 mg/dl; postprandial plasma glucose <180 mg/dl; and HbA1c < 7% [30].

Given the pivotal role of the immune system in T1DM pathogenesis, there has been enhanced interest in the research and development of immunotherapeutic medications. Teplizumab, an FDA-approved monoclonal antibody in 2022, is intended to delay the onset of stage 3 T1DM in adults and pediatric patients ($\geq$ eight years) with stage 2 T1DM [6]. Teplizumab binds to CD3 on the surface of T lymphocytes and inhibits the activation of autoreactive T lymphocytes in pancreatic β-cells. It is given by intravenous infusion once a day for 14 days.

Notably, the FDA recently approved the first cellular therapy to treat T1DM [7]. Donislecel, an allogeneic pancreatic islet cellular suspension derived from deceased donors, was approved by the FDA in 2023 to treat T1DM adults with recurrent severe hypoglycemia. The mechanism of action of donislecel is insulin secretion from infused allogeneic β-cells [31]. Immunosuppressive therapy is recommended to be administered concurrently with donislecel treatment.

TYPE 1 DIABETES MELLITUS AND HERBS

In this section, the results of induced animal models of T1DM and clinical trials in T1DM patients with various herbs or herbal products are discussed. The results of the preclinical studies are presented in Table **1**, and the results of the clinical studies are presented in Table **2**.

Table 1. Preclinical studies with herbs or herbal products in T1DM.

Compounds	Administration Dose and Protocol	Main Findings Related to Antidiabetic Effect	Refs.
Fenugreek	4-hydroxyisoleucine (50 mg/kg/day by intubation) for four weeks in male Wistar rats.	↓ plasma glucose levels No effect on plasma insulin levels.	[32]
	Aqueous fenugreek seed extract (0.87 g/kg and 1.74 g/kg) in male Wistar rats.	↓ plasma glucose levels	[33]
	Fenugreek oil (10% in the diet) for four weeks in male Wistar rats.	↓ plasma glucose levels ↑ plasma insulin levels Protected pancreatic β-cells ↓ pancreatic WBC and lymphocyte count and IL-6 levels.	[34]
	Soluble dietary fibre fraction of fenugreek (0.5 g/kg by gavage) in male Long-Evans rats.	No effect on FBG levels. Improved glucose tolerance.	[35]
	Trigonelline (70 mg/kg by gavage) for four weeks in male C57BL/6j mice.	↓ blood glucose levels ↑ serum and pancreatic insulin content ↓ serum inflammatory markers Antioxidant activity in pancreas tissue. Restored pancreas morphology. and protected pancreatic β-cells.	[36]
	Fenugreek seed powder (5% in the diet) for eight weeks in female Wistar rats.	Slightly ↓ blood glucose levels	[37]
	Fenugreek seed powder (5% in the diet) for 21 days in female Wistar rats.	↓ blood glucose levels	[38, 39]
	Fenugreek seed powder (5% in the diet) for 21 days in female Wistar rats.	↓ blood glucose levels	[40]
	Fenugreek seed powder (0.5 and 1.0 g/kg orally) for four weeks in male Wistar rats.	↓ serum glucose levels	[41]

(Table 1) cont.....

Compounds	Administration Dose and Protocol	Main Findings Related to Antidiabetic Effect	Refs.
Ficus extracts	*Ficus carica* leaf extract (200 mg/kg, orally), bud extract (200 mg/kg, orally) and their combination treatment (100+100 mg/kg, orally) for 30 days in male Wistar rats.	↓ blood glucose level Antioxidant activity in pancreas tissue.	[42]
	Ficus deltoidea petroleum ether, chloroform, and methanol extracts (250, 500, 1000 mg/kg, orally) for 14 days in female Sprague Dawley rats.	↓ blood glucose levels (250, 500 and1000 mg/kg methanol extract) ↑ plasma insulin levels (250, 500 and1000 mg/kg methanol extract) Protected pancreatic β-cell against STZ (1000 mg/kg methanol extract).	[43]
	Aqueous extract of *Ficus bengalensis* bark (500 mg/kg by oral intubation) in male Wistar rats.	↓ plasma glucose levels at 5 hours	[44]
	Ficus hispida leaf methanol extract (100, 200, and 400 mg/kg, oral) for 21 days in male Wistar rats.	↓ blood glucose levels ↑ serum insulin levels (200 and 400 mg/kg)	[45]
Cinnamon	Cinnamaldehyde (20 mg/kg, orally) for 60 days in male Wistar rats.	↓ FBG levels ↑ serum insulin levels ↓ HbA1c levels ↑ β-cell insulin release *in vitro*	[46]
	Cinnamon extract (100, 200, and 400 mg/kg, orally) for six weeks in male Wistar rats.	↓ FBG levels	[47]
	Cinnamon oil (100 mg/kg, oral liquid-loadable tablets (1), a self-emulsifying formulation (2) and formulated in normal saline (3)) for 45 days in male Wistar rats.	↓ blood glucose levels ((1) and (2)) ↓ HbA1c levels ((1) and (2)) ↑ serum insulin levels ((1) and (2)) Improved pancreatic β-cell recovery ((1) and (2))	[48]
	Cinnamon extract (30 mg/kg and 100 mg/kg in water) for 22 days in male Wistar rats.	↓ blood glucose levels	[49]

(Table 1) cont.....

Compounds	Administration Dose and Protocol	Main Findings Related to Antidiabetic Effect	Refs.
Berberine	Berberine (50, 150 and 500 mg/kg by tube feeding) for 14 weeks in female NOD mice (NOD/ShiLtJ).	↑ pancreatic cell numbers and serum insulin levels.	[50]
		No effect on blood glucose levels.	[51]
	Berberine (200 mg/kg by gavage) for two weeks in female NOD mice.	↓ cytokine levels Inhibited the differentiation of Th1 and Th17 cells. Prevented T1DM progression.	[52]
	Berberine (100 and 200 mg/kg, orally) for three weeks in female NOD/LtJ mice.	No effect on FBG or fasting serum insulin levels.	[53]
	Berberine (50 mg/kg, orally) for 4 weeks in female Wistar rats.	No effect on non-FBG levels.	[54]
	Berberine (50, 100, and 200 mg/kg intragastrically) for eight weeks in male Sprague Dawley rats.	↓ FBG levels	[55]
	Berberine (100 mg/kg) for 21 days in male Kunming mice.	No effect on blood glucose levels.	[56]
Silymarin	Silymarin (50 mg/kg, orally, for 28 days) in male Wistar rats.	↓ blood glucose levels Improved the diabetes-induced cellular vacuolation and β-cells depletion.	[57]
	Silymarin (50 and 100 mg/kg, intragastric tube, for four weeks) in male Wistar rats.	No effect on the level of blood glucose and insulin.	[58]
Silibinin	Silibinin (50 mg/kg/day, intramuscular injection, for eight weeks) in female and male Kunming mice.	↓ HbA1c and blood glucose ↓ apoptosis ratio of pancreatic β-cells. Improved the downregulation of SIRT1.	[59]
	Silibinin (100-200 mg/kg/day, orally, for 4 weeks) in male Wistar rats.	No effect on the level of blood glucose. ↓ DNA damage.	[60]

(Table 1) cont.....

Compounds	Administration Dose and Protocol	Main Findings Related to Antidiabetic Effect	Refs.
Curcumin	Curcumin (5-25-50 mg/kg, 95%, daily i.p. for seven days and every other day until the 60th day) in female NOD, NODscid and NOD.BDC2·5 transgenic T-cell receptor (tgTCR) (BDC2·5) mice.	↓ diabetes incidence due to dose-related effects. Delayed the onset of diabetes. Prevented insulitis. ↓ T-cell proliferation.	[61]
	Curcumin (100 mg/kg/day) orally for six weeks in male Sprague Dawley Rats.	↓ blood glucose levels ↓ cardiac oxidative stress and fibrosis.	[62]
	Curcumin (30 mg/kg/day, i.p.) for 14 days in C57BL /6 mice.	↓ FBG levels ↓ IL-6, IL-17, IFN-γ levels ↑ IL-10 levels ↑ plasma insulin levels	[63]
	Curcumin (80 and 130 mg/kg/day) by gavage for 60 days in male Wistar rats.	↓ FBG levels ↓ oxidative stress markers	[64]
	Curcumin (100 mg/kg/day, oral) and metformin (200 mg/kg/day, po) for six weeks in male Wistar rats.	No effect on blood glucose levels ↓ TGF-β levels ↓ oxidative stress Inhibited JAK2/STAT3 and Improved inflammatory state Inhibited cardiac injury.	[65]
	Curcumin (1.0%, weight ratio) mixed diet for 21 days in male Sprague-Dawley rats.	↓ blood glucose levels ↑ insulin levels ↓ oxidative stress marker	[66]
	Curcumin (1500 mg/kg/day) within diet in male C57BL/6 J mice.	No effect on plasma glucose or insulin levels. Inhibited NF-κB activation ↓ TNF-α and IL-1β levels. Inhibited oxidative stress.	[67]

(Table 1) cont.....

Compounds	Administration Dose and Protocol	Main Findings Related to Antidiabetic Effect	Refs.
	Curcumin (100 mg/kg/day, orally) for 12 weeks in male Sprague-Dawley rats.	No effect on plasma glucose or insulin levels. ↓ inflammatory cytokines and reactive oxygen species levels	[68]
	Curcumin (100 mg/kg/day) by oral gavage for eight weeks in male Sprague–Dawley rats.	↓ plasma glucose levels	[69]
	Curcumin (100 mg/kg/day) by oral gavage for eight weeks in male Sprague–Dawley rats.	↓ plasma glucose levels ↓ oxidative stress	[70]
Resveratrol	Resveratrol (250 mg/kg/day) or Mega resveratrol (99% purity) by gavage. Resveratrol (25 mg/kg, s.c.) every other day in NOD (H-2g7), NOD.BDC2.5 and NOD/SCID mice.	Delayed T1DM particularly by s.c. injection ↓ CCR6 expression which is a critical mediator in pathogenic lymphocyte migration	[71]
	Resveratrol (20mg/kg) for eight weeks in rats.	↓ FBG and HbA1c levels ↑ antioxidant enzymes activities Inhibited lipid peroxidation	[72]
	Resveratrol (50 mg/kg, i.p.) for 12 days in male BALB/c albino mice.	↓ FBG, WBC count, serum NO, and TNF-α levels ↓ CXCL16 cleavage by ADAM10 ↑ fasting insulin levels	[73]
	Resveratrol (50 mg/kg, i.p.) for 12 days in male BALB/c albino mice.	↓ blood glucose and glucose intolerance Improved fasting insulin levels and insulin tolerance ↓ CXCL16, ox-LDL, and TF levels in pancreatic β-cells Inhibited the expression of CXCL16/NF p65 in pancreatic islets	[74, 75]

(Table 1) cont.....

Compounds	Administration Dose and Protocol	Main Findings Related to Antidiabetic Effect	Refs.
	Resveratrol (10 mg/kg, i.p.) combined with NPH insulin (5 U/day, s.c.) for 30 days in male Wistar rats.	↓ glucosuria ↓ fructosamine levels ↑ SIRT1 in liver	[76]
	Resveratrol (15 mg/kg twice a day, i.p.) for one week and then one hour before STZ injection in male Sprague Dawley rats.	Inhibited the activation of caspase-3 and PARP Protected β-cells *via* inhibited apoptosis	[77]
	Resveratrol (200 mg/kg/day) by gavage on the 3rd day following T1DM onset in female NOD mice.	↓ blood glucose ↓ inflammatory factors expression (RAGE, NF-κB (P65) and NOX4)	[78]
	Resveratrol (0.5 mg/kg, three times a day) by gastric intubation for 14 days in male Sprague-Dawley rats.	Hypoglycemic activities No effect on plasma insulin levels Proposed insulin-like effect	[79]
	Resveratrol (0.75 mg/kg, three times a day) by gastric intubation for eight weeks in male Sprague-Dawley rats.	↓ diabetic ketoacidosis Activated AMPK and SIRT1 in the liver ↓ NF-kB, IL-6, IL-β	[80]
Catechins	Epicatechin (purity>90%, 0.5% in drinking water) for 28 weeks in female NOD/LtJ mice.	↑ plasma insulin levels ↓ HbA1c concentrations ↑ IL-10 and IL-12 levels Improved pancreatic insulitis and islet mass	[81]
	Epigallocatechin gallate (0.05% in drinking-water) for 27 weeks in female NOD/LtJ mice.	↑ plasma insulin levels ↓ HbA1c ↑ IL-10 levels No effect on insulitis	[82]
	Epigallocatechin gallate (100 mg/kg/day) for 10 days in male C57BL/KsJ mice.	↓ blood glucose levels ↓ iNOS Ameliorated pancreatic islet mass	[83]
	(-)-epicatechin-3-β-O-D-allopyranoside (10, 20, or 40 mg/kg/day) by oral gavage for four weeks in male C57BL/6J mice.	↓ blood glucose levels and HbA1c ↓ leptin levels ↑ insulin and adiponectin levels Ameliorated size and number of islets cells Activated AMPK Regulated insulin pathway (Akt)	[84]

(Table 1) cont.....

Compounds	Administration Dose and Protocol	Main Findings Related to Antidiabetic Effect	Refs.
Ginseng	Korean red ginseng extract (25, 100, 1000 mg/kg/day) for two weeks prior to the STZ injection and thereafter every other day for four more weeks in female C57BL/6J mice.	↓ blood glucose levels Improved pancreatic tissue and insulin secretion ↑ lymphocyte counts in the spleen	[85]
	Diol ginsenoside fraction (1 mg/g/day, orally) for eight weeks in female DP-BB rats.	↓ insulitis ↑ plasma and pancreatic insulin levels ↓ cytokine production ↑ β-cell resistance	[86]
	Panaxadiol (50 mg/kg/day) for 25 days in male wild-type C57BL/6 J mice.	Inhibited IL-17A production Ameliorated pancreatic islet β cell function	[87]
	North American ginseng (200 mg/kg/day) by oral gavage for four-eight weeks in male C57BL/6 mice.	↓ blood glucose levels and HbA1c ↑ insulin and C-peptide levels ↑ islet/pancreas ratio	[88]
	Panax ginseng alcohol extract (0.66 mg/ml/day) in drinking water for 20 weeks in male New Zealand white rabbits.	Ameliorated serum glucose, insulin, and HBA1c levels	[89]
Olive leaf	Olive leaf powder (0.3, and 0.6%) in diet for four weeks in male mice.	↓ plasma glucose levels ↑ insulin levels, superoxide dismutase, glutathione peroxidase, and catalase activities, and TH2 cytokine levels ↓ NO, iNOS, interferon-γ, IL-17, TH1 and TH17 cytokine levels	[90]
	Dried leaf extract of *Olea europaea* (100 mg/kg/day, by gavage or 40 mg/kg, i.p.) for 15 days in male C57BL/6 and CBA/H mice and female non-obese diabetic mice.	↓ plasma glucose levels Prevented changes in pancreatic islets Ameliorated insulin expression and release ↓ IFN-γ, IL-17, TNF-α	[91]

(Table 1) cont.....

Compounds	Administration Dose and Protocol	Main Findings Related to Antidiabetic Effect	Refs.
Allicin	Allicin (16 mg/kg/day by gavage for 30 days in male Wister rats.	↓ blood glucose levels ↑ plasma insulin levels	[92]
	Allicin (4, 8, and 16 mg/kg, i.p.) for 28 days in male Wister rats.	↓ blood glucose levels (8 and 16 mg/kg)	[93]
	Allicin (15, 30 and 45 mg/kg by gavage) for 12 weeks in Sprague Dawley rats.	↓ blood glucose levels (30 and 45 mg/kg)	[94]
	Allicin (8 and 16 mg/kg, i.p.) for 30 days in male Sprague Dawley rats.	↓ FBG levels ↑ serum insulin levels ↓ anti-islet cell antibodies Protected Langerhans islet cells	[95]
	Allicin (10 and 30 mg/kg by gavage) for six weeks in male BALB/c mice.	↓ FBG levels (starting from day 28) (30 mg/kg) ↑ serum insulin levels and pancreatic insulin-positive area (30 mg/kg) Improved pancreatic islet structure and reduced β-cell apoptosis (10 and 30 mg/kg)	[96]
Thymoquinone	Thymoquinone (5 mg/kg, i.p., for 30 days in male Sprague-Dawley rats.	Suppressed lipid peroxidation in pancreatic tissue ↑ antioxidant enzyme levels	[97]
	Thymoquinone (3 mg/kg/day, i.p.) for three days in male Wister rats.	Inhibited hyperglycemia Prevented inhibition of serum insulin levels by STZ	[98]
Mangiferin	Mangiferin (40 mg/kg orally) for 30 days in male Wister rats.	↓ plasma glucose levels Inhibited oxidative stress Protected from apoptosis	[99]

Abbreviations: ADAM10: A disintegrin and metalloprotease domain 10, AMPK: Adenosine monophosphate-activated protein kinase, CCR6: C-C chemokine receptor type 6, CXCL16: CXC chemokine ligand 16, DP-BB: Diabetes-prone biobreeding, FBG: Fasting blood glucose, G6pc: Glucose-6-phosphatase catalytic subunit, GLUT: Glucose transporter, HbA1c: Hemoglobin A1c, iNOS: Inducible nitric oxide synthase, i.p.: Intraperitoneal, IFN-γ: Interferon-gamma, IL: Interleukin, JAK2: Janus kinase 2, MLD-STZ: Multiple low dose-streptozotocin, NF-κB: Nuclear factor kappa B, NO: Nitric oxide, NOD: Non-obese diabetic, NPH: Neutral Protamine Hagedorn, NOX4: NADPH oxidase 4, ox-LDL: Oxidized low-density lipoprotein, PARP: Poly-ADP ribose polymerase, Pck1: Phosphoenolpyruvate carboxykinase, RAGE: Receptor for advanced glycation end product, Ref: References, Slc2a2: Solute carrier family 2 member 2, SIRT1: Sirtuin 1, STAT3: Signal transducer and activator of transcription 3, STZ: Streptozotocin, T1DM: Type 1 diabetes mellitus, TGF-β: Transforming growth factor-β, TH: T helper, TNF-α: Tumor necrosis factor-alpha, WBC: White blood cell.

Table 2. Clinical studies on herbs or herbal products in T1DM.

Compounds	Study Design	Population	Administration dose and Protocol	Proposed Effects	Refs.
Ficus extracts	-	Female (*n* =6) and male (*n* =4) patients with T1DM	*Ficus carica* leaf decoction (13 g sachet of leaves) for two months with a cleansing period after one month.	Improved glycemic control	[103]
Cinnamon	Prospective, double-blind, placebo-controlled study	72 adolescents with T1DM	Cinnamon (1g/day) for 90 days.	No effect on HbA1c levels, daily insulin requirement and the number of hypoglycemic episodes.	[102]
Resveratrol	An exploratory, single-centre clinical trial	Female (*n* =5) and male (*n* = 8) patients with T1DM	Resveratrol 500 mg capsules (99% pure, Biotivia, Bioceuticals International, SRL, Verona, Italy), twice daily for 60 days.	↓ FBG and HbA1c ↓ oxidative stress markers No effect on insulin levels, HOMA-IR, HOMA-β, markers of hepatic-renal and inflammatory (c-reactive protein, TNF-α, and IL-1β).	[100]
Olive leaf	A randomized, double-blind, placebo-controlled trial	77 healthy overweight/obese adults	Olive leaf extract 500 mg (*n* = 39) or placebo (*n* = 38) for eight weeks.	No significant effect on blood glucose and insulin levels.	[101]

Abbreviations: FBG: Fasting blood glucose, HbA1c: Hemoglobin A1c, HOMA-IR: Homeostatic Model Assessment for Insulin Resistance, IL: Interleukin, Ref: References, T1DM: Type 1 diabetes mellitus, TNF-α: Tumor necrosis factor-alpha.

Fenugreek

Fenugreek (*Trigonella foenum-graecum*) is used for antioxidant, glucose-lowering and cholesterol-lowering effects [104]. Acute treatment with the soluble dietary fibre fraction of fenugreek (0.5 g/kg) did not affect FBG levels but significantly ameliorated glucose tolerance in streptozotocin (STZ)-induced diabetic rats [35]. Treatment with aqueous fenugreek seed extract at both doses (0.87 g/kg and 1.74 g/kg) reduced plasma glucose levels in STZ-induced diabetic rats [33].

Treatment with 4-hydroxyisoleucine, the major constituent of fenugreek seeds (50 mg/kg/day) for four weeks, markedly decreased plasma glucose levels in STZ-diabetic rats. However, the treatment failed to reverse the STZ-induced decrease in plasma insulin levels [32]. In this study, the antidiabetic activity of 4-hydroxyisoleucine was suggested to be insulin-independent [32]. However, trigonelline (70 mg/kg), the active compound of fenugreek, was used for four weeks that restored pancreatic morphology, reduced β-cell apoptosis, increased β-islet area and increased both pancreatic insulin content and serum insulin concentration in STZ-induced diabetic mice, leading to reduced blood glucose levels in a time-dependent manner [36]. In addition, trigonelline reduced elevated serum inflammatory markers and showed antioxidant activity in pancreatic tissues [36]. Histological analysis showed that treatment with fenugreek oil (10% in the diet) for four weeks protected against pancreatic β-cell damage caused by alloxan-induced diabetes in rats [34]. This effect was attributed to reduced pancreatic white blood cell and lymphocyte counts and IL-6 levels. Its beneficial effect on pancreatic β-cell resulted in increased plasma insulin levels and consequently lower plasma glucose levels [34].

HbA1c levels in alloxan-diabetic rats were markedly reduced by an 8-week treatment with 5% fenugreek seed powder [37]. While the blood glucose levels were reduced compared to diabetic animals, statistical significance was not shown in this study [37]. Conversely, a shorter treatment period (21 days) with fenugreek seed powder (5%) substantially decreased blood glucose levels in alloxan diabetic rats [38 - 40]. Supporting that, treatment with fenugreek seed powder (0.5 and 1.0 g/kg) for four weeks reduced serum glucose levels in a dose-dependent manner in alloxan-diabetic rats [41].

Preclinical studies suggest that fenugreek has both glycemic and insulinotropic effects in T1DM. However, clinical studies investigating the antidiabetic activity of fenugreek have mostly been conducted in T2DM patients. Therefore, more comprehensive studies are needed to elucidate its antidiabetic effect in T1DM and T2DM [104].

Ficus Extracts

Ficus species have been shown to regulate blood glucose levels through several mechanisms, including regeneration of β-cells and their function and increased insulin secretion in T1DM [105]. In a clinical setting, fig leaf decoction supplementation improved glycemic control in patients with T1DM [103]. Patients who received the supplementation required less insulin and had lower mean capillary glucose levels [103].

Aqueous extract of *Ficus bengalensis* bark administration at 500 mg/kg markedly decreased plasma glucose levels at 5 hours in all fasted, fed and glucose-fed STZ-induced diabetic rats [44]. *Ficus carica* leaf extract (200 mg/kg), bud extract (200 mg/kg) and their combination treatment (100+100 mg/kg) for 30 days reduced blood glucose levels in a time-dependent manner in alloxan diabetic rats [42]. In addition, all treatments showed antioxidant effects in pancreatic tissues [42].

It is important to use solvents that are appropriate for the desired effect when preparing plant extracts. The antidiabetic effects of *Ficus deltoidea* leaf extracts in petroleum ether, chloroform and methanol were investigated in STZ-induced diabetic rats. Only methanol extract showed a blood glucose-lowering effect. In addition, 14-day treatment with methanol extract at doses of 250 and 500 showed a time- and dose-dependent decrease in blood glucose levels [43]. Treatment with methanol extract at 250, 500, and 1000 mg/kg increased plasma insulin levels in a dose-dependent manner. The treatment of 1000 mg/kg of methanol extract protected pancreatic β-cells against STZ by reducing GLUT2 mRNA levels [43]. Similarly, treatment with *Ficus hispida* leaf methanol extract at 100, 200 and 400 mg/kg for 21 days increased serum insulin levels, but only the medium and high doses produced a marked reduction in blood glucose levels from day seven [45].

Cinnamon

Cinnamon is a widely used spice that contains chemicals such as cinnamaldehyde, cinnamate and cinnamic acid, which have various beneficial effects, including antidiabetic [106]. Treatment with cinnamon (1 g/day) for 90 days did not significantly change HbA1c levels, daily insulin requirements or the number of hypoglycemic episodes in adolescents with T1DM [102]. However, clinical studies had a high risk of bias and were inconclusive in showing the beneficial effects of cinnamon treatment in T1DM and T2DM [107].

Cinnamon extract (100, 200 and 400 mg/kg) treatment for six weeks significantly reduced FBG levels in STZ-diabetic rats, and the glucose-lowering effect of treatment was higher at 200 and 400 mg/kg doses of the extract [47]. Treatment with aqueous cinnamon extract (30 mg/kg and 100 mg/kg) for 22 days reduced blood glucose levels in STZ diabetic rats through insulin-independent pathways [49].

Treatment with cinnamaldehyde, an active substance of cinnamon (20 mg/kg) for 60 days, reduced FBG levels and enhanced serum insulin levels in a time-dependent manner compared to STZ-diabetic animals. The effect of this compound on insulin was further supported by increased *in vitro* insulin release [46]. In addition, HbA1c levels increased significantly from baseline in diabetic and cinnamaldehyde-treated diabetic animals. However, an increase in HbA1c was dramatically higher in the diabetic group, and cinnamaldehyde treatment markedly reduced HbA1c compared to diabetic animals at the end of the study [46].

Oral liquid-loadable cinnamon oil tablets and a self-emulsifying cinnamon oil formulation and cinnamon oil formulated in normal saline at 100 mg/kg were administered to the alloxan diabetic rats for 45 days [48]. The first two formulations markedly reduced blood glucose and HbA1c levels and augmented serum insulin levels compared to diabetic animals. This finding was consistent with the pancreatic β-cell recovery effect of these two cinnamon oil formulations [48].

Berberine

Berberine is a quaternary benzylisoquinoline alkaloid found in various plants such as barberry, Oregon grape, turmeric, and many others, and has been used in inflammatory disorders, and microbial pathologies. There is growing experimental evidence of its ameliorative effect on diabetes [108].

Non-obese diabetic (NOD) mice have been widely used in studies investigating the antidiabetic effects of berberine. Berberine treatment (200 mg/kg) for two weeks prevented the progression of T1DM in NOD mice by reducing cytokine levels and inhibiting the differentiation of Th1 and Th17 cells [52]. Prolonged treatment (14 weeks) with 50, 150, and 500 mg/kg berberine increased pancreatic cell numbers in a dose-dependent manner and increased the serum insulin levels in NOD mice [50]. In addition, a slight positive correlation was found between serum berberine concentration and pancreatic islet cell number, suggesting that berberine supplementation partially protects pancreatic tissue [50]. In a following study by the same research group, blood glucose levels in NOD mice were not affected by berberine supplementation. However, the improper progression of T1DM in NOD mice does not allow a definitive conclusion in this study [51]. Moreover, 100 and 200 mg/kg berberine treatment for three weeks did not affect either FBG or fasting serum insulin levels in type 1 diabetic NOD/LtJ mice [53].

The effect of berberine has also been studied using an STZ-induced diabetes model. 50 mg/kg berberine treatment for four weeks did not affect non-FBG levels [54]. Similarly, 100 mg/kg berberine for 21 days did not affect blood glucose levels in STZ-diabetic mice [56]. Unlike the two studies mentioned, 50, 100 and 200 mg/kg berberine treatment for eight weeks showed a blood glucose-lowering effect in a dose-dependent manner in STZ-diabetic rats [55].

Silymarin and Silibinin

Silymarin is the active constituent found in *Silybum marianum* (commonly known as milk thistle), and silibinin is the main component of silymarin. In particular, both silymarin and silibinin recognized for their hepatoprotective properties [109], have attracted attention for their potential effects. Silymarin is generally safe and well-tolerated in clinical studies [110]. In the context of experimental rat models using STZ to simulate T1DM, silymarin administration at 50 mg/kg was observed to yield beneficial outcomes [57]. These include an augmentation in the β-cells quantity, a slight decline in glucose levels, and an enhancement in insulin levels.

In mice with STZ-induced T1DM, an eight weeks regimen of silibinin injection at 50 mg/kg/day exhibited a decline in HbA1c and blood glucose, an improvement of sirtuin 1 (SIRT1) downregulation, and a reduction in pancreatic β-cell apoptosis [59]. Conversely, oral administration of silibinin at 100 and 200 mg/kg/day over four weeks to STZ-induced T1DM rats did not manifest alterations in blood glucose levels [60]. However, a reduction in DNA damage was observed as a result of this intervention. In an STZ-induced T1DM rat model, intragastric tube administration of silymarin for four weeks at 50 and 100 mg/kg did not induce changes in blood glucose and insulin levels [58].

Curcumin

Curcumin, chemically referred to as diferuloylmethane, is an antioxidant compound isolated from the *Curcuma longa* [111]. Curcumin, known for its anti-inflammatory and antioxidant properties, has been postulated to have favorable outcomes on diabetes and its associated complications [112]. Nevertheless, the translation of these therapeutic benefits into clinical practice is hampered by poor bioavailability. Consequently, strategies encompassing the development of delivery systems for curcumin are under investigation [113].

In murine models, curcumin administration has exhibited the potential to mitigate the progression of autoimmune diabetes. Specifically, curcumin intervention in cyclophosphamide-induced NOD mice and adoptive transfer of diabetogenic spleen cells into NOD-scid mice, an accelerated autoimmune diabetes model, has demonstrated the capacity to delay disease onset and protect against autoimmune diabetes [61].

Oral administration of curcumin at 100 mg/kg/day to STZ-induced T1DM rats was associated with notable reductions in blood glucose levels and ameliorative effects on oxidative stress and cardiac fibrosis [62]. Similarly, intraperitoneal administration of curcumin at 30 mg/kg/day to STZ-induced T1DM mice was shown to reduce FBG, increase plasma insulin and C-peptide levels, and exert anti-inflammatory effects by influencing cytokine profiles [63]. This study further suggests that the action of curcumin involves attenuating pancreatic β-cell destruction through decreasing proinflammatory cytokines (IL-6, IL-17, and IFN-γ) and increasing the anti-inflammatory cytokine IL-10. In another study, curcumin was shown to reduce oxidative stress and lower FBG in the STZ-induced rat model of T1DM [64]. Moreover, curcumin may protect against diabetic nephropathy by potentially benefiting renal tissue [64]. The addition of curcumin to the diet of STZ-induced T1DM rats increased insulin levels while reducing blood glucose and markers of oxidative stress [66]. However, it is noteworthy to consider the potential limitations of the study, such as the fact that insulin was administered until the animals were harvested, which reduced mortality in diabetic rats. In the STZ-induced T1DM rat model, curcumin administration at 100 mg/kg/day demonstrated the ability to reduce plasma glucose levels and potentially prevent renal and cardiac fibrosis processes, attributed to its antioxidant effects [69, 70].

Contrasting observations emerge from investigations involving cardiac and fibrotic parameters. Curcumin administration did not affect blood glucose levels in STZ-induced T1DM rats [65]. Nevertheless, the same study suggests the potential of curcumin to mitigate cardiac fibrosis through the modulation of oxidative stress and anti-inflammatory pathways. Dietary curcumin supplementation at 1500 mg/kg/day in STZ-induced T1DM mice did not affect plasma glucose or insulin levels but reduced inflammation, oxidative stress, and skeletal muscle atrophy [67]. In another study, curcumin (100 mg/kg/day) did not affect plasma glucose or insulin levels in the STZ-induced rat model of T1DM. However, it has been suggested that it may prevent nephropathy by reducing the levels of inflammatory cytokines and reactive oxygen species [68].

Resveratrol

Resveratrol (3,5,4'-trihydroxystilbene) is found in strawberries, grapes and peanuts and has anti-inflammatory, antioxidant, and organ-protective properties [114, 115]. Resveratrol augments the activity of the protein SIRT1, which exerts an inhibitory effect on T-cell activation [116].

An exploratory, single-centre clinical trial was conducted to assess the efficacy and safety of resveratrol in patients with T1DM [100]. Thirteen participants diagnosed with T1DM who had been on oral antidiabetic therapy and/or insulin injections for at least six months, were enrolled in this study. Over a span of two months, these individuals were administered 500 mg resveratrol capsules twice daily. A comprehensive analysis of serum samples was performed at baseline and the end of the first and second months. The results of this trial revealed that short-term administration of resveratrol has been shown to reduce FBG and HbA1c levels, as well as diminished oxidative markers. The findings of this study suggest that resveratrol may have a beneficial effect as an adjuvant therapy in the treatment of T1DM [100].

The potential of resveratrol to modulate the development of T1DM has been investigated in murine models. Resveratrol administration at 200 mg/kg/day in NOD mice significantly decreased blood glucose levels and expression of inflammatory factors and improved renal function [78]. In NOD mice, administration of resveratrol at 25 mg/kg every other day led to downregulation of C-C chemokine receptor type 6 (CCR6) expression and subsequently delayed the onset of T1DM [71]. Similarly, in the STZ-induced T1DM mice models, resveratrol doses of 50 mg/kg (i.p.) for 12 days revealed a reduction in FBG levels and an increase in insulin concentrations [73, 74]. Resveratrol has been suggested to reduce tissue factor (TF) activation and autophagic β-cell destruction in T1DM through the inhibition of CXCL16/ox-LDL signaling and suppression of CXCL16/NF-κB p65 expression in the pancreas [74, 75].

The potential of resveratrol to protect pancreatic β-cells and its effects on metabolic parameters has been studied in rats. Resveratrol (15 mg/kg twice daily, i.p.) has been proposed to protect β-cells by inhibiting apoptosis in STZ-induced T1DM rats [77]. Resveratrol administration at 20 mg/kg for eight weeks decreased FBG and HbA1c levels and increased antioxidant enzyme activities in STZ-induced T1DM rats [72]. Oral resveratrol (1.5 mg/kg) for 14 days produced hypoglycemic and hypolipidemic effects in STZ-induced T1DM rats. Although resveratrol did not affect plasma insulin levels in this study, it was suggested that it may have an insulin-like effect [79]. In the field of therapeutic combinations, the synergy between resveratrol and insulin has attracted attention. Administration of resveratrol (10 mg/kg, i.p.) in addition to NPH insulin to STZ-induced T1DM rats was shown to further reduce glucosuria and fructosamine levels, accompanied by improvements in glycemic control [76]. Mechanistically, this was linked to the downregulation of Solute carrier family 2 member 2 (Slc2a2)/GLUT2, phosphoenolpyruvate carboxykinase (Pck1) and glucose-6-phosphatase catalytic subunit (G6pc) expression and increased SIRT1 levels in the liver [76]. Oral administration of resveratrol (2.25 mg/kg) to STZ-induced T1DM rats for eight weeks reduced diabetic ketoacidosis. In addition, activation of adenosine monophosphate-activated protein kinase (AMPK) and SIRT1 in the liver and reduced inflammation were suggested [80].

Catechins

Catechins constitute the active compounds found in green tea (*Camellia sinensis*), including epigallocatechin gallate, epigallocatechin, epicatechin gallate, and epicatechin [117]. Epigallocatechin gallate is the most abundant of these catechins and has antioxidant, anti-inflammatory, and glucose-lowering effects [118].

Administration of epigallocatechin gallate at 100 mg/kg/day for ten days to low-dose STZ-induced T1DM mice reduced blood glucose and improved pancreatic islet mass [83]. This study suggests that epigallocatechin gallate may play a role in preventing the onset of diabetes by protecting pancreatic islets [83]. Oral administration of epicatechin and epigallocatechin gallate to NOD mice increased plasma insulin levels and decreased HbA1c concentrations, thereby improving glucose tolerance [81, 82]. Furthermore, these catechins showed the ability to increase circulating IL-10 levels and may protect pancreatic islets against autoimmune destruction [81, 82]. Oral administration of (-)-epicatechin-3-β-O-D-allopyranoside to mice with an STZ-induced T1DM model reduced blood glucose, triglycerides, leptin, and HbA1c levels and increased insulin and adiponectin levels [84]. An improvement in the number and size of pancreatic islet cells was observed. Mechanistically, this study proposed that the observed improvements could be attributed to AMPK activation and regulation of the Akt (protein kinase B) pathway.

Ginseng

The genus Panax contains more than twelve species, the two best known being Asian (*Panax ginseng Meyer*) and American (*Panax quinquefolius L.*), whose effects on cognition, fatigue and glucose metabolism have been investigated in clinical trials [119].

Korean red ginseng extract (25, 100, 1000 mg/kg/day) administered prophylactically to STZ-induced T1DM mice reduced blood glucose levels and improved pancreatic tissue and insulin secretion [85]. Notable increases in splenic lymphocyte counts highlighted the immunomodulatory potential of Korean red ginseng. These observed hypoglycemic and immunoregulatory effects of Korean red ginseng underline its prospective utility in the management of T1DM.

In a distinct murine model of C57BL/6J mice with STZ-induced T1DM, ginseng-derived panaxadiol at 50 mg/kg/day inhibited IL-17A production and improved the pancreatic islets β-cells function [87]. This suggests the potential of ginseng-derived compounds to ameliorate immune-mediated β-cell dysfunction.

The influence of North American ginseng was investigated in STZ-induced T1DM mouse models. Oral administration of North American ginseng at 200 mg/kg/day for 4-8 weeks to STZ-induced T1DM mice resulted in a decrease in blood glucose and HbA1c levels, while insulin and C-peptide levels were increased [88]. A significant improvement in the islet/pancreas ratio was also observed [88]. This study suggested that North American ginseng may enhance insulin secretion through β-cell regeneration [88].

Administration of the diol ginsenoside fraction of Korean red ginseng to diabetes-prone biobreeding (DP-BB) rats displayed multiple benefits, including preservation of insulin levels, reduction of cytokine production, elevated β-cell resistance, and potential attenuation of insulitis [86]. These findings suggest that Korean red ginseng may have the potential to delay T1DM onset. Furthermore, oral administration of Panax ginseng extract (0.66 mg/ml/day) for 20 weeks to rabbits with alloxan-induced T1DM resulted in improvements in serum glucose, insulin, and HBA1c levels, suggesting its potential to improve markers of diabetes [89].

Olive Leaf

Olive leaves contain phenolic compounds that have been reported to have antioxidant, hypoglycemic and anti-inflammatory properties, such as oleuropein, hydroxytyrosol, verbascoside, apigenin-7-glucoside, and luteolin-7-glucoside [120 - 122].

A randomized, double-blind, placebo-controlled study was performed to examine the effect of olive leaf extract on cardiovascular health [101]. In overweight/obese adults, an 8-week regimen of olive leaf extract (500 mg) showed no significant effect on blood glucose or insulin levels [101].

Administration of olive leaf powder (0.3% and 0.6%) in the diet of STZ-induced T1DM mice for four weeks reduced plasma glucose and elevated insulin levels [90]. Olive leaf powder also led to a reduction in oxidative stress and proinflammatory cytokines levels [90]. In another study, the dried leaf extract of *Olea europaea* was administered at 100 mg/kg/day (gavage) or 40 mg/kg (i.p.) for 15 days to multiple low-dose (MLD)-STZ-induced T1DM mice and cyclophosphamide-accelerated T1DM mice [91]. These interventions lowered plasma glucose levels, improved insulin levels, decreased proinflammatory markers, and prevented changes in pancreatic islets.

Allicin

Allicin (diallyl thiosulfinate), the main active compound of *Allium sativum* (garlic), exhibits antioxidant and anti-inflammatory activity, contributing to its beneficial effect on various diseases. Although the effect of allicin on diabetes has been relatively less studied, it has been shown to have hypoglycemic activity [123].

Treatment with 8 and 16 mg/kg, but not 4 mg/kg, of allicin for 28 days reduced blood glucose levels [93] and 16 mg/kg allicin for 30 days significantly diminished blood glucose levels and enhanced plasma insulin levels in STZ-diabetic rats [92]. Treatment with 8 and 16 mg/kg allicin for 30 days resulted in a reduction in FBG levels in STZ diabetic rats and, interestingly this reduction was slightly higher with the lower dose of allicin [95]. Allicin treatment led to enhanced serum insulin levels and reduced anti-islet cell antibodies in a dose-dependent manner compared to the diabetic group. Furthermore, allicin treatment dose-dependently reversed deleterious changes in Langerhans islet cells [95].

Higher doses of this component have also been used in some of the studies that have investigated the antidiabetic activity of allicin. STZ diabetic rats were treated with 15, 30 and 45 mg/kg allicin for 12 weeks as a preventive setting. Medium and high doses of allicin significantly decreased FBG levels from week 4 of treatment. However, blood glucose levels were still markedly higher than the control group [94]. There was a downward trend in FBG levels from day 28 of treatment with a high dose (30 mg/kg) but not a low dose (10 mg/kg) of allicin treatment for six weeks in STZ diabetic mice. Blood glucose levels were significantly lower from day 35 of treatment [96]. High-dose allicin increased serum insulin levels and pancreatic insulin-positive area. These findings were supported by increased insulin protein expression with high-dose allicin [96]. Both doses improved pancreatic islet structure and attenuated pancreatic β-cell apoptosis [96].

Others

Thymoquinone is an active constituent derived from *Nigella sativa*. Administration of thymoquinone at 5 mg/kg to STZ-induced T1DM rats attenuated pancreatic lipid peroxidation and concurrently elevated levels of antioxidant enzymes [97]. In this study, thymoquinone was suggested to affect inflammation in diabetes pathology and the preservation of pancreatic β-cells. Notably, the pathogenesis of STZ-induced pancreatic β-cell impairment has been linked to the involvement of nitric oxide [124]. Pretreatment of T1DM rats with thymoquinone reduced serum glucose concentrations and prevented the insulin-suppressive effect induced by STZ [98].

Mangiferin is found in several plant species, including the mango tree (*Mangifera indica*). Oral administration of mangiferin at 40 mg/kg over a 30-day period to rats afflicted with STZ-induced T1DM [99]. These interventions yielded a notable reduction in plasma glucose levels and protective effects against oxidative stress and apoptosis.

CONCLUSION AND FUTURE PERSPECTIVES

The antidiabetic effects and possible underlying mechanisms of action have mainly been studied in animal models of T1DM and a limited number of clinical trials. These diverse studies demonstrate the potential effects of various herbs and herbal products in lowering blood glucose levels, increasing insulin secretion, reducing inflammation and oxidative stress, modulating the immune system, and protecting pancreatic islet β-cells in T1DM (Fig. **3**). At the same time, T1DM in animal studies is often induced by different concentrations of chemical agents, which may affect the severity of diabetes and, subsequently, the outcome and conclusion of the study on the antidiabetic activity of herbal medicines. In conclusion, the emerging evidence for the potential benefits of herbs and herbal products in T1DM models underscores the need for further mechanistic studies and well-designed clinical trials to establish their therapeutic efficacy and safety for the management of T1DM in humans.

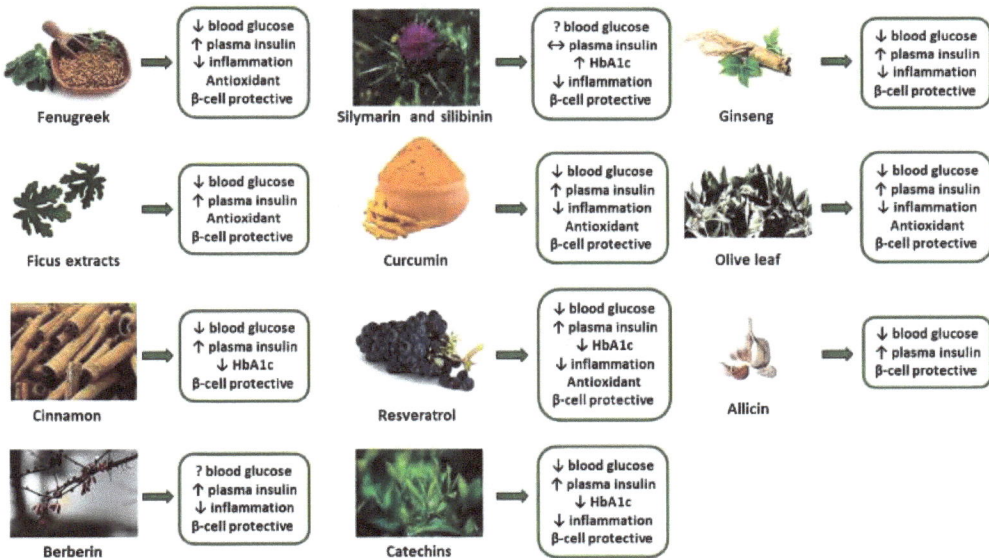

Fig. (3). Antidiabetic mechanisms of action of herbal medicines in type 1 diabetes. ?:inconsistent findings, ↔:no change,↓:decreased,↑:increased. The figure has been prepared using the Pixabay website (https://pixabay.com/tr/).

LIST OF ABBREVIATIONS

ADAM10	A Disintegrin and Metalloprotease domain 10
AMPK	Adenosine Monophosphate-activated Protein Kinase
CCR6	C-C chemokine Receptor type 6
CXCL16	CXC Chemokine Ligand 16
DP-BB	Diabetes-prone Biobreeding
FBG	Fasting Blood Glucose
G6pc	Glucose-6-phosphatase Catalytic subunit
GADA	Glutamatic Acid Decarboxylase Antibody
GLUT	Glucose Transporter
HbA1c	Hemoglobin A1c
HLA	Human Leukocyte Antigen
HOMA-IR	Homeostatic Model Assessment for Insulin Resistance
IAA	Insulin Autoantibodies
IA-2A	Insulinoma-associated-2 Autoantibodies
IDF	International Diabetes Federation
IFN-γ	Interferon-gamma
IL	Interleukin
IRS	Insulin Receptor Substrates
iNOS	Inducible Nitric Oxide Synthase
i.p.	Intraperitoneal
i.v.	Intravenous
JAK2	Janus Kinase 2
MLD-STZ	Multiple Low Dose-streptozotocin
NADPH	Nicotinamide Adenine Dinucleotide Phosphate
NF-κB	Nuclear Factor kappa B
NO	Nitric Oxide
NOD	Non-obese Diabetic
NOX4	NADPH Oxidase 4
NPH	Neutral Protamine Hagedorn
ox-LDL	Oxidized Low-density Lipoprotein
PARP	Poly-ADP Ribose Polymerase
Pck1	Phosphoenolpyruvate carboxykinase
RAGE	Receptor for Advanced Glycation end product
SIRT1	Sirtuin 1

Slc2a2	Solute carrier family 2 member 2
STAT3	Signal Transducer and Activator of Transcription 3
STZ	Streptozotocin
T1DM	Type 1 Diabetes Mellitus
T2DM	Type 2 Diabetes Mellitus
TGF-β	Transforming Growth Factor-β
TF	Tissue Factor
TH	T Helper
TNF-α	Tumor Necrosis Factor-alpha
WBC	White Blood Cell
ZnT8A	Zinc Transporter 8 Antibody

AUTHORS' CONTRIBUTIONS

BRE and ZSA were involved in the conceptualization, investigation, resources, writing-original draft preparation-reviewing and editing of the chapter.

REFERENCES

[1]　Atkinson MA, Eisenbarth GS, Michels AW. Type 1 diabetes. Lancet 2014; 383(9911): 69-82.
[http://dx.doi.org/10.1016/S0140-6736(13)60591-7] [PMID: 23890997]

[2]　Sun H, Saeedi P, Karuranga S, *et al.* IDF Diabetes Atlas: Global, regional and country-level diabetes prevalence estimates for 2021 and projections for 2045. Diabetes Res Clin Pract 2022; 183: 109119.
[http://dx.doi.org/10.1016/j.diabres.2021.109119] [PMID: 34879977]

[3]　ElSayed NA, Aleppo G, Aroda VR, *et al.* 2. Classification and Diagnosis of Diabetes: *Standards of Care in Diabetes—2023*. Diabetes Care 2023; 46 (Suppl. 1): S19-40.
[http://dx.doi.org/10.2337/dc23-S002] [PMID: 36507649]

[4]　Thomas NJ, Lynam AL, Hill AV, *et al.* Type 1 diabetes defined by severe insulin deficiency occurs after 30 years of age and is commonly treated as type 2 diabetes. Diabetologia 2019; 62(7): 1167-72.
[http://dx.doi.org/10.1007/s00125-019-4863-8] [PMID: 30969375]

[5]　Thomas NJ, Jones SE, Weedon MN, Shields BM, Oram RA, Hattersley AT. Frequency and phenotype of type 1 diabetes in the first six decades of life: a cross-sectional, genetically stratified survival analysis from UK Biobank. Lancet Diabetes Endocrinol 2018; 6(2): 122-9.
[http://dx.doi.org/10.1016/S2213-8587(17)30362-5] [PMID: 29199115]

[6]　Beran D, Abidha C, Adler A, *et al.* Teplizumab approval for type 1 diabetes in the USA. Lancet Diabetes Endocrinol 2023; 11(2): 78-80.
[http://dx.doi.org/10.1016/S2213-8587(22)00384-9] [PMID: 36623522]

[7]　Affan M, Dar MS. Donislecel-the first approved pancreatic islet cell therapy medication for type 1 diabetes: a letter to the editor. Ir J Med Sci 2023.
[PMID: 37450257]

[8]　Diaz-Valencia PA, Bougnères P, Valleron AJ. Global epidemiology of type 1 diabetes in young adults and adults: a systematic review. BMC Public Health 2015; 15(1): 255.
[http://dx.doi.org/10.1186/s12889-015-1591-y] [PMID: 25849566]

[9]　Magliano DJ, Boyko EJ. IDF DIABETES ATLAS. IDF Diabetes Atlas. 10th ed Brussels 2021. 2021.

[10]   Mobasseri M, Shirmohammadi M, Amiri T, Vahed N, Hosseini Fard H, Ghojazadeh M. Prevalence and incidence of type 1 diabetes in the world: a systematic review and meta-analysis. Health Promot Perspect 2020; 10(2): 98-115.
[http://dx.doi.org/10.34172/hpp.2020.18] [PMID: 32296622]

[11]   Green A, Hede SM, Patterson CC, *et al.* Type 1 diabetes in 2017: global estimates of incident and prevalent cases in children and adults. Diabetologia 2021; 64(12): 2741-50.
[http://dx.doi.org/10.1007/s00125-021-05571-8] [PMID: 34599655]

[12]   Quattrin T, Mastrandrea LD, Walker LSK. Type 1 diabetes. Lancet 2023; 401(10394): 2149-62.
[http://dx.doi.org/10.1016/S0140-6736(23)00223-4] [PMID: 37030316]

[13]   Insel RA, Dunne JL, Atkinson MA, *et al.* Staging presymptomatic type 1 diabetes: a scientific statement of JDRF, the Endocrine Society, and the American Diabetes Association. Diabetes Care 2015; 38(10): 1964-74.
[http://dx.doi.org/10.2337/dc15-1419] [PMID: 26404926]

[14]   Ramachandran A. Know the signs and symptoms of diabetes. Indian J Med Res 2014; 140(5): 579-81.
[PMID: 25579136]

[15]   Ehrmann D, Kulzer B, Roos T, Haak T, Al-Khatib M, Hermanns N. Risk factors and prevention strategies for diabetic ketoacidosis in people with established type 1 diabetes. Lancet Diabetes Endocrinol 2020; 8(5): 436-46.
[http://dx.doi.org/10.1016/S2213-8587(20)30042-5] [PMID: 32333879]

[16]   Ilonen J, Lempainen J, Veijola R. The heterogeneous pathogenesis of type 1 diabetes mellitus. Nat Rev Endocrinol 2019; 15(11): 635-50.
[http://dx.doi.org/10.1038/s41574-019-0254-y] [PMID: 31534209]

[17]   Wållberg M, Cooke A. Immune mechanisms in type 1 diabetes. Trends Immunol 2013; 34(12): 583-91.
[http://dx.doi.org/10.1016/j.it.2013.08.005] [PMID: 24054837]

[18]   Todd JA. Etiology of type 1 diabetes. Immunity 2010; 32(4): 457-67.
[http://dx.doi.org/10.1016/j.immuni.2010.04.001] [PMID: 20412756]

[19]   Esposito S, Toni G, Tascini G, Santi E, Berioli MG, Principi N. Environmental Factors Associated With Type 1 Diabetes. Front Endocrinol (Lausanne) 2019; 10: 592.
[http://dx.doi.org/10.3389/fendo.2019.00592] [PMID: 31555211]

[20]   Lampasona V, Liberati D. Islet Autoantibodies. Curr Diab Rep 2016; 16(6): 53.
[http://dx.doi.org/10.1007/s11892-016-0738-2] [PMID: 27112957]

[21]   Ziegler AG, Rewers M, Simell O, *et al.* Seroconversion to multiple islet autoantibodies and risk of progression to diabetes in children. JAMA 2013; 309(23): 2473-9.
[http://dx.doi.org/10.1001/jama.2013.6285] [PMID: 23780460]

[22]   Bach JF. Insulin-dependent diabetes mellitus as an autoimmune disease. Endocr Rev 1994; 15(4): 516-42.
[http://dx.doi.org/10.1210/edrv-15-4-516] [PMID: 7988484]

[23]   Anderson AM, Landry LG, Alkanani AA, *et al.* Human islet T cells are highly reactive to preproinsulin in type 1 diabetes. Proc Natl Acad Sci USA 2021; 118(41): e2107208118.
[http://dx.doi.org/10.1073/pnas.2107208118] [PMID: 34611019]

[24]   Lu J, Liu J, Li L, Lan Y, Liang Y. Cytokines in type 1 diabetes: mechanisms of action and immunotherapeutic targets. Clin Transl Immunology 2020; 9(3): e1122.
[http://dx.doi.org/10.1002/cti2.1122] [PMID: 32185024]

[25]   Melloul D. Role of NF-κB in β-cell death. Biochem Soc Trans 2008; 36(3): 334-9.
[http://dx.doi.org/10.1042/BST0360334] [PMID: 18481952]

[26]   Banting FG, Best CH, Collip JB, Campbell WR, Fletcher AA. Pancreatic Extracts in the Treatment of

Diabetes Mellitus. Can Med Assoc J 1922; 12(3): 141-6.
[PMID: 20314060]

[27]   Donnor T, Sarkar S. Insulin- Pharmacology, Therapeutic Regimens and Principles of Intensive Insulin
        Therapy. In: Feingold KR, Anawalt B, Blackman MR, Boyce A, Chrousos G, Corpas E, Eds.
        Endotext. South Dartmouth, MA 2000.

[28]   Pessin JE, Saltiel AR. Signaling pathways in insulin action: molecular targets of insulin resistance. J
        Clin Invest 2000; 106(2): 165-9.
        [http://dx.doi.org/10.1172/JCI10582] [PMID: 10903329]

[29]   Mathieu C, Gillard P, Benhalima K. Insulin analogues in type 1 diabetes mellitus: getting better all the
        time. Nat Rev Endocrinol 2017; 13(7): 385-99.
        [http://dx.doi.org/10.1038/nrendo.2017.39] [PMID: 28429780]

[30]   ElSayed NA, Aleppo G, Aroda VR, *et al.* 6. Glycemic Targets: *Standards of Care in Diabetes—2023.*
        Diabetes Care 2023; 46 (Suppl. 1): S97-S110.
        [http://dx.doi.org/10.2337/dc23-S006] [PMID: 36507646]

[31]   Harris E. FDA Greenlights First Cell Therapy for Adults With Type 1 Diabetes. JAMA 2023; 330(5):
        402.
        [http://dx.doi.org/10.1001/jama.2023.12542] [PMID: 37436739]

[32]   Haeri MR, Limaki HK, White CJB, White KN. Non-insulin dependent anti-diabetic activity of (2S,
        3R, 4S) 4-hydroxyisoleucine of fenugreek (*Trigonella foenum graecum*) in streptozotocin-induced
        type I diabetic rats. Phytomedicine 2012; 19(7): 571-4.
        [http://dx.doi.org/10.1016/j.phymed.2012.01.004] [PMID: 22397995]

[33]   Haghani K, Bakhtiyari S, Doost Mohammadpour J. Alterations in plasma glucose and cardiac
        antioxidant enzymes activity in streptozotocin-induced diabetic rats: effects of trigonella foenum-
        graecum extract and swimming training. Can J Diabetes 2016; 40(2): 135-42.
        [http://dx.doi.org/10.1016/j.jcjd.2015.08.012] [PMID: 26778682]

[34]   hamden K, Masmoudi H, Carreau S, elfeki A. Immunomodulatory, β-cell, and neuroprotective actions
        of fenugreek oil from alloxan-induced diabetes. Immunopharmacol Immunotoxicol 2010; 32(3): 437-
        45.
        [http://dx.doi.org/10.3109/08923970903490486] [PMID: 20100065]

[35]   Hannan JMA, Ali L, Rokeya B, *et al.* Soluble dietary fibre fraction of *Trigonella foenum-graecum*
        (fenugreek) seed improves glucose homeostasis in animal models of type 1 and type 2 diabetes by
        delaying carbohydrate digestion and absorption, and enhancing insulin action. Br J Nutr 2007; 97(3):
        514-21.
        [http://dx.doi.org/10.1017/S0007114507657869] [PMID: 17313713]

[36]   Liu L, Du X, Zhang Z, Zhou J. Trigonelline inhibits caspase 3 to protect β cells apoptosis in
        streptozotocin-induced type 1 diabetic mice. Eur J Pharmacol 2018; 836: 115-21.
        [http://dx.doi.org/10.1016/j.ejphar.2018.08.025] [PMID: 30130525]

[37]   Preet A, Siddiqui MR, Taha A, *et al.* Long-term effect of Trigonella foenum graecum and its
        combination with sodium orthovanadate in preventing histopathological and biochemical
        abnormalities in diabetic rat ocular tissues. Mol Cell Biochem 2006; 289(1-2): 137-47.
        [http://dx.doi.org/10.1007/s11010-006-9156-0] [PMID: 16718375]

[38]   Raju J, Gupta D, Rao AR, Yadava PK, Baquer NZ. Trigonellafoenum graecum (fenugreek) seed
        powder improves glucose homeostasis in alloxan diabetic rat tissues by reversing the altered
        glycolytic, gluconeogenic and lipogenic enzymes. Mol Cell Biochem 2001; 224(1/2): 45-51.
        [http://dx.doi.org/10.1023/A:1011974630828] [PMID: 11693199]

[39]   Thakran S. Salimuddin, Baquer NZ. Oral administration of orthovanadate and Trigonella foenum
        graecum seed powder restore the activities of mitochondrial enzymes in tissues of alloxan-induced
        diabetic rats. Mol Cell Biochem 2003; 247(1/2): 45-53.
        [http://dx.doi.org/10.1023/A:1024188600523] [PMID: 12841630]

[40]   Yadav UCS, Moorthy K, Baquer NZ. Effects of sodium-orthovanadate andTrigonella foenum-graecum seeds on hepatic and renal lipogenic enzymes and lipid profile during alloxan diabetes. J Biosci 2004; 29(1): 81-91.
[http://dx.doi.org/10.1007/BF02702565] [PMID: 15286407]

[41]   Ramadan G, El-Beih NM, Abd El-Kareem HF. Anti-metabolic syndrome and immunostimulant activities of Egyptian fenugreek seeds in diabetic/obese and immunosuppressive rat models. Br J Nutr 2011; 105(7): 995-1004.
[http://dx.doi.org/10.1017/S0007114510004708] [PMID: 21205429]

[42]   El Ghouizi A, Ousaaid D, Laaroussi H, *et al. Ficus carica* (Linn.) Leaf and Bud Extracts and Their Combination Attenuates Type-1 Diabetes and Its Complications *via* the Inhibition of Oxidative Stress. Foods 2023; 12(4): 759.
[http://dx.doi.org/10.3390/foods12040759] [PMID: 36832834]

[43]   Farsi E, Ahmad M, Hor SY, *et al.* Standardized extract of Ficus deltoidea stimulates insulin secretion and blocks hepatic glucose production by regulating the expression of glucose-metabolic genes in streptozitocin-induced diabetic rats. BMC Complement Altern Med 2014; 14(1): 220.
[http://dx.doi.org/10.1186/1472-6882-14-220] [PMID: 24993916]

[44]   Gayathri M, Kannabiran K. Antidiabetic and ameliorative potential of Ficus bengalensis bark extract in streptozotocin induced diabetic rats. Indian J Clin Biochem 2008; 23(4): 394-400.
[http://dx.doi.org/10.1007/s12291-008-0087-2] [PMID: 23105795]

[45]   Ravichandra V, Paarakh PM. Evaluation of Anti-diabetic Potentials of Methanol Extract of Ficus hispida Linn. Leaves Against Alloxan Induced Diabetic Rats. Br J Pharm Res 2014; 4(3): 315-24.
[http://dx.doi.org/10.9734/BJPR/2014/5187]

[46]   Anand P, Murali KY, Tandon V, Murthy PS, Chandra R. Insulinotropic effect of cinnamaldehyde on transcriptional regulation of pyruvate kinase, phosphoenolpyruvate carboxykinase, and GLUT4 translocation in experimental diabetic rats. Chem Biol Interact 2010; 186(1): 72-81.
[http://dx.doi.org/10.1016/j.cbi.2010.03.044] [PMID: 20363216]

[47]   Farazandeh M, Mahmoudabady M, Asghari AA, Niazmand S. Diabetic cardiomyopathy was attenuated by cinnamon treatment through the inhibition of fibro-inflammatory response and ventricular hypertrophy in diabetic rats. J Food Biochem 2022; 46(8): e14206.
[http://dx.doi.org/10.1111/jfbc.14206] [PMID: 35474577]

[48]   Han C, Cui B. Improvement of the bioavailability and glycaemic metabolism of cinnamon oil in rats by liquid loadable tablets. The Scientific World Journal 2012; 2012.
[http://dx.doi.org/10.1100/2012/681534]

[49]   Shen Y, Fukushima M, Ito Y, *et al.* Verification of the antidiabetic effects of cinnamon (Cinnamomum zeylanicum) using insulin-uncontrolled type 1 diabetic rats and cultured adipocytes. Biosci Biotechnol Biochem 2010; 74(12): 2418-25.
[http://dx.doi.org/10.1271/bbb.100453] [PMID: 21150113]

[50]   Chueh WH, Lin JY. Berberine, an isoquinoline alkaloid in herbal plants, protects pancreatic islets and serum lipids in nonobese diabetic mice. J Agric Food Chem 2011; 59(14): 8021-7.
[http://dx.doi.org/10.1021/jf201627w] [PMID: 21696141]

[51]   Chueh WH, Lin JY. Protective effect of berberine on serum glucose levels in non-obese diabetic mice. Int Immunopharmacol 2012; 12(3): 534-8.
[http://dx.doi.org/10.1016/j.intimp.2012.01.003] [PMID: 22266065]

[52]   Cui G, Qin X, Zhang Y, Gong Z, Ge B, Zang YQ. Berberine differentially modulates the activities of ERK, p38 MAPK, and JNK to suppress Th17 and Th1 T cell differentiation in type 1 diabetic mice. J Biol Chem 2009; 284(41): 28420-9.
[http://dx.doi.org/10.1074/jbc.M109.012674] [PMID: 19661066]

[53]   Kong WJ, Zhang H, Song DQ, *et al.* Berberine reduces insulin resistance through protein kinase

C–dependent up-regulation of insulin receptor expression. Metabolism 2009; 58(1): 109-19.
[http://dx.doi.org/10.1016/j.metabol.2008.08.013] [PMID: 19059538]

[54]   Londzin P, Kocik S, Kisiel-Nawrot E, *et al.* Lack of berberine effect on bone mechanical properties in rats with experimentally induced diabetes. Biomed Pharmacother 2022; 146: 112562.
[http://dx.doi.org/10.1016/j.biopha.2021.112562] [PMID: 35062058]

[55]   Ni WJ, Ding HH, Zhou H, Qiu YY, Tang LQ. Renoprotective effects of berberine through regulation of the MMPs/TIMPs system in streptozocin-induced diabetic nephropathy in rats. Eur J Pharmacol 2015; 764: 448-56.
[http://dx.doi.org/10.1016/j.ejphar.2015.07.040] [PMID: 26192633]

[56]   Sun J, Bao H, Peng Y, *et al.* Improvement of intestinal transport, absorption and anti-diabetic efficacy of berberine by using Gelucire44/14: *In vitro, in situ* and *in vivo* studies. Int J Pharm 2018; 544(1): 46-54.
[http://dx.doi.org/10.1016/j.ijpharm.2018.04.014] [PMID: 29654898]

[57]   Amniattalab A, Malekinejad H, Rezabakhsh A, Rokhsartalab-Azar S, Alizade-Fanalou S. Silymarin: A Novel Natural Agent to Restore Defective Pancreatic β Cells in Streptozotocin (STZ)-induced Diabetic Rats. Iran J Pharm Res 2016; 15(3): 493-500.
[PMID: 27980584]

[58]   Borymska W, Zych M, Dudek S, Kaczmarczyk-Sedlak I. Silymarin from Milk Thistle Fruits Counteracts Selected Pathological Changes in the Lenses of Type 1 Diabetic Rats. Nutrients 2022; 14(7): 1450.
[http://dx.doi.org/10.3390/nu14071450] [PMID: 35406062]

[59]   Wang Q, Liu M, Liu WW, *et al. In vivo* recovery effect of silibinin treatment on streptozotocin-induced diabetic mice is associated with the modulations of sirt-1 expression and autophagy in pancreatic β-cell. J Asian Nat Prod Res 2012; 14(5): 413-23.
[http://dx.doi.org/10.1080/10286020.2012.657180] [PMID: 22423887]

[60]   Toğay VA, Sevimli TS, Sevimli M, Çelik DA, Özçelik N. DNA damage in rats with streptozotocin-induced diabetes; protective effect of silibinin. Mutat Res Genet Toxicol Environ Mutagen 2018; 825: 15-8.
[http://dx.doi.org/10.1016/j.mrgentox.2017.11.002] [PMID: 29307371]

[61]   Castro CN, Barcala Tabarrozzi AE, Winnewisser J, *et al.* Curcumin ameliorates autoimmune diabetes. Evidence in accelerated murine models of type 1 diabetes. Clin Exp Immunol 2014; 177(1): 149-60.
[http://dx.doi.org/10.1111/cei.12322] [PMID: 24628444]

[62]   Gbr AA, Abdel Baky NA, Mohamed EA, Zaky HS. Cardioprotective effect of pioglitazone and curcumin against diabetic cardiomyopathy in type 1 diabetes mellitus: impact on CaMKII/NF-κB/TGF-β1 and PPAR-γ signaling pathway. Naunyn Schmiedebergs Arch Pharmacol 2021; 394(2): 349-60.
[http://dx.doi.org/10.1007/s00210-020-01979-y] [PMID: 32984914]

[63]   Jafari Khataylou Y, Ahmadiafshar S, Rezaei R, Parsamanesh S, Hosseini G. Curcumin Ameliorate Diabetes type 1 Complications through Decreasing Pro-inflammatory Cytokines in C57BL/6 Mice. Iran J Allergy Asthma Immunol 2020; 19(S1): 55-62.
[http://dx.doi.org/10.18502/ijaai.v19i(s1.r1).2854] [PMID: 32534511]

[64]   Ghasemi H, Einollahi B, Kheiripour N, Hosseini-Zijoud SR, Farhadian Nezhad M. Protective effects of curcumin on diabetic nephropathy *via* attenuation of kidney injury molecule 1 (KIM-1) and neutrophil gelatinase-associated lipocalin (NGAL) expression and alleviation of oxidative stress in rats with type 1 diabetes. Iran J Basic Med Sci 2019; 22(4): 376-83.
[PMID: 31168341]

[65]   Abdelsamia EM, Khaleel SA, Balah A, Abdel Baky NA. Curcumin augments the cardioprotective effect of metformin in an experimental model of type I diabetes mellitus; Impact of Nrf2/HO-1 and JAK/STAT pathways. Biomed Pharmacother 2019; 109: 2136-44.

[http://dx.doi.org/10.1016/j.biopha.2018.11.064] [PMID: 30551471]

[66] Xie Z, Wu B, Shen G, Li X, Wu Q. Curcumin alleviates liver oxidative stress in type 1 diabetic rats. Mol Med Rep 2018; 17(1): 103-8.
[http://dx.doi.org/http://dx.doi.org/10.3892/mmr.2017.7911] [PMID: 29115468]

[67] Ono T, Takada S, Kinugawa S, Tsutsui H. Curcumin ameliorates skeletal muscle atrophy in type 1 diabetic mice by inhibiting protein ubiquitination. Exp Physiol 2015; 100(9): 1052-63.
[http://dx.doi.org/10.1113/EP085049] [PMID: 25998196]

[68] AlFaris NA, Al-Farga AM, Alshammari GM, BinMowyna MN, Yahya MA. Curcumin reverses diabetic nephropathy in streptozotocin-induced diabetes in rats by inhibition of PKCbeta/p(66)Shc axis and activation of FOXO-3a. J Nutr Biochem 2021; 87: 108515.
[http://dx.doi.org/10.1016/j.jnutbio.2020.108515] [PMID: 33017608]

[69] Soetikno V, Watanabe K, Sari FR, et al. Curcumin attenuates diabetic nephropathy by inhibiting PKC-α and PKC-β $_1$ activity in streptozotocin-induced type I diabetic rats. Mol Nutr Food Res 2011; 55(11): 1655-65.
[http://dx.doi.org/10.1002/mnfr.201100080] [PMID: 22045654]

[70] Soetikno V, Sari FR, Sukumaran V, et al. Curcumin prevents diabetic cardiomyopathy in streptozotocin-induced diabetic rats: Possible involvement of PKC–MAPK signaling pathway. Eur J Pharm Sci 2012; 47(3): 604-14.
[http://dx.doi.org/10.1016/j.ejps.2012.04.018] [PMID: 22564708]

[71] Lee SM, Yang H, Tartar DM, et al. Prevention and treatment of diabetes with resveratrol in a non-obese mouse model of type 1 diabetes. Diabetologia 2011; 54(5): 1136-46.
[http://dx.doi.org/10.1007/s00125-011-2064-1] [PMID: 21340626]

[72] Bashir SO. Concomitant administration of resveratrol and insulin protects against diabetes mellitus type-1-induced renal damage and impaired function *via* an antioxidant-mediated mechanism and up-regulation of Na$^+$/K$^+$-ATPase. Arch Physiol Biochem 2019; 125(2): 104-13.
[http://dx.doi.org/10.1080/13813455.2018.1437752] [PMID: 29436859]

[73] Abdel-Bakky MS, Alqasoumi A, Altowayan WM, Amin E, Darwish MA. Resveratrol Inhibited ADAM10 Mediated CXCL16-Cleavage and T-Cells Recruitment to Pancreatic β-Cells in Type 1 Diabetes Mellitus in Mice. Pharmaceutics 2022; 14(3): 594.
[http://dx.doi.org/10.3390/pharmaceutics14030594] [PMID: 35335970]

[74] Darwish MA, Abdel-Bakky MS, Messiha BAS, Abo-Saif AA, Abo-Youssef AM. Resveratrol mitigates pancreatic TF activation and autophagy-mediated beta cell death *via* inhibition of CXCL16/ox-LDL pathway: A novel protective mechanism against type 1 diabetes mellitus in mice. Eur J Pharmacol 2021; 901: 174059.
[http://dx.doi.org/10.1016/j.ejphar.2021.174059] [PMID: 33794215]

[75] Darwish MA, Abo-Youssef AM, Messiha BAS, Abo-Saif AA, Abdel-Bakky MS. Resveratrol inhibits macrophage infiltration of pancreatic islets in streptozotocin-induced type 1 diabetic mice *via* attenuation of the CXCL16/NF-κB p65 signaling pathway. Life Sci 2021; 272: 119250.
[http://dx.doi.org/10.1016/j.lfs.2021.119250] [PMID: 33631174]

[76] Yonamine CY, Pinheiro-Machado E, Michalani ML, et al. Resveratrol improves glycemic control in insulin-treated diabetic rats: participation of the hepatic territory. Nutr Metab (Lond) 2016; 13(1): 44.
[http://dx.doi.org/10.1186/s12986-016-0103-0] [PMID: 27366200]

[77] Ku CR, Lee HJ, Kim SK, Lee EY, Lee MK, Lee EJ. Resveratrol prevents streptozotocin-induced diabetes by inhibiting the apoptosis of pancreatic β-cell and the cleavage of poly (ADP-ribose) polymerase. Endocr J 2012; 59(2): 103-9.
[http://dx.doi.org/10.1507/endocrj.EJ11-0194] [PMID: 22068111]

[78] Xian Y, Gao Y, Lv W, et al. Resveratrol prevents diabetic nephropathy by reducing chronic inflammation and improving the blood glucose memory effect in non-obese diabetic mice. Naunyn Schmiedebergs Arch Pharmacol 2020; 393(10): 2009-17.

[http://dx.doi.org/10.1007/s00210-019-01777-1] [PMID: 31970441]

[79]   Su HC, Hung LM, Chen JK. Resveratrol, a red wine antioxidant, possesses an insulin-like effect in streptozotocin-induced diabetic rats. Am J Physiol Endocrinol Metab 2006; 290(6): E1339-46.
[http://dx.doi.org/10.1152/ajpendo.00487.2005] [PMID: 16434553]

[80]   Chen KH, Cheng ML, Jing YH, Chiu DTY, Shiao MS, Chen JK. Resveratrol ameliorates metabolic disorders and muscle wasting in streptozotocin-induced diabetic rats. Am J Physiol Endocrinol Metab 2011; 301(5): E853-63.
[http://dx.doi.org/10.1152/ajpendo.00048.2011] [PMID: 21791624]

[81]   Fu Z, Yuskavage J, Liu D. Dietary flavonol epicatechin prevents the onset of type 1 diabetes in nonobese diabetic mice. J Agric Food Chem 2013; 61(18): 4303-9.
[http://dx.doi.org/10.1021/jf304915h] [PMID: 23578364]

[82]   Fu Z, Zhen W, Yuskavage J, Liu D. Epigallocatechin gallate delays the onset of type 1 diabetes in spontaneous non-obese diabetic mice. Br J Nutr 2011; 105(8): 1218-25.
[http://dx.doi.org/10.1017/S0007114510004824] [PMID: 21144096]

[83]   Song EK, Hur H, Han MK. Epigallocatechin gallate prevents autoimmune diabetes induced by multiple low doses of streptozotocin in mice. Arch Pharm Res 2003; 26(7): 559-63.
[http://dx.doi.org/10.1007/BF02976881] [PMID: 12934649]

[84]   Lin CH, Wu JB, Jian JY, Shih CC. (−)-Epicatechin-3-O-β-D-allopyranoside from Davallia formosana prevents diabetes and dyslipidemia in streptozotocin-induced diabetic mice. PLoS One 2017; 12(3): e0173984.
[http://dx.doi.org/10.1371/journal.pone.0173984] [PMID: 28333970]

[85]   Hong YJ, Kim N, Lee K, *et al.* Korean red ginseng (Panax ginseng) ameliorates type 1 diabetes and restores immune cell compartments. J Ethnopharmacol 2012; 144(2): 225-33.
[http://dx.doi.org/10.1016/j.jep.2012.08.009] [PMID: 22925946]

[86]   Ju C, Jeon SM, Jun HS, Moon CK. Diol-ginsenosides from Korean Red Ginseng delay the development of type 1 diabetes in diabetes-prone biobreeding rats. J Ginseng Res 2020; 44(4): 619-26.
[http://dx.doi.org/10.1016/j.jgr.2019.06.001] [PMID: 32617042]

[87]   Tian S, Chen S, Feng Y, He J, Li Y. Ginseng-derived panaxadiol ameliorates STZ-induced type 1 diabetes through inhibiting RORγ/IL-17A axis. Acta Pharmacol Sin 2023; 44(6): 1217-26.
[http://dx.doi.org/10.1038/s41401-022-01042-x] [PMID: 36650291]

[88]   Sen S, Querques MA, Chakrabarti S. North American Ginseng (Panax quinquefolius) prevents hyperglycemia and associated pancreatic abnormalities in diabetes. J Med Food 2013; 16(7): 587-92.
[http://dx.doi.org/10.1089/jmf.2012.0192] [PMID: 23875898]

[89]   Adam GO, Kim GB, Lee SJ, *et al.* Long-term oral intake of *Panax ginseng* improves hypomagnesemia, hyperlactatemia, base deficit, and metabolic acidosis in an alloxan-induced rabbit model. Iran J Basic Med Sci 2019; 22(6): 703-9.
[PMID: 31231500]

[90]   Park JH, Jung JH, Yang JY, Kim HS. Olive leaf down-regulates the oxidative stress and immune dysregulation in streptozotocin-induced diabetic mice. Nutr Res 2013; 33(11): 942-51.
[http://dx.doi.org/10.1016/j.nutres.2013.07.011] [PMID: 24176234]

[91]   Cvjetićanin T, Miljković D, Stojanović I, Dekanski D, Stošić-Grujičić S. Dried leaf extract of *Olea europaea* ameliorates islet-directed autoimmunity in mice. Br J Nutr 2010; 103(10): 1413-24.
[http://dx.doi.org/10.1017/S0007114509993394] [PMID: 20025835]

[92]   Arellano-Buendía AS, Castañeda-Lara LG, Loredo-Mendoza ML, *et al.* Effects of allicin on pathophysiological mechanisms during the progression of nephropathy associated to diabetes. Antioxidants 2020; 9(11): 1134.
[http://dx.doi.org/10.3390/antiox9111134] [PMID: 33203103]

[93]   Huang W, Wang Y, Cao YG, *et al.* Antiarrhythmic effects and ionic mechanisms of allicin on

myocardial injury of diabetic rats induced by streptozotocin. Naunyn Schmiedebergs Arch Pharmacol 2013; 386(8): 697-704.
[http://dx.doi.org/10.1007/s00210-013-0872-1] [PMID: 23604291]

[94]   Huang H, Jiang Y, Mao G, *et al.* Protective effects of allicin on streptozotocin□induced diabetic nephropathy in rats. J Sci Food Agric 2017; 97(4): 1359-66.
[http://dx.doi.org/10.1002/jsfa.7874] [PMID: 27363537]

[95]   Osman M, Adnan A, Bakar NS, Alashkham F. Allicin has significant effect on autoimmune anti-islet cell antibodies in type 1 diabetic rats. Pol J Pathol 2012; 4(4): 248-54.
[http://dx.doi.org/10.5114/pjp.2012.32772] [PMID: 23359194]

[96]   Qian R, Chen H, Lin H, *et al.* The protective roles of allicin on type 1 diabetes mellitus through AMPK/mTOR mediated autophagy pathway. Front Pharmacol 2023; 14: 1108730.
[http://dx.doi.org/10.3389/fphar.2023.1108730] [PMID: 36817124]

[97]   Al Wafai RJ. Nigella sativa and thymoquinone suppress cyclooxygenase-2 and oxidative stress in pancreatic tissue of streptozotocin-induced diabetic rats. Pancreas 2013; 42(5): 841-9.
[http://dx.doi.org/10.1097/MPA.0b013e318279ac1c] [PMID: 23429494]

[98]   El-Mahmoudy A, Shimizu Y, Shiina T, Matsuyama H, El-Sayed M, Takewaki T. Successful abrogation by thymoquinone against induction of diabetes mellitus with streptozotocin *via* nitric oxide inhibitory mechanism. Int Immunopharmacol 2005; 5(1): 195-207.
[http://dx.doi.org/10.1016/j.intimp.2004.09.001] [PMID: 15589481]

[99]   Pal PB, Sinha K, Sil PC. Mangiferin attenuates diabetic nephropathy by inhibiting oxidative stress mediated signaling cascade, TNFα related and mitochondrial dependent apoptotic pathways in streptozotocin-induced diabetic rats. PLoS One 2014; 9(9): e107220.
[http://dx.doi.org/10.1371/journal.pone.0107220] [PMID: 25233093]

[100] Movahed A, Raj P, Nabipour I, *et al.* Efficacy and Safety of Resveratrol in Type 1 Diabetes Patients: A Two-Month Preliminary Exploratory Trial. Nutrients 2020; 12(1): 161.
[http://dx.doi.org/10.3390/nu12010161] [PMID: 31935938]

[101] Stevens Y, Winkens B, Jonkers D, Masclee A. The effect of olive leaf extract on cardiovascular health markers: a randomized placebo-controlled clinical trial. Eur J Nutr 2021; 60(4): 2111-20.
[http://dx.doi.org/10.1007/s00394-020-02397-9] [PMID: 33034707]

[102] Altschuler JA, Casella SJ, MacKenzie TA, Curtis KM. The effect of cinnamon on A1C among adolescents with type 1 diabetes. Diabetes Care 2007; 30(4): 813-6.
[http://dx.doi.org/10.2337/dc06-1871] [PMID: 17392542]

[103] Serraclara A, Hawkins F, Pérez C, Domínguez E, Campillo JE, Torres MD. Hypoglycemic action of an oral fig-leaf decoction in type-I diabetic patients. Diabetes Res Clin Pract 1998; 39(1): 19-22.
[http://dx.doi.org/10.1016/S0168-8227(97)00112-5] [PMID: 9597370]

[104] Haber SL, Keonavong J. Fenugreek use in patients with diabetes mellitus. Am J Health Syst Pharm 2013; 70(14): 1196-203.
[http://dx.doi.org/10.2146/ajhp120523] [PMID: 23820455]

[105] Deepa P, Sowndhararajan K, Kim S, Park SJ. A role of Ficus species in the management of diabetes mellitus: A review. J Ethnopharmacol 2018; 215: 210-32.
[http://dx.doi.org/10.1016/j.jep.2017.12.045] [PMID: 29305899]

[106] Rao PV, Gan SH. Cinnamon: a multifaceted medicinal plant. Evidence-Based Complementary and Alternative Medicine. 2014; 2014.
[http://dx.doi.org/10.1155/2014/642942]

[107] Leach MJ, Kumar S. Cinnamon for diabetes mellitus. Cochrane database of systematic reviews. 2012; (9): CD007170.
[http://dx.doi.org/10.1002/14651858.CD007170.pub2]

[108] Neag MA, Mocan A, Echeverría J, *et al.* Berberine: Botanical occurrence, traditional uses, extraction

methods, and relevance in cardiovascular, metabolic, hepatic, and renal disorders. Front Pharmacol 2018; 9: 557.
[http://dx.doi.org/10.3389/fphar.2018.00557] [PMID: 30186157]

[109] Federico A, Dallio M, Loguercio C. Silymarin/Silybin and Chronic Liver Disease: A Marriage of Many Years. Molecules 2017; 22(2): 191.
[http://dx.doi.org/10.3390/molecules22020191] [PMID: 28125040]

[110] Soleimani V, Delghandi PS, Moallem SA, Karimi G. Safety and toxicity of silymarin, the major constituent of milk thistle extract: An updated review. Phytother Res 2019; 33(6): 1627-38.
[http://dx.doi.org/10.1002/ptr.6361] [PMID: 31069872]

[111] Fujisawa S, Atsumi T, Ishihara M, Kadoma Y. Cytotoxicity, ROS-generation activity and radical-scavenging activity of curcumin and related compounds. Anticancer Res 2004; 24(2B): 563-9.
[PMID: 15160995]

[112] Parsamanesh N, Moossavi M, Bahrami A, Butler AE, Sahebkar A. Therapeutic potential of curcumin in diabetic complications. Pharmacol Res 2018; 136: 181-93.
[http://dx.doi.org/10.1016/j.phrs.2018.09.012] [PMID: 30219581]

[113] Anchi P, Khurana A, Swain D, Samanthula G, Godugu C. Dramatic improvement in pharmacokinetic and pharmacodynamic effects of sustain release curcumin microparticles demonstrated in experimental type 1 diabetes model. Eur J Pharm Sci 2019; 130: 200-14.
[http://dx.doi.org/10.1016/j.ejps.2019.02.002] [PMID: 30731237]

[114] Ghanim H, Sia CL, Abuaysheh S, *et al.* An antiinflammatory and reactive oxygen species suppressive effects of an extract of Polygonum cuspidatum containing resveratrol. J Clin Endocrinol Metab 2010; 95(9): E1-8.
[http://dx.doi.org/10.1210/jc.2010-0482] [PMID: 20534755]

[115] Schmatz R, Perreira LB, Stefanello N, *et al.* Effects of resveratrol on biomarkers of oxidative stress and on the activity of delta aminolevulinic acid dehydratase in liver and kidney of streptozotocin-induced diabetic rats. Biochimie 2012; 94(2): 374-83.
[http://dx.doi.org/10.1016/j.biochi.2011.08.005] [PMID: 21864646]

[116] Malaguarnera L. Influence of Resveratrol on the Immune Response. Nutrients 2019; 11(5): 946.
[http://dx.doi.org/10.3390/nu11050946] [PMID: 31035454]

[117] Musial C, Kuban-Jankowska A, Gorska-Ponikowska M. Beneficial Properties of Green Tea Catechins. Int J Mol Sci 2020; 21(5): 1744.
[http://dx.doi.org/10.3390/ijms21051744] [PMID: 32143309]

[118] Miyoshi N, Pervin M, Suzuki T, *et al.* Green tea catechins for well-being and therapy: Prospects and opportunities. 2015; 85-96.

[119] Mancuso C, Santangelo R. Panax ginseng and Panax quinquefolius: From pharmacology to toxicology. Food Chem Toxicol 2017; 107: 362-72.
[http://dx.doi.org/http://dx.doi.org/10.1016/j.fct.2017.07.019] [PMID: 28698154]

[120] Khalatbary AR, Zarrinjoei GR. Anti-inflammatory effect of oleuropein in experimental rat spinal cord trauma. Iran Red Crescent Med J 2012; 14(4): 229-34.
[PMID: 22754686]

[121] Kontogianni VG, Charisiadis P, Margianni E, Lamari FN, Gerothanassis IP, Tzakos AG. Olive leaf extracts are a natural source of advanced glycation end product inhibitors. J Med Food 2013; 16(9): 817-22.
[http://dx.doi.org/10.1089/jmf.2013.0016] [PMID: 24044491]

[122] Benavente-García O, Castillo J, Lorente J, Ortuño A, Del Rio JA. Antioxidant activity of phenolics extracted from Olea europaea L. leaves. Food Chem 2000; 68(4): 457-62.
[http://dx.doi.org/10.1016/S0308-8146(99)00221-6]

[123] Savairam VD, Patil NA, Borate SR, Ghaisas MM, Shete RV. Allicin: A review of its important

pharmacological activities. Pharmacological Research-Modern Chinese Medicine 2023; p. 100283.

[124] Tanaka Y, Shimizu H, Sato N, Mori M, Shimomura Y. Involvement of spontaneous nitric oxide production in the diabetogenic action of streptozotocin. Pharmacology 1995; 50(2): 69-73.
[http://dx.doi.org/10.1159/000139268] [PMID: 7716177]

CHAPTER 4

Traditional Medicine and Modern Drug Delivery Systems: Promising Roles of Phyto-Nanotechnology in Rheumatoid Arthritis Treatment

Miray Ilhan[1,*] and **Maide Ozturk**[1]

[1] Department of Pharmaceutical Technology, Faculty of Pharmacy, Duzce University, Duzce 81620, Turkiye

Abstract: Phyto-nanotechnology presents a promising avenue for revolutionizing rheumatoid arthritis (RA) treatment. By integrating plant-derived compounds with nanotechnology, this approach addresses the limitations of conventional RA therapies. Nanoformulations of phytochemicals, such as curcumin, resveratrol, and quercetin, enable targeted drug delivery to inflamed joints, optimizing therapeutic efficacy while minimizing systemic side effects. Enhanced bioavailability, attributed to the encapsulation of phytochemicals within nanoparticles, facilitates improved pharmacokinetics and delivery across biological barriers. The immunomodulatory and anti-inflammatory properties of phytochemicals are harnessed more effectively through nanoparticle-mediated sustained release, offering the potential to suppress inflammatory processes and mitigate joint damage. Furthermore, the cartilage-protective and regenerative capabilities of certain plant-derived compounds can be optimized with nanotechnology, promoting joint health. The versatility of phyto-nanotechnology allows for combination therapies, synergizing the benefits of multiple compounds and conventional drugs within nanoparticles. While these advancements hold substantial promise, further research is imperative to refine nanoparticle formulations, assess safety, and validate efficacy through preclinical and clinical studies, ultimately paving the way for transformative RA treatments in clinical practice. In this chapter, phyto-nano drug delivery systems that can increase the effectiveness of medicinal plants in RA treatment are focused on.

Keywords: Green synthesis, Herbal medicine, Modern drug delivery systems, Nanoparticles, Nanocarriers, Phyto-nanotechnology, Rheumatoid arthritis, Traditional medicine.

* **Corresponding author Miray Ilhan:** Department of Pharmaceutical Technology, Faculty of Pharmacy, Duzce University, Duzce 81620, Turkiye; Tel: +90 3805421415; E-mail: mirayilhan@duzce.edu.tr

INTRODUCTION

Rheumatoid arthritis (RA) is a chronic autoimmune disease characterized by progressive inflammation of the joints and damage to many organs, including the heart, kidneys, lungs, digestive tract, eyes, skin, and nervous system [1, 2]. While only a few of the joints are affected at the beginning of the disease, symptoms in other organs, particularly bone and cartilage, are encountered in the later stages of RA. While around 350 million people worldwide experience one type of arthritis, RA has the highest incidence [3]. Apart from RA, the types with the highest incidence among more than a hundred different types of arthritis are osteoarthritis, inflammatory arthritis, and psoriatic arthritis. Inflammation, synovial swelling, monocyte infiltration, joint stiffness, pannus development, and deterioration of articular cartilage are the general features of all types of arthritis. The specific cause and permanent treatment of arthritis are still under investigation. However, it is entirely known that many risk factors such as environmental variables, genetic variables, and lifestyle also trigger the pathogenesis of RA [4, 5]. Various bacterial and viral infections, gout, smoking, red meat and coffee consumption, air pollution, decreased antioxidant and vitamin D consumption are thought to play a role in the exacerbation of RA in vulnerable individuals. Symptoms can be treated with medication, but no successful treatment approach has been found for its etiology [6]. If the patient's condition becomes severe enough to cause loss of function, it can be restored by surgical intervention. Although the most commonly used drugs for treatment are anti-inflammatories, their notable side effects such as heart attack and bleeding in the gastrointestinal tract limit the use of these active pharmaceutical ingredients for most individuals [7]. Also, the administration of biological agents, corticosteroids, and disease-modifying anti-rheumatic drugs does not promote complete recovery [8]. Due to the limitations encountered in conventional treatments such as serious side effects, allergic reactions, and hematological disorders, adjunctive therapies, including herbal medicines, are being studied for the treatment of RA. Although there are many herbal phytocomponents effective in the treatment of RA, they lack the desired physical, chemical, and pharmacokinetic properties. It is inevitable to develop new nano drug delivery systems loaded with phytocomponents that are stable and have increased therapeutic efficacy [9, 10].

In this chapter, the etiology and pathophysiology RA, RA treatment approaches, RA treatment with plants, preparation and characterization techniques of phyto-nano drug delivery systems and improving the properties of herbal medicines effective in RA with nano drug delivery systems will be discussed.

Aetiology of RA

RA is the most common chronic inflammatory polyarticular autoimmune disease in the world. In addition, women suffer from RA 2-3 times more than men [1, 11]. It is characterized by arthralgia due to chronic synovitis which leads to cartilage and bone defects [12]. Early clinical symptoms of rheumatoid arthritis include fatigue, flu-like feeling, swollen and tender joints, and morning stiffness. In the advanced stage, pleural effusions, lung nodules and interstitial lung disease, lymphomas, vasculitis of small or medium-sized arteries, keratoconjunctivitis, atherosclerosis, hematological abnormalities, joint misalignment, immobility, bone erosion, cartilage destruction, and rheumatic nodules occur [1].

RA is a multifactorial disease and the severity and course of the disease depend on both genetic and environmental factors [13]. The diagnosis of RA is made by evaluating and detecting the patient's symptoms, physician examination results, evaluation of risk factors, family history, joint evaluation with ultrasound sonography, and laboratory markers such as elevated C-reactive protein (CRP) and erythrocyte sedimentation rate levels in serum. Although there is no definitively accepted biomolecular hypothesis regarding the pathophysiology of RA, it has been proven that innate and acquired immune reactions play a role in its pathological mechanism [12]. As hypothesized for other autoimmune diseases, the early onset of RA occurs through two separate situations. The first one is the patient's genetic predisposition resulting in the generation of autoreactive T and B cells, and the second one is a triggering condition such as viral and bacterial infections or tissue damage. Smoking, obesity, exposure to UV light, sex hormones, drugs, changes in gut, mouth and lung microbiomes, periodontal disease (periodontitis) and infections are risk factors for the development of RA [14]. More than 100 loci associated with RA have been identified through genomic studies. Moreover, epigenetic modifications are also associated with disease etiology. Factors such as infection and smoking lead to the development of the disease. Smoking induces the formation of free radicals, causes increased cell death, increases the level of monocytes and macrophages in the alveoli, and triggers synovial inflammation. It also causes higher expression of fibrinogen, CRP, interleukin (IL)-1, IL-6 and IL-8. Increased alcohol consumption is associated with a lower risk of RA, while red meat is associated with increased risk and disease severity. Dietary habits such as the Mediterranean diet and intermittent fasting have been proven to reduce RA activity score and inflammation [13, 15].

Autoimmune tissue destruction in RA manifests as synovitis, an inflammation of the joint capsule (Fig. **1**). Excessive activation of fibroblast-like synoviocytes (FLSs) is the central event of RA synovial hyperplasia [16]. This state is initiated and maintained by the complex interaction between different dendritic cell subtypes, T cells, macrophages, B cells, neutrophils, fibroblasts, and osteoclasts [17]. Because RA-specific autoantigens cannot be completely cleared, this sustained immune cell activation causes a self-sustaining, chronic inflammatory state in the joint and swelling of the synovial membrane, which is recognized by affected patients as pain and joint swelling. This chronic inflammatory environment in the arthritic joint, in turn, leads to expansion of the synovial membrane called the "pannus" invading the periarticular bone at the cartilage-bone junction, resulting in bone erosion and cartilage degradation [14].

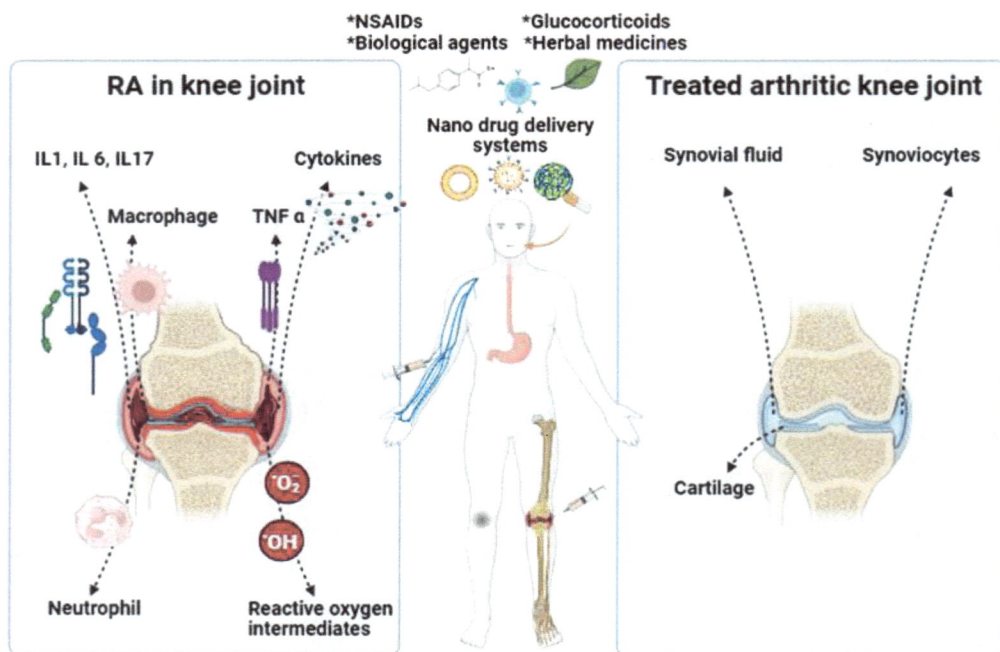

Fig. (1). Pathogenesis and treatment of RA (This figure was created with BioRender.com).

Conventional Therapy in RA

Although early diagnosis and treatment of RA contribute to better outcomes, there is no permanent cure for RA. Therefore, the main purpose of treatment is to reduce joint inflammation, relieve pain, and prevent or reduce bone and cartilage destruction that occurs as a result of immunogenic destructive mechanisms. Irreversible deformations can be prevented by rapid and aggressive therapeutic intervention [18]. The only treatment available with the current knowledge is to inhibit the autoimmune response. Therefore, pharmacotherapeutic management of RA includes the use of non-steroidal anti-inflammatory drugs (NSAIDs), glucocorticoids (GCs), and disease-modifying anti-rheumatic drugs (DMARDs) (Fig. **2**). However, each therapeutic option used has its own inadequacy for the treatment of RA. NSAIDs fail to prevent joint injury and internal bleeding. GCs have systemic side effects that cause osteoporosis and hypertension. DMARDs have disadvantages such as causing liver and kidney failure, delayed response and high infection risk [12].

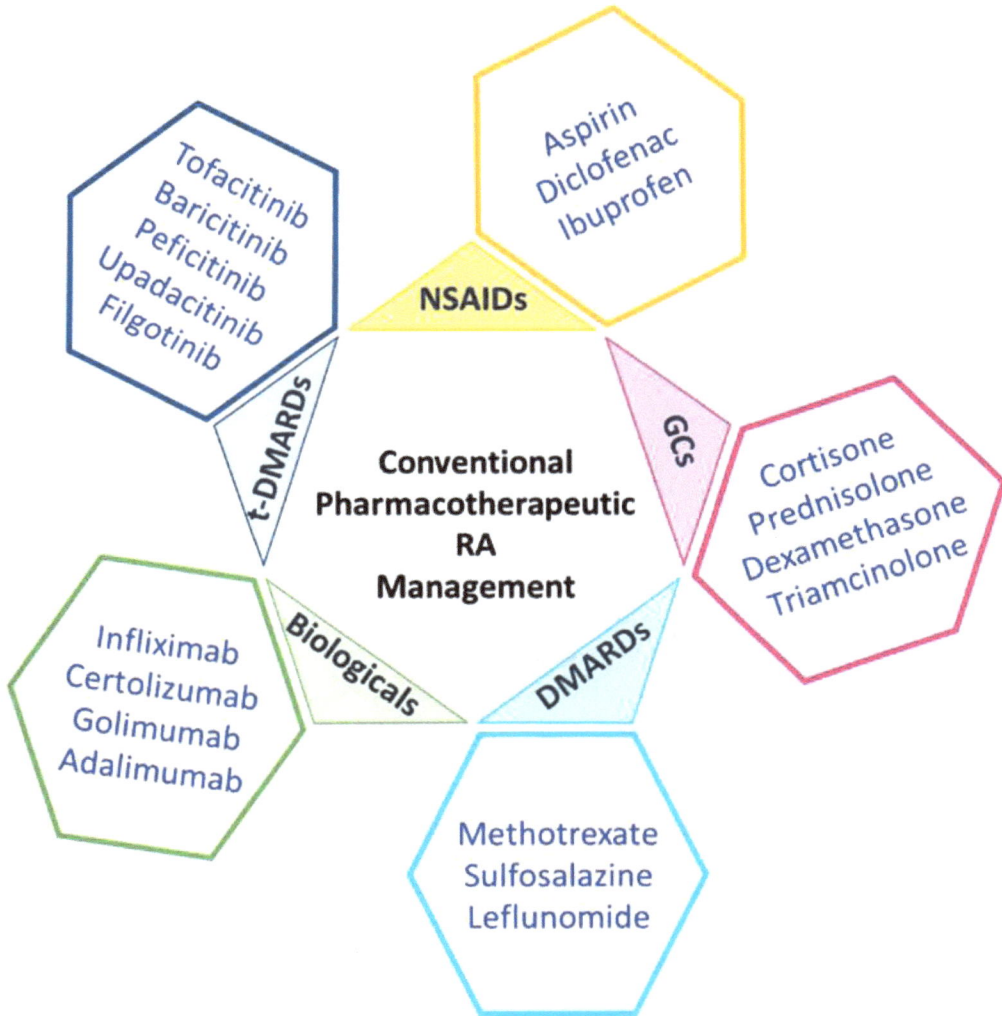

Fig. (2). Conventional drugs used in the treatment of RA (Non-steroidal anti-inflammatory drugs (NSAIDs), glucocorticoids (GCs), disease-modifying antirheumatic drugs (DMARDs), targeted DMARDs (t-DMARDs)).

NSAIDs are used to reduce pain by reducing inflammation in the acute phase response. They exert their pharmacological effects by inhibiting cyclooxygenase (COX), especially COX-2, which increases during inflammation. NSAIDs such as aspirin, diclofenac, or ibuprofen may be useful as transitional therapy in the weeks at the onset of RA clinical symptoms and before the onset of slow-acting DMARDs. The action mechanism of NSAIDs is to inhibit COX enzymes that function in arachidonic acid metabolism to produce pro-inflammatory prostaglandins. Drugs in this pharmacological group effectively reduce pain and swelling and improve joint function. However, NSAIDs cannot change the course of the disease, as they do not prevent additional joint damage. Continued use of NSAIDs causes gastrointestinal abnormalities such as ulcers and perforation. In addition, since the vascular structure in the glomerulus is controlled by thromboxanes and prostaglandins in the arteries that control glomerular pressure, NSAIDs can also cause kidney damage. In order to reduce the risk of side effects, there has been an increasing trend recently for NSAIDs that selectively inhibit COX-2. Compared to traditional NSAIDs, the risk of gastrointestinal complications is lower with COX-2 targeted therapy [1, 19, 20].

GCs reduce inflammation by suppressing the immune response. GCs act by reducing the activation, proliferation, differentiation and survival of various cells involved in the production of inflammatory mediators in RA patients. GCs such as cortisone, cortisol, methylprednisolone, prednisolone, triamcinolone, dexamethasone are used in treatment. GCs can suppress the function and proliferation of T helper 1 cells and thus cause decreased production of proinflammatory cytokines such as IL-1β, IL-2, IL-3, IL-6, tumor necrosis factor. With GC treatment, it is aimed to prevent joint damage and to relieve symptoms immediately by changing the course of the disease. Despite their beneficial effects, long-term use of GCs causes serious multisystemic side effects such as gastrointestinal bleeding, osteoporosis and ulcer formation [1, 20].

DMARDs suppress autoimmune activity and promote remission by delaying or preventing joint degeneration. DMARDs are drugs that target rheumatoid inflammation and thus prevent further joint damage. Methotrexate interferes with the activity of dihydrofolate reductase, inhibits the metabolism of hydrochloroquine deoxyribonucleotide and enhances the stabilization of the lysosomal membrane by impairing antigen presentation. Sulfasalazine reduces immunoglobulin levels by inhibition of neutrophil function. On the other hand, leflunomide provides an anti-inflammatory effect by interfering with the synthesis of pyrimidines required for lymphocyte activation. However, side effects such as nausea, vomiting and diarrhea are common in the use of drugs in this pharmacological drug group. In addition to these side effects, patients are more likely to experience more serious side effects such as cirrhosis and hepatitis.

Biological DMARDs are one of the new drug groups used for the last 15 years in the treatment of RA. These drugs act by targeting inflammatory processes, pro-inflammatory cytokines, the involvement of specific cells and molecules, and various pathways at the molecular level. It is aimed to stop the progression of RA in mechanisms such as tumor necrosis factor inhibition, B-cell depletion, T-cell targeting, and inhibition of different interleukin species. Targeted synthetic DMARDs emerged after the discovery of the use of the signal transducer and activator of transcription (STAT) and Janus kinase (JAK) pathway by various cytokines to perform their biological activities [21]. Small molecular agents that provide the inhibition of JAK have been developed. Treatments of biological and targeted synthetic DMARDs are more costly than the other three classes. Biological DMARDs are produced with recombinant DNA technology. They are designed to target inflammatory molecules, cells and pathways that cause tissue damage in RA patients. Targeted synthetic DMARDs act by targeting intracellular enzyme groups that play a role in RA progression [1, 20].

Traditional Herbal Medicine in RA Treatment

It has been proven that herbal sources and phytochemicals isolated from plants can be effective in the treatment of RA with many mechanisms. Different plant species are used in the treatment of RA with activities such as anti-inflammatory, chondroprotective, immunomodulatory, antiangiogenic, and antioxidant properties. Phytochemicals with potential efficacy in RA are examined under the classes of phenolic compounds, carotenoids, and alkaloids [22].

Numerous studies have shown the beneficial effects of phenolic compounds such as flavonoids, resveratrol, emodin, rosmarinic acid, and mangiferin in the treatment of RA. Accordingly, these compounds have been reported to act through modulation of pro-inflammatory pathways. Flavonoids show antioxidant activity by reducing the production of reactive oxygen species (ROS) in RA. Carotenoids such as β-cryptoxanthin, lycopene, β-carotene, α-carotene, zeaxanthin, and lutein exhibit antioxidant activities through the inhibition of ROS and thus have a protective effect in the management of RA. Carotenoids found in fruits and vegetables such as sweet potatoes, carrots, red peppers, zucchini, avocados and watermelons have been reported to reduce C-reactive protein levels, thus protecting against RA-related inflammation. It has been shown that alkaloidal compounds such as piperlongumine, oxymatrine, and cynomenin inhibit the progression of RA in different ways, such as the suppression of cluster of differentiation (CD), suppression of ROS, T cell proliferation, TNF-a, IL-6, IL-12 [23].

Curcuma longa, which belongs to the Zingiberaceae family, is a plant with active components such as curcumin, campesterol, stigmasterol, B-sitosterol, cholesterol and fatty acids. It has various pharmacological properties such as anti-inflammatory, antimicrobial, antioxidant and anticancer activities. In various studies, it has been proven that curcumin inhibits interleukins and TNF-α expression, resulting in a decrease in RA severity [24]. However, the use of curcumin is limited due to its hydrophobic nature, solubility in toxic organic solvents, poor gastrointestinal absorption, first-pass metabolism, and stability problems with light and temperature changes [25, 26].

Withania somnifera from the Solanaceae family called the winter cherry of the tropical region, is widely used in the treatment of RA. Withanin, a component of *Withania somnifera*, has been found to suppress the nuclear factor kappa beta (NFkB) transcriptor factor, pain mediators, proinflammatory cytokines, TNF-α, and reduced levels of receptor activator of nuclear factor kappa beta ligand (RANKL), which is necessary for osteoclast differentiation [23].

Celastrus paniculatus is a therapeutic herb belonging to the Celastraceae family, traditionally used for its anti-inflammatory, antioxidant and antipyretic activity. It contains many analgesic and anti-inflammatory components such as sesquiterpenoids, alkaloids, sterols and polyalcohol [27].

Terminalia chebula Retz. is a tree belonging to the family Combretaceae. It has been reported that the plant has anti-arthritis, anti-inflammatory, antioxidant, antibacterial, anticancer, antidiabetic, antimicrobial, and hypocholesterolemic activities thanks to its phytochemical components such as flavonoids, terpenes, anthocyanins, polyphenols, and glycosides. In particular, chebulagic acid and chebulinic acid are known to be responsible for anti-inflammatory and antioxidant effects [28].

Centella asiatica (L.), also known as Gotu Kola, is a medicinal plant belonging to the Apiaceae family. It is rich in saponins and the therapeutic efficacy is attributed to madecassoside and asiaticoside. This herb is used to treat fever, skin diseases, injuries and inflammation-related diseases. Madecassoside has been proven to play an important role in regulating various immune responses, as well as suppressing inflammation and oxidative stress [29].

Gardenia jasminoides J. Ellis is a plant from the Rubiaceae family. Dried and ripe fruits of the plant have been traditionally used in Chinese medicine for their various pharmacological activities. Studies have found that the crude polysaccharides found in the fruit have a certain immunomodulatory effect. Geniposide, an iridoid glycoside, is extracted from the fruits of this plant and induces apoptosis by reducing the abnormal proliferation of FLSs [16, 30].

Polygonum cuspidatum is a plant from the Polygonaceae family. Stilbene compounds (resveratrol and polydatin), anthraquinone compounds (emodin and derivatives), and flavonoids (quercetin) are the primary active phytochemicals of the plant. *In vivo* experiments showed that the ethanol extract of this plant has the potential to treat RA thanks to the primary anti-inflammatory phytochemical components polydatin, resveratrol, and emodin. It has also been confirmed that the plant can be used in the treatment of arthritis, as resveratrol regulates the expression of type II collagen in chondrocytes [31].

Citrus sp. is a plant belonging to the Rutaceae family. Citrus peels' ethanol extract is rich in hesperidin content and has promising anti-inflammatory activity. Studies have confirmed the anti-arthritic profile of citrus species by down-regulation of the levels of pro-inflammatory cytokines such as TNF-α, IL-6 and IL-17 and CRP by the application of hesperidin-containing extract [32].

Paeonia lactiflora Pall. is a plant from the Paeoniaceae family. It is a perennial flowering plant and well-known medicinal plant in China. The decoction of the root has been used in the treatment of RA more than 1000 years. Paeoniflorin, paeonin, paeonolide, paeonol, albiflorin, lactiflorin, and its derivatives found in the water or ethanol extract of the plant root are known as peony total glycosides (TGP). More than 90% of TGP content is water-soluble paeoniflorin and it has been proven by studies to be the compound responsible for pharmacological effects. For this reason, paeoniflorin is used for standardization in the dosing of formulations containing TGP. In 1998, a drug containing paeoniflorin was approved by the Chinese State Food and Drug Administration for use in the treatment of RA [33].

Roles of Nanotechnology in RA

Therapeutic agents have to overcome many physiological barriers to reach the inflamed areas and the effective dose. Reasons such as rapid half-life of active ingredients, poor bioavailability and insufficient solubility, and low patient compliance in conventional treatment cause ineffective results in treatment. With the developments in drug technology, the use of new drug delivery systems has increased to overcome the problems in current treatment [34, 35]. Nano-sized drug delivery systems have helped overcome the difficulties in transporting the active ingredient to bones and cartilages [11].

The synovial fluid in inflamed joints becomes abnormally enlarged, accompanied by angiogenesis and inflammatory cell infiltration. Thus, nanoparticles can be targeted to diseased tissue by the emergence of endothelial spaces in the microenvironment of RA, the formation of leaky vasculature and increased interstitial pressure. This passive targeting mechanism is similar to the enhanced permeability and retention (EPR) effect that occurs in tumor tissues due to similar leaky vessels presented at disease sites. Unlike EPR in tumors, the retention mechanism in RA is mainly based on the sequestration of local inflammatory cells [34, 36].

DMARDs and GCs, which are frequently used in the treatment of RA today, cause many adverse effects as well as reduce the efficacy of treatment with their low solubility, untargeted distribution and poor bioavailability. With appropriate nanocarrier systems, systems with high drug carrying capacity and drug release in the inflamed area can be produced [37].

Clinical studies show that gene therapy, which is a new approach to the treatment of RA, provides effective results in healing the inflamed area. Due to the high molecular weight, negative charge and instability of nucleic acids such as siRNA, mRNA, microRNA and plasmid DNA, it is almost impossible to apply them directly in clinical applications. For this reason, studies have focused on nanoparticle drug delivery systems in order to protect the nucleic acid and ensure its delivery to the target tissue [37].

In addition to passive targeting, active targeting can also be done through ligands attached to the nanoparticle surface. The use of ligands that can bind specifically to receptors on immune cells or enzymes that cause RA-related inflammation and joint deformation are specifically targeted at the damaged area. Folic acid targeting the folate receptor β, hyaluronic acid targeting the CD44 receptor, and sialic acid targeting the E-selectin receptor are some of the ligands used for active targeting of nanoparticles [37].

Phyto-nanotechnology in RA Therapy

Herbal components have a wide potential for the treatment of arthritis, but limitations such as poor water solubility, stability, low bioavailability and first pass metabolism lead to a decrease in the therapeutic efficacy of these drugs. To overcome these limitations of herbal medicines, nanotechnology provides great advantages. Many nanotechnology-based drug delivery systems such as polymer-based nanoparticles, nanoemulsions, liposomes, and metal nanoparticles are used to transport herbal components. Controlled delivery of both hydrophobic and hydrophilic components is preferred for its high drug-carrying capacity, high stability, and suitability for different dosage forms. In addition, as explained in the previous section, nanotechnological drug delivery systems also provide significant improvements in the biodistribution and pharmacokinetic properties of the therapeutic agent it carries [27, 38].

Curcumin, the main component of turmeric, plays a role in inducing cytokines and chemokines, causing interaction between endothelial and inflammatory cells, thereby preventing bone degradation and cartilage erosion. In a clinical study, it was shown that its use in combination with phenylbutazone reduces morning stiffness and swelling in the joints. However, its poor bioavailability, low solubility in aqueous media, instability in body fluids and high degradation rate have limited the therapeutic applications of this component. In order to overcome these problems, nanotechnological applications have been directed. In the study of Zheng *et al.*, a nanoemulsion formulation of curcumin was prepared. Oral administration of the prepared nanoemulsion and IV administration of free curcumin were compared. Compared to free curcumin, the nanoemulsion formulation has been proven to increase the plasma concentration of curcumin threefold and reduce TNF-a and IL-1β levels twofold in both synovial fluid and serum [39, 40]. In addition, curcumin has been recognized as GRAS (Generally Recognized as Safe) by the FDA [24, 26, 41].

TGP, extracted from the roots of Paeonia lactiflora Pall, is an FDA-approved drug for the treatment of RA. It acts as an anti-inflammatory and immunomodulatory, improving clinical symptoms and signs of RA. Studies have shown that the clinical effects of TGP are just as good. However, its oral bioavailability is 3-4%. Therefore, its stability and bioavailability in the gastrointestinal tract were increased by preparing a microemulsion formulation of TGP [42].

Preparation Techniques of Phyto-nano Drug Delivery Systems

Phyto-nano drug delivery systems are nano-sized drug delivery systems that contain plant constituents as building blocks of nanostructure or as active pharmaceutical ingredients. Thanks to many unique features of nano drug delivery systems such as small particle size, high surface area, and adjustment of hydrophilic and lipophilic properties, treatment efficiency can be increased by improving poor solubility and/or permeation problems of herbal medicines. Moreover, the nano drug delivery systems are also useful in improving the stability and minimizing the side effects of the plant extract and constituents [43].

Nano-precipitated Nanoparticles

In the nanoprecipitation method, an organic phase containing an organic solvent such as ethanol, isopropanol or acetone, in which the active substance is dissolved, and a surfactant with a low HLB, and a phase that cannot dissolve the active substance (usually water) are used. When the organic phase is properly mixed with the aqueous phase, the nanoparticles are formed by precipitation. The properties of the nano-sized system produced by the nanoprecipitation method are related to the formulation-dependent parameters. The interfacial turbulence and mechanical mixing, which occurs as a result of the changing interfacial tensions of the organic and water phases with the Marangoni effect, allows the organic phase to disperse in the aqueous phase as droplets. As a result, the particles become insoluble and precipitate. The standardization of the nanoprecipitation method is difficult. For this reason, a wide and asymmetrical particle size distribution is usually obtained with this method [44].

Polymer-based Nanoparticles

Polymeric nanoparticles are nano-sized solid particles in which the active pharmaceutical ingredients are encapsulated in a biocompatible and biodegradable natural or synthetic polymeric matrix. Chitosan, alginate and albumin from natural polymers are the most preferred ones for the production of polymeric nanoparticles, while the most widely used synthetic polymers are poly-D, L-lactic-co-glycolic acid (PLGA), poly-D, L-lactic acid (PLA) and poly (ε-caprolactone) (PCL) [43]. They are generally manufactured by ionotropic gelation and double emulsion solvent evaporation methods [45, 46].

Solid Lipid Nanoparticles

The solid lipid nano particles are dispersions of drugs entrapped inside the solid lipid core. Solid lipid nanoparticles are spherical in shape and average particle size is between 10 and 1000 nm. In the preparation of solid lipid nanoparticles, methods such as emulsification/evaporation, ultrasonication, high speed homogenization, high pressure homogenization, and supercritical liquid extraction of emulsions are used. Solid lipid nanoparticles are basically composed of a lipid carrier such as glycerides, triglycerides, waxes, fatty acids and steroids. Generally, biocompatible surfactants poloxamer and polysorbate are preferred for formulation preparation. Drugs with permeability problems pass through the lipid bilayer with a lipid carrier and therapeutic efficacy is achieved [43]. The use of biodegradable lipids confers them low toxicity and high biocompatibility [47].

Nanoemulsions

Nanoemulsions are heterogeneous mixtures in which the lipid phase is dispersed in the aqueous phase as droplets of 100 to 600 nm in size using suitable surfactants. Nanoemulsions are thermodynamically stable. Through a lipophilic internal phase, they can transport lipophilic components more easily than liposomes. Nanoemulsions are prepared by solvent evaporation, high-pressure homogenisation, and microfluidization techniques. The use of the nanoemulsion formulations as drug delivery systems is limited because of the stability problems and higher cost of manufacturing [43].

Liposomes

Liposomes are bilayer and spherical lipid-based drug carriers composed of cholesterol and phospholipids [48]. The particle size of the liposomes is between 50 nm and 5 μm. The hydrophilic drug is surrounded by a self-assembled lipid bilayer and entrapped in the hydrophilic core. Thin film hydration method is generally used for liposome production. With its lipophilic nature, the liposome has a unique ability to pass through the lipid bilayer of biologic membranes [43, 49].

Phytosomes

Phytosome drug delivery systems are mostly prepared to increase the lipophilicity of drugs to increase their permeability and bioavailability. In the production of phytosome drug delivery systems, water-soluble polar phytocomponents are complexed with the polar head of phospholipids by hydrogen bonding to increase lipid solubility. Thus, the permeability of herbal medicines through the cell membrane can be increased with amphiphilic phospholipids [43, 48].

Green Synthesized Metal Nanoparticles

The environmentally friendly synthesis of nanomaterials using natural resources has become very popular with the green synthesis method. The use of plant extracts, algae, fungi, and even bacteria in the green synthesis of metallic nanoparticles is among the very current topics in terms of materials science. Potent phytochemicals such as flavonoids, phenols, ketones, terpenoids, and aldehydes are suitable phytochemical components for the production of metallic nanoparticles by green synthesis [44]. Metal nanoparticles can be used in RA therapy as therapeutic agents or drug carriers. They are generally made of silver, gold, copper or iron [50].

Physical Characterization of Phyto-nano Drug Delivery Systems

The characterization of nano drug delivery systems is integral at every stage, from the design of the formulation to the final product. The commonly used physical characterization studies include many different experiments such as particle size, polydispersity index, zeta potential, nuclear magnetic resonance (NMR), Fourier transform infrared spectroscopy (FTIR), scanning electron microscopy (SEM), transmission electron microscopy (TEM), and atomic force microscopy (AFM) [43].

NMR and FTIR analyses are used to identify hydrogen bonds and functional groups in the molecules being analyzed [43]. The size and size distribution of a nano drug delivery system are the most important parameters that affect many properties of the active pharmaceutical ingredient, such as solubility, permeability, stability, encapsulation, *in vitro* drug release rate and distribution to tissues. The particle size of the properly prepared nanoparticles should be in the range of 100-200 nm. Particle size below 100 nm increases the toxicity risk of nanoparticles [43]. The polydispersity index (PDI) indicates the size distribution of the population within a sample, and the value of the particle size is in the range of 0-1. Generally, 0.3-0.7 is an acceptable range for lipid-based and polymeric particulate systems [43, 45]. Particle size can be determined by dynamic light scattering (DLS), SEM and TEM analysis. With the DLS method, the PDI value can also be determined. SEM, TEM, and AFM are methods used to examine the surface morphology of nanoparticles. The zeta potential is the electrostatic potential in the shear plane. In zeta potential analysis, the surface charge of nanoparticles in a colloidal solution is measured. The zeta potential is important for nano-sized drug delivery systems as it reflects colloidal stability. In order to ensure high stability in nano drug delivery systems, the zeta potential value should be >+30 mV or <−30 mV [43].

Advantages of Phyto-nanotechnology in Treatment of RA

Formulating phytocomponents as a nano drug carrier system and combining the positive properties of both components bring various advantages for biological applications (Fig. 3). With this conjunction, solubility and toxicity problems are eliminated, while disease-focused designs such as drug targeting can be created. These advantages are given in detail under the following headings.

Stability

Stability problems are generally observed during storage due to the sensitive contents of herbal medicines to various stimuli such as light, heat or humidity. Major stability problems, such as the formation of toxic metabolites and loss of biological activity, pose question marks in the safe consumption of patients. In addition, stability problems can occur due to *in vivo* conditions. Phyto-nanotechnology can largely solve the stability problems in traditional herbal medicines [43]. Various nano drug delivery systems are being studied to increase the stability and efficacy of essential oils, which are generally easily volatile and chemically unstable in the presence of oxygen, light and/or heat [51].

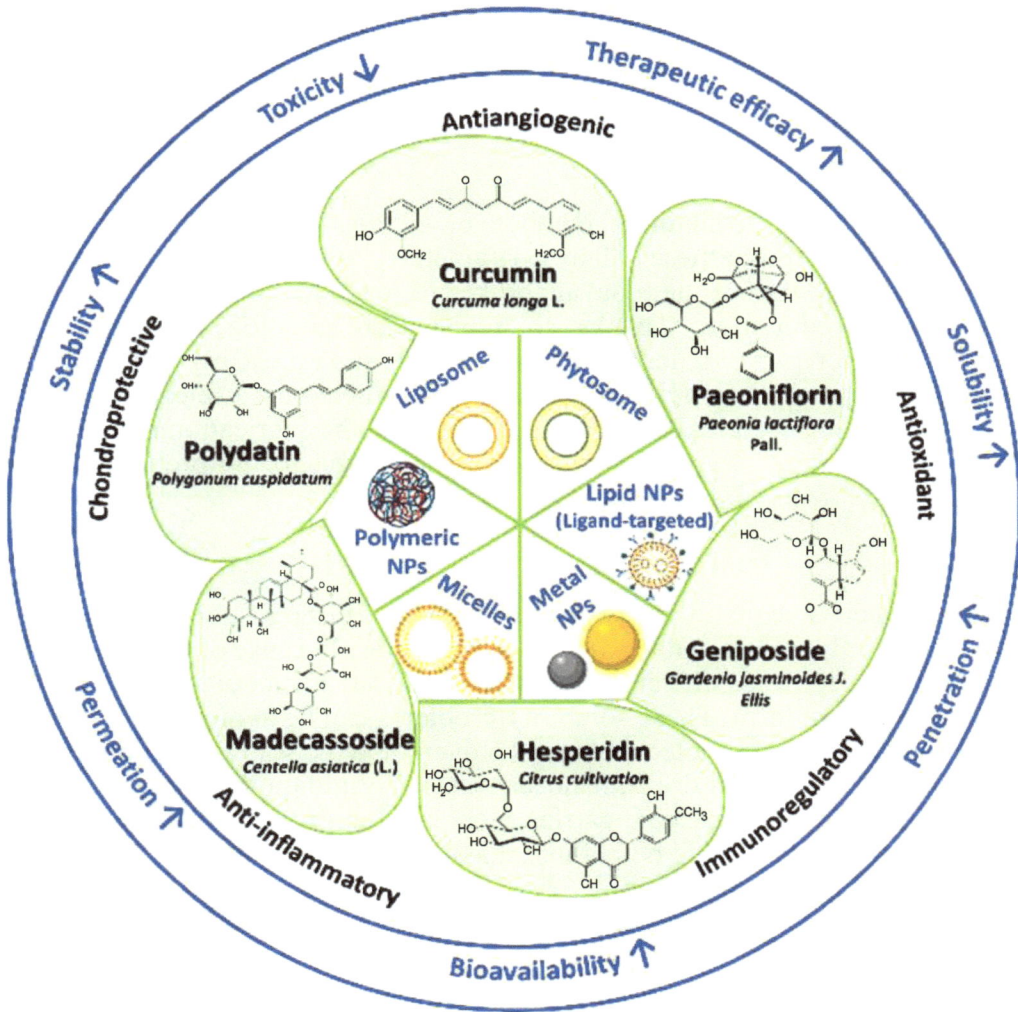

Fig. (3). Advantages of phyto-nano drug delivery systems in the treatment of RA.

Toxicity

Nanotechnology has paved the way for similar or better therapeutic effects to occur in a non-toxic manner by applying low-dose bioactive components that are effective at high doses [43]. With the controlled release of phytocompounds by the nano drug delivery systems, the fluctuation of drug concentration in the blood is regulated and the safety of the phytocomponents is increased. The increase in the absorption of the phytocomponent thanks to the nano drug carrier systems also makes it possible to reduce the toxic and side effects by reducing the dose [51].

However, safety and biocompatibility of nanosystems should be evaluated with appropriate *in vitro*, *ex vivo*, and *in vivo* studies to prevent non-IgE-mediated hypersensitivity or pseudo-allergy reactions [43].

Bioavailability and Regulation of Traditional Herbal Medicine in Microcirculation

Plant-derived drugs contain a number of phytocomponents with different physicochemical properties. Many parameters, particularly solubility and permeability, can reduce the bioavailability of bioactive compounds by limiting their *in vivo* activities. Thanks to phyto-nanotechnology, solubility and permeability increase with decreasing particle size and increasing surface area. In addition, it is possible to produce controlled or targeted drug release systems as well as increasing the bioavailability by modifying the fabrication materials and components of nano drug delivery systems according to the properties of the bioactive ingredients [43].

Solubility

Herbal medicines contain many molecules with different solubility, such as water-soluble glycosides and lipid-soluble terpenoids. Because of these significant differences, it is always difficult to formulate various plant components together in a single dosage form. These solubility problems can be avoided by combining phytoconstituents and nanotechnology. To overcome the solubility complications of water-insoluble herbal drugs, nanosuspension formulations can be developed, acting as endogenous molecule carrier such as albumin, or nanocrystals can be produced from hydrophobic herbal ingredients. In addition, for herbal medicines that are very soluble in water, lipid-based nanocarriers can be used to reduce the solubility and prolong the drug release [52].

Permeation and Penetration

The first obstacle that drug delivery systems have to overcome after administration is biological barriers. Many biological barriers, for example, the gastrointestinal tract and blood-brain barrier, restrict the permeation of the active pharmaceutical ingredient by many factors such as polarity of the drugs, large or small molecular structure, surface charge, and/or the stability of the drug in the acidic environment [43, 51].

Targeted Drug Delivery

Targeted drug delivery systems are at the forefront for effective treatment. In particular, drug delivery systems sensitive to the tumor microenvironment are milestones in the field of medicine in terms of eliminating the damage caused by chemotherapeutics in healthy tissues. However, it is a very difficult process to design the structure that can complete this important mission. Nanotechnology offers a wide design field for the production of drug targeting systems [43].

Therapeutic Efficacy

Nano drug delivery systems prolong drug circulation time and maintain stability, attenuate systemic toxicity, allow controlled and targeted drug release, and increase therapeutic efficacy. For this reason, it is advantageous to administer drugs such as anti-inflammatory drugs or biological agents, which have many causes that limit their use, to patients using nanotechnology-based drug delivery systems [52, 53].

Limitations of Phyto-nanotechnology

The combination of phytocomponents and nanodrug delivery systems can further increase RA treatment effectiveness and reduce side effects. Nanoscale drug delivery systems such as liposomes, phytosomes, micelles, polymeric nanoparticles, and inorganic systems have been developed for the delivery of therapeutic phytochemicals. Nowadays, there are rare reports of drug therapy using nano drug delivery systems for the treatment of RA in the clinic. There are still some uncertainties in biosafety, mechanism of action, allergic reactions, and drug interactions that hinder its therapeutic efficacy and clinical use. However, we believe that phyto-nanotechnological drug delivery systems, which are formed by combining phytochemical and nanoparticulate systems, will be promising for the treatment of RA and many other diseases in the clinical environment by further development.

CONCLUDING REMARKS

In conclusion, phyto-nanotechnology emerges as a promising frontier in revolutionizing RA treatment. This innovative approach, amalgamating plant-derived compounds with nanotechnology, addresses key limitations of traditional therapies. The targeted drug delivery capabilities of nanoformulations enhance therapeutic efficacy while minimizing systemic side effects. Improved bioavailability, facilitated by encapsulation within nanoparticles, optimizes pharmacokinetics and biological barrier penetration. By leveraging immunomodulatory and anti-inflammatory properties, phyto-nanotechnology holds potential for suppressing inflammation and mitigating joint damage in RA [52]. Additionally, the application of nanotechnology in delivering cartilage-protective compounds may contribute to joint health and regeneration. The adaptability of phyto-nanotechnology allows for synergistic combination therapies, offering a comprehensive approach to RA management. While these advancements hold great promise, further research is essential to refine formulations, ensure safety, and validate efficacy in clinical settings. Ultimately, the integration of phyto-nanotechnology into RA treatment protocols has the potential to reshape therapeutic landscapes and improve outcomes for patients grappling with this chronic autoimmune disorder.

REFERENCES

[1]   Lin YJ, Anzaghe M, Schülke S. Update on the pathomechanism, diagnosis, and treatment options for rheumatoid arthritis. Cells 2020; 9(4): 880.
[http://dx.doi.org/10.3390/cells9040880] [PMID: 32260219]

[2]   Radu AF, Bungau SG. Management of rheumatoid arthritis: An overview. Cells 2021; 10(11): 2857.
[http://dx.doi.org/10.3390/cells10112857] [PMID: 34831081]

[3]   Vijeta B, Namrata M, Alagusundaram M. Ultra deformable vesicular system loaded bioactive/phytoconstituents for targeted drug delivery for the treatment of rheumatoid arthritis– an overview. Lat Am J Pharm 2023; 42(1).

[4]   Logesh K, Raj B, Bhaskaran M, *et al.* Nanoparticulate drug delivery systems for the treatment of rheumatoid arthritis: A comprehensive review. J Drug Deliv Sci Technol 2023; 81: 104241.
[http://dx.doi.org/10.1016/j.jddst.2023.104241]

[5]   Conigliaro P, Triggianese P, De Martino E, *et al.* Challenges in the treatment of rheumatoid arthritis. Autoimmun Rev 2019; 18(7): 706-13.
[http://dx.doi.org/10.1016/j.autrev.2019.05.007] [PMID: 31059844]

[6]   Almutairi K, Nossent J, Preen D, Keen H, Inderjeeth C. The global prevalence of rheumatoid arthritis: a meta-analysis based on a systematic review. Rheumatol Int 2021; 41(5): 863-77.
[http://dx.doi.org/10.1007/s00296-020-04731-0] [PMID: 33175207]

[7]   Vasdev N, Pawar B, Gupta T, Mhatre M, Tekade RK. A bird's eye view of various cell-based biomimetic nanomedicines for the treatment of arthritis. Pharmaceutics 2023; 15(4): 1150.
[http://dx.doi.org/10.3390/pharmaceutics15041150] [PMID: 37111636]

[8]   Libánská A, Randárová E, Skoroplyas S, *et al.* Size-switchable polymer-based nanomedicines in the advanced therapy of rheumatoid arthritis. J Control Release 2023; 353: 30-41.
[http://dx.doi.org/10.1016/j.jconrel.2022.11.027] [PMID: 36403682]

[9]   Maity S, Wairkar S. Dietary polyphenols for management of rheumatoid arthritis: Pharmacotherapy and novel delivery systems. Phytother Res 2022; 36(6): 2324-41.
[http://dx.doi.org/10.1002/ptr.7444] [PMID: 35318759]

[10]   Zhang Z, Yu Y, Zhu G, *et al.* The emerging role of plant-derived exosomes-like nanoparticles in immune regulation and periodontitis treatment. Front Immunol 2022; 13: 896745.
[http://dx.doi.org/10.3389/fimmu.2022.896745] [PMID: 35757759]

[11]   Vyawahare A, Ahmad A, Kanika , *et al.* Autophagy targeting nanoparticles in rheumatoid arthritis and osteoarthritis. Materials Advances 2022; 3(9): 3820-34.
[http://dx.doi.org/10.1039/D2MA00011C]

[12]   Radu AF, Bungau SG. Nanomedical approaches in the realm of rheumatoid arthritis. Ageing Res Rev 2023; 87: 101927.
[http://dx.doi.org/10.1016/j.arr.2023.101927] [PMID: 37031724]

[13]   Prasad P, Verma S, Surbhi , Ganguly NK, Chaturvedi V, Mittal SA. Rheumatoid arthritis: advances in treatment strategies. Mol Cell Biochem 2023; 478(1): 69-88.
[http://dx.doi.org/10.1007/s11010-022-04492-3] [PMID: 35725992]

[14] Scherer HU, Häupl T, Burmester GR. The etiology of rheumatoid arthritis. J Autoimmun 2020; 110: 102400.
[http://dx.doi.org/10.1016/j.jaut.2019.102400] [PMID: 31980337]

[15] Kondo Y, Abe S, Toko H, *et al.* Effect of climatic environment on immunological features of rheumatoid arthritis. Sci Rep 2023; 13(1): 1304.
[http://dx.doi.org/10.1038/s41598-022-27153-3] [PMID: 36693893]

[16] Ran D, Yan W, Yanhong B, Hong W. Geniposide augments apoptosis in fibroblast-like synoviocytes by restoring hypoxia-enhanced JNK-BNIP3-mediated autophagy. Inflamm Res 2023; 72(8): 1745-60.
[http://dx.doi.org/10.1007/s00011-023-01782-4] [PMID: 37624402]

[17] Jain S, Tran TH, Amiji M. Macrophage repolarization with targeted alginate nanoparticles containing IL-10 plasmid DNA for the treatment of experimental arthritis. Biomaterials 2015; 61: 162-77.
[http://dx.doi.org/10.1016/j.biomaterials.2015.05.028] [PMID: 26004232]

[18] Deshmukh R. Rheumatoid arthritis: Pathophysiology, current therapeutic strategies and recent advances in targeted drug delivery system. Mater Today Commun 2023; 35: 105877.
[http://dx.doi.org/10.1016/j.mtcomm.2023.105877]

[19] Rotpenpian N, Wanasuntronwong A, Tapechum S, *et al.* Standardized Centella asiatica (ECa 233) extract decreased pain hypersensitivity development in a male mouse model of chronic inflammatory temporomandibular disorder. Sci Rep 2023; 13(1): 6642.
[http://dx.doi.org/10.1038/s41598-023-33769-w] [PMID: 37095163]

[20] Abbasi M, Mousavi MJ, Jamalzehi S, *et al.* Strategies toward rheumatoid arthritis therapy; the old and the new. J Cell Physiol 2019; 234(7): 10018-31.
[http://dx.doi.org/10.1002/jcp.27860] [PMID: 30536757]

[21] Köhler BM, Günther J, Kaudewitz D, Lorenz HM. Current therapeutic options in the treatment of rheumatoid arthritis. J Clin Med 2019; 8(7): 938.
[http://dx.doi.org/10.3390/jcm8070938] [PMID: 31261785]

[22] Li X, Zhang S. Herbal compounds for rheumatoid arthritis: Literatures review and cheminformatics prediction. Phytother Res 2020; 34(1): 51-66.
[http://dx.doi.org/10.1002/ptr.6509] [PMID: 31515874]

[23] Sharma D, Chaubey P, Suvarna V. Role of natural products in alleviation of rheumatoid arthritis—A review. J Food Biochem 2021; 45(4): e13673.
[http://dx.doi.org/10.1111/jfbc.13673] [PMID: 33624882]

[24] Bose S, Sarkar N, Banerjee D. Natural medicine delivery from biomedical devices to treat bone disorders: A review. Acta Biomater 2021; 126: 63-91.
[http://dx.doi.org/10.1016/j.actbio.2021.02.034] [PMID: 33657451]

[25] Silvestre ALP, dos Santos AM, de Oliveira AB, *et al.* Evaluation of photodynamic therapy on nanoparticles and films loaded-nanoparticles based on chitosan/alginate for curcumin delivery in oral biofilms. Int J Biol Macromol 2023; 240: 124489.
[http://dx.doi.org/10.1016/j.ijbiomac.2023.124489] [PMID: 37076077]

[26] Epstein J, Sanderson IR, MacDonald TT. Curcumin as a therapeutic agent: the evidence from *in vitro*, animal and human studies. Br J Nutr 2010; 103(11): 1545-57.
[http://dx.doi.org/10.1017/S0007114509993667] [PMID: 20100380]

[27] Singh S, Singh TG, Mahajan K, Dhiman S. Medicinal plants used against various inflammatory biomarkers for the management of rheumatoid arthritis. J Pharm Pharmacol 2020; 72(10): 1306-27.
[http://dx.doi.org/10.1111/jphp.13326] [PMID: 32812250]

[28] Tiwari M, Barooah MS. A comprehensive review on the ethno-medicinal and pharmacological properties of terminalia chebula fruit. Phytochem Rev 2023; 23(1): 1-21.
[http://dx.doi.org/10.1007/s11101-023-09878-9]

[29]   Bandopadhyay S, Mandal S, Ghorai M, *et al.* Therapeutic properties and pharmacological activities of asiaticoside and madecassoside: A review. J Cell Mol Med 2023; 27(5): 593-608.
[http://dx.doi.org/10.1111/jcmm.17635] [PMID: 36756687]

[30]   Shao J, Li T, Zeng S, *et al.* The structures of two acidic polysaccharides from Gardenia jasminoides and their potential immunomodulatory activities. Int J Biol Macromol 2023; 248: 125895.
[http://dx.doi.org/10.1016/j.ijbiomac.2023.125895] [PMID: 37481185]

[31]   Ke J, Li MT, Xu S, Ma J, Liu MY, Han Y. Advances for pharmacological activities of *Polygonum cuspidatum* - A review. Pharm Biol 2023; 61(1): 177-88.
[http://dx.doi.org/10.1080/13880209.2022.2158349] [PMID: 36620922]

[32]   Babu V, Binwal M, Ranjana , *et al.* Hesperidin-rich ethanol extract from waste peels of *Citrus limetta* mitigates rheumatoid arthritis and related complications. Phytother Res 2021; 35(6): 3325-36.
[http://dx.doi.org/10.1002/ptr.7053] [PMID: 33624898]

[33]   He DY, Dai SM. Anti-inflammatory and immunomodulatory effects of paeonia lactiflora pall, a traditional chinese herbal medicine. Front Pharmacol 2011; 2: 10.
[http://dx.doi.org/10.3389/fphar.2011.00010] [PMID: 21687505]

[34]   Rabiei M, Kashanian S, Samavati SS, Derakhshankhah H, Jamasb S, McInnes SJP. Nanotechnology application in drug delivery to osteoarthritis (OA), rheumatoid arthritis (RA), and osteoporosis (OSP). J Drug Deliv Sci Technol 2021; 61: 102011.
[http://dx.doi.org/10.1016/j.jddst.2020.102011]

[35]   Nasra S, Bhatia D, Kumar A. Recent advances in nanoparticle-based drug delivery systems for rheumatoid arthritis treatment. Nanoscale Adv 2022; 4(17): 3479-94.
[http://dx.doi.org/10.1039/D2NA00229A] [PMID: 36134349]

[36]   Siddique R, Mehmood MH, Haris M, Saleem A, Chaudhry Z. Promising role of polymeric nanoparticles in the treatment of rheumatoid arthritis. Inflammopharmacology 2022; 30(4): 1207-18.
[http://dx.doi.org/10.1007/s10787-022-00997-x] [PMID: 35524837]

[37]   Wang Q, Qin X, Fang J, Sun X. Nanomedicines for the treatment of rheumatoid arthritis: State of art and potential therapeutic strategies. Acta Pharm Sin B 2021; 11(5): 1158-74.
[http://dx.doi.org/10.1016/j.apsb.2021.03.013] [PMID: 34094826]

[38]   Thajuddin N, Mathew S. Phytonanotechnology. Elsevier 2020.

[39]   Cai H, Zheng Z, Sun Y, Liu Z, Zhang M, Li C. The effect of curcumin and its nanoformulation on adjuvant-induced arthritis in rats. Drug Des Devel Ther 2015; 9: 4931-42.
[http://dx.doi.org/10.2147/DDDT.S90147] [PMID: 26345159]

[40]   Esmaeili Y, Khavani M, Bigham A, *et al.* Mesoporous silica@chitosan@gold nanoparticles as "on/off" optical biosensor and pH-sensitive theranostic platform against cancer. Int J Biol Macromol 2022; 202: 241-55.
[http://dx.doi.org/10.1016/j.ijbiomac.2022.01.063] [PMID: 35041881]

[41]   Del Prado-Audelo M, Caballero-Florán I, Meza-Toledo J, *et al.* Formulations of curcumin nanoparticles for brain diseases. Biomolecules 2019; 9(2): 56.
[http://dx.doi.org/10.3390/biom9020056] [PMID: 30743984]

[42]   Zheng YQ, Wei W. Total glucosides of paeony suppresses adjuvant arthritis in rats and intervenes cytokine-signaling between different types of synoviocytes. Int Immunopharmacol 2005; 5(10): 1560-73.
[http://dx.doi.org/10.1016/j.intimp.2005.03.010] [PMID: 16023608]

[43]   Teja PK, Mithiya J, Kate AS, Bairwa K, Chauthe SK. Herbal nanomedicines: Recent advancements, challenges, opportunities and regulatory overview. Phytomedicine 2022; 96: 153890.
[http://dx.doi.org/10.1016/j.phymed.2021.153890] [PMID: 35026510]

[44]   Bhattacharya T, Soares GAB, Chopra H, *et al.* Applications of phyto-nanotechnology for the treatment

of neurodegenerative disorders. Materials (Basel) 2022; 15(3): 804.
[http://dx.doi.org/10.3390/ma15030804] [PMID: 35160749]

[45]   Ilhan M, Kilicarslan M, Alcigir ME, Bagis N, Ekim O, Orhan K. Clindamycin phosphate and bone morphogenetic protein-7 loaded combined nanoparticle-graft and nanoparticle-film formulations for alveolar bone regeneration – An *in vitro* and *in vivo* evaluation. Int J Pharm 2023; 636: 122826.
[http://dx.doi.org/10.1016/j.ijpharm.2023.122826] [PMID: 36918117]

[46]   Gungor Ak A, Turan I, Sayan Ozacmak H, Karatas A. Chitosan nanoparticles as promising tool for berberine delivery: Formulation, characterization and *in vivo* evaluation. J Drug Deliv Sci Technol 2023; 80: 104203.
[http://dx.doi.org/10.1016/j.jddst.2023.104203]

[47]   Teixeira MI, Lopes CM, Gonçalves H, *et al.* Formulation, characterization, and cytotoxicity evaluation of lactoferrin functionalized lipid nanoparticles for riluzole delivery to the brain. Pharmaceutics 2022; 14(1): 185.
[http://dx.doi.org/10.3390/pharmaceutics14010185] [PMID: 35057079]

[48]   Gültekin HE, Oner E, İlhan M, Karpuz M. Nanovesicles for intravenous drug delivery 2022. Available from: https://doi.org/https://doi.org/10.1016/B978-0-323-91865-7.00018-3
[http://dx.doi.org/10.1016/B978-0-323-91865-7.00018-3]

[49]   Karpuz M, İlhan M, Gültekin HE, Ozgenc E, Şenyiğit Z, Atlihan-Gundogdu E. Nanovesicles for tumor-targeted drug delivery 2022. Available from: https://doi.org/https://doi.org/10.1016/B978--323-91865-7.00017-1
[http://dx.doi.org/10.1016/B978-0-323-91865-7.00017-1]

[50]   Li Y, Liang Q, Zhou L, Liu J, Liu Y. Metal nanoparticles: a platform integrating diagnosis and therapy for rheumatoid arthritis. J Nanopart Res 2022; 24(4): 84.
[http://dx.doi.org/10.1007/s11051-022-05469-5]

[51]   Zhang J, Hu K, Di L, *et al.* Traditional herbal medicine and nanomedicine: Converging disciplines to improve therapeutic efficacy and human health. Adv Drug Deliv Rev 2021; 178: 113964.
[http://dx.doi.org/10.1016/j.addr.2021.113964] [PMID: 34499982]

[52]   Jose A. 2022.
[http://dx.doi.org/10.1016/B978-0-323-88450-1.00010-7]

[53]   He R, Li L, Zhang T, *et al.* Recent advances of nanotechnology application in autoimmune diseases – A bibliometric analysis. Nano Today 2023; 48: 101694.
[http://dx.doi.org/10.1016/j.nantod.2022.101694]

CHAPTER 5

The Effects of Herbal Medicines on the Management of Inflammatory Bowel Disease

Aybala Temel[1,*]

[1] *Department of Pharmaceutical Microbiology, Faculty of Pharmacy, Izmir Katip Celebi University, Izmir 35620, Türkiye*

Abstract: Inflammatory bowel disease (IBD) that affects a large population worldwide, is a gastrointestinal disorder that includes Crohn's disease and ulcerative colitis. The genetic factors, immunological, and microbial factors play critical roles in the pathogenesis of IBD. However, there is still no pharmacological therapy providing the definitive treatment of the disease. Gastrointestinal symptoms of IBD significantly reduce the patient's quality of life and IBD patients often tend to use herbal medicines as an alternative and complementary therapy for improving the symptoms. Among herbal medicines used for IBS, *Andrographis paniculata*, *Boswellia serrata*, and *Aloe vera* are prominent plant species, and catechins and curcumin are the commonly investigated phytochemicals. Here, we summarized the main factors in the pathogenesis of IBD, the current treatment strategies, and commonly used natural compounds and herbs with evidence-based data. The findings pointed out that further clinical trials having a higher sample size are required prior to the recommended use of these herbal medicines in therapy.

Keywords: *Andrographis paniculata*, *Aloe vera*, *Boswellia serrata*, Catechins, Crohn's disease, Curcumin, Herbal medicine, Inflammatory Bowel Disease, Ulcerative colitis.

INTRODUCTION

Inflammatory bowel disease (IBD), which is divided into two types ulcerative colitis (UC) and Crohn's disease (CD), is one of the chronic inflammatory diseases of the gastrointestinal tract that is common especially in adolescence and young adulthood [1]. The onset of IBD is dependent on the effects of genetic and environmental parameters on the immune system [2].

[*] **Corresponding author Aybala Temel:** Department of Pharmaceutical Microbiology, Faculty of Pharmacy, Izmir Katip Celebi University, Izmir 35620, Türkiye; Tel: +90 2323293535; E-mail: aybala.temel@ikcu.edu.tr

Cennet Ozay & Gokhan Zengin (Eds.)

The symptoms of IBD generally present early in life, and approximately 25% of IBD patients are diagnosed before the age of twenty years [3]. Even though the incidence rate of IBD has started to decline in Western countries since 1990, the incidence rate continues to increase rapidly in newly industrialized countries [4, 5]. While the European countries with the highest prevalence of IBS are reported to be Norway and Germany, the disease is more common in Canada, and USA [5]. Inflammatory bowel disease directly or indirectly affects the patients' quality of life, mental health, work productivity and overall health [6 - 8]. The diagnosis of IBD, its treatment and follow-up of the patients bring a great economic burden to the national health systems of the countries. The estimated annual treatment costs for IBS patients in the United States alone, are more than USD 6.8 billion [6, 9]. Therefore, it is necessary to understand the pathogenesis of this disease and develop new evidence-based diagnosis and treatment strategies for IBD disease.

PATHOGENESIS OF IBD

The reason why and how IBS occurs is not yet fully understood, but it was known that the dysregulated mucosal immune response against commensal gut microbiota of the host is responsible for the pathogenesis of the diseases. Host genetic factors and enviromental conditions have been identified as the main reasons for this dysregulation in recent studies [1, 2, 10]. Inflammatory bowel disease is classified into two predominant groups, ulcerative colitis and Crohn's Disease, which have similar symptoms. A healthy colon consists of a loose outer layer suitable for bacterial growth, a firmer and sterile inner layer and a continuous mucus coating. There is a marked increase in bacteria associated with the adherent mucus layer of the colon when IBD occurs, particularly in CD [11 - 13]. Some of these similar symptoms of CD and UC are diarrhea, weight loss, abdominal pain, and rectal bleeding. The main characteristic feature of CD and UC is inflammation in the gastrointestinal tract and its gradual exacerbation [2, 14, 15]. On the other hand, there are certain variations between the symptoms of patients suffering from CD and UC.

Crohn's disease is more common in patients at the ages of 15-35 and directly affects the mouth, the stomach, the esophagus, the anus and the intestinal mucosa in the body. Differently, ulcerative colitis is mostly confined to the colon and affects parts of the large intestine, including the rectum [16]. Ulcerative colitis mostly causes damage to the internal parts of the body and isassociated with osteoporosis and colon cancer. Crohn's disease, which affects the entire intestine, mostly cause skin diseases and biliary stones in the later stages of the disease [17]. The four main components of IBD pathogenesis characterized by a chronic inflammation in gut may be listed as genetic, environmental, microbial and immunological factors [11].

Genetic Factors

Thanks to the technological developments in recent years, new important informationhas been obtained regarding the interaction between the pathogenesis of IBD and the genetic characteristics of the host [11, 18]. By using genome-wide association studies (GWAS), which identify single nucleotide polymorphisms, 200 IBD-associated risk alleles have been identified until nowadays [19]. The findings of recent studies on the genetic factors associated with IBD, provided noteworthy clues about the underlying mechanism of the disease [11]. A total of 163 IBD-associated gene loci were detected, of which 30 were CD-specific, 23 were specific for UC, and 110 were associated with both diseases [11, 20]. NOD2 (nucleotide-binding oligomerization domain containing 2 domains) was the first gene discovered to be associated with CD, in 2001 [21]. The protein that performs encoding by NOD2 was described as an intracellular receptor, which recognizes the muramyl dipeptide (MDP) in the peptidoglycan layer of the bacterial cell membrane [22]. Autophagy contributes to the removal of intracellular microbes by the degradation of cytosolic contents and organelles [10]. The autophagy-associated genes (ATG16L1 and IRGM) relate with the risk of CD. CD-associated polymorphisms and various mutations in these genes cause defects in antibacterial autophagy [23, 24].

One of the most important genetic findings related to IBD is the determination of the relation between the IL23R gene and the proinflammatory cytokines encoded by this gene. IL-23 is a receptor peptide playing a role in Th17 cell generation. It is well known that Th17 cells and interleukin IL-23, a pro-inflammatory cytokine, have a detrimental effect on CD and UC progression [25 - 27]. These risk-associated gene loci show heterogenicity between populations; NOD2 and IL23R variants are present in the majority of European patients, but rare in East Asian ancestry patients. Additionally, some individuals having IBD-associated gene loci, may not even develop the symptoms of the disease [28]. Various environmental factors and the interactions between the gut microbiota and host immune system are critical for the pathogenesis of IBD, in addition to genetic parameters [4].

Environmental Factors

External environmental factors have direct or indirect effects on IBD as in almost every disease. Smoking, diet and nutrition, drug usage, air pollution, demographic properties, and stress conditions are prominent environmental prompters associated with the development of IBD [29]. High-stress levels have been paid attention to as a predisposing factor the pathogenesis of both CD and UC for many years [30, 31]. It has been reported that individuals with low stress levels have a lower risk of the onset of the disease and different stress conditions such as depression and anxiety can exacerbate the clinical progress of the IBD [32, 33]. Goodhand *et al.* indicated a reduction in symptomatic relapses of IBD patients being treated with antidepressants. Contrarily, Cochrane database findings showed no significant impact of psychological interventions in IBD [32, 33]. Medications and dietary habits are the two most determining environmental factors in IBS. They have undeniable effects on both the intestines and the whole body of the host. Evidence-based studies on aspirin, non-steroidal anti-inflammatory drugs (NSAIDs), antibiotics, and antispasmodics that are used for the treatment of IBS symptoms are found in the literature [11].

Aspirin and NSAIDs are commonly prescribed drugs for many different diseases. No association was detected between the dose of aspirin use and the risk for IBD by Ananthakrishnan *et al.* However, the high dose and prolonged use of NSAIDs have been related to higher risk for CD/UC [34, 35]. Antibiotic exposure, particularly in early childhood, is associated with IBD and many gastrointestinal disorders. It has been clarified that antibiotics may alter the intestinal microbiota composition by declining the diversity of microorganisms and this effect can trigger the susceptibility to IBD [19]. In a cohort study on the interaction between antibiotic usage in childhood and IBD progress, it was reported that a dose dependent effect associated with antibiotics was found only in CD [36]. Intriguingly, C Ng *et al.* reported that antibiotic exposure was associated with a lower risk of CD or UC, in their population-based case-control study in Asia-Pacific [37].

Microbial Factors

The bidirectional interactions between the host immune system and the gut microbiota maintain homeostasis in the human body [38]. The human microbiota which begins to be colonized by microorganisms at birth, shows significant differences depending on predisposing factors and life periods [39, 40]. Four main bacterial phyla dominating the gut microbiota that contains more than 1000 different species are Furmicutes (~49–76%), Bacteroidetes (~16–23%), Actinobacteria (<5%), and Proteobacteria (<10%) [38, 41]. An imbalance in gut microbial diversity, also defined as 'dysbiosis', can result in the occurrence of metabolic, chronic or infectious diseases, such as IBD, irritable bowel diseases, colon cancer, hypertension, autism, and asthma [38, 42 - 44]. A healthy host–microorganism balance in the intestines is a requirement for sustaining intestinal homeostasis and function, protecting the host from the diseases, especially infections and inflammation [4, 38]. Commensal microorganisms in the gut have a protective role against enteric pathogenic infections *via* colonization resistance phenomenon or regulating the immune system components [39, 40].

Microbes that enter the human body can be caught by pattern recognition receptors (PRRs) of pathogen-associated molecular patterns (PAMPs), which are found in many bacteria species. This recognition process is performed by the host's immune system cells, and then pro-inflammatory cytokines and chemokines are produced that provide the inflammatory response against the pathogens [40]. The association between the changes in the microbiota and IBD has been first established with research on animal models. Animal studies have demonstrated that the intestinal microbiota members play pro-inflammatory and anti-inflammatory roles in IBD. Within the animal colitis models, it was noticed that the intestinal microbiota composition is a crucial driver for the development and progress of this disease and its symptoms [45, 46]. Since studies on humans and animal models of infection are not fully compatible, it seems unlikely that a single infection can cause IBD in humans. However, it has been clearly noticed that there is an interaction between the development of IBD and the intestinal microbiota [39, 40].

Melgar *et al.* reported that *Mycobacterium avium* subsp. *paratuberculosis* and invasive *Escherichia coli* species is increased in CD patients while *Clostridium difficile* has been increased in both CD and UC patients in remission conditions [47]. In summary, microbial factors directly affect the gut microbiota and their promoter role in the host immune system must be kept in mind in the pathogenesis of IBD.

Immunological Factors

The dysregulations of innate and adaptive immune pathways triggers the aberrant intestinal inflammatory response in patients with IBD. The evidence-based investigations on the interaction between IBD and immunity has been mostly focused on the T cell response [11]. The innate immune response, which is the primary line of defense of the host against pathogens, is non-specific and is stimulated in a short time. Neutrophils, epithelial cells, monocytes, macrophages and natural killer cells are the mediators cell types responsible for innate immune response [48]. The innate immune response is initiated by the recognition of microbial antigens, which are mediated by Toll-like receptors (TLRs) on the surface of cells. Recent immunological research works have shown that the activation of the cells rolling in innate immunity are altered significantly in IBD patients, depending on the expression and function of TLRs [11, 49]. Marks *et al.* found that the production of IL-1β and IL-8 is selectively decreased in CD patients [50]. IL-23 is another key cytokine, possessing a central role in both early immune responses against pathogens and chronic bowel inflammation. It is understood that IL23R polymorphisms have been associated IBD. Recent studies have demonstrated that IL-23 has an inductive effect on Th17 cytokine production by innate lymphoid cells [51]. GWAS research revealed that the NOD2 mutations are frequently associated with the defects in the intestine to provide defence against bacterial LPS, and this may be one of the reasons that contribute to disease susceptibility in IBD patients [52]. It is suggested that the underlying mechanism, mutation and function loss of NOD2, may cause a lack of TLR2 inhibition [53, 54]. Other studies suggest that the functional loss of NOD2 may result in the lack of inhibition of TLR2 stimulation, leading to the activation of inflammatory pathways and excessive Th-1 responses [53, 54]. An abnormal Th1 response is thought to exacerbate intestinal inflammation in CD and may also activate components of adaptive immunity [55]. The adaptive immune responses are more specific, and IFN-γ induced by Th1 and interleukins (IL-2, IL-4, IL-5, IL-13) released from Th2 cells come into play [56]. In the studies investigating immunological factors on IBD, CD is mostly associated with Th1 cell response, while Th2-mediated immune mechanisms have a role in the prognosis of UC [57]. The high levels of IFN-γ were found by Rovedatti et al., in the study conducted on the biopsies of CD and UC patients cultured *in vitro* release [58]. It has also been observed that IL-13 levels in the intestinal biopsies cultured *in vitro* are lower than IFN-γ concentration among CD, UC and control groups [59]. These data from previous studies have led researchers to rethink the Th1/Th2 paradigm in CD and UC, which is still controversial [57]. Further studies are required for a better understanding of the immunological mechanisms in IBD pathogenesis.

TREATMENT STRATEGIES

Clinicians generally do not prefer using pharmacologic therapy for an initial management strategy for IBD patients with mild/intermittent symptoms. Lifestyle and dietary habits (low FODMAP diet, lactose avoidance) are modified for improving the symptoms [60]. If these modifications are not sufficient, adjunctive pharmacologic therapy is applied to the patients. The main management strategies of IBD include antibiotics, corticosteroids, anti-tumor necrosis factor, antibodies, and aminosalicylates [61]. The treatment of IBD with these drugs targets to induce and maintain remission in the progress of the disease.

HERBAL MEDICINES FOR IBD

The main management strategies of IBD includes antibiotics, corticosteroids, anti-tumor necrosis factor-antibodies, and aminosalicylates. However current pharmacological therapies provide limited symptomatic improvement to IBD patients and no certain successful treatment is still currently available for IBD. Hence, the use of complementary and alternative therapeutic approaches by patients has increased to prevent the symptoms from decreasing the quality of life [62]. Herbal therapies have been used for a variety of health conditions and diseases since ancient times in different regions worldwide, especially in Asian and Eastern countries [62, 63]. Intriguingly, some natural compounds and herbal medicines have shown efficacy for IBD in experimental animal models and clinical trials [64]. Evidence-based research have pointed out that herbal medicines, including natural compounds such as curcumin, berberine, cannabinoids, catechines and certain plants such as *Aloe vera*, *Boswellia serrata*, and *Andrographis paniculata* may exhibit efficacy on amelioreting IBD.

Curcuma Species

The genus *Curcuma* belonging to Zingiberaceae, has been used for several purposes such as wound healing, liver and skin diseases, jaundice treatment in different traditional medicines since ancient times [65, 66]. Two species of Curcuma genus, *Curcuma longa* and *Curcuma xanthorrhiza* which are the main source of curcumin, draw attention for the improvement of gastrointestinal symptoms with their pharmacological properties and active ingredients [66]. Chemical studies have shown that *Curcuma* species have various phenolic compounds, essential oils, alkaloids and steroids. Among them, curcuminoids (including curcumin and curcumin derivates) belonging to the group of diarylheptanoids, are major phenolic compounds in *Curcuma* [65, 66]. Curcumin (called diferuloyl methane) is an arylheptanoid pigment derived from the rhizomes of *Curcuma longa* and is an active ingredient in turmeric. Curcumin which is poorly absorbed orally, reaches high concentrations in the gastrointestinal lumen [67, 68].

Curcuma longa has shown potential effects against IBS symptoms by reducing various pro-inflammatory cytokines (TNF-α, IFN-γ, IL-12) in several trials [69 - 71]. Deguchi *et al.* reported that nuclear factor-kappa (NF-κB) activation was blocked in the mucosa in dextran sulfate sodium (DSS) + curcumin-treated experimental mice with colitis. It was indicated that cellular infiltration and epithelial disruption were much more severe in DSS-treated mice than in DSS + curcumin-treated mice, in the same study [72]. Another study focused on the protective role of curcumin in chronic colonic inflammation suggesting that curcumin could reduce COX-2 and Inducible nitric oxide synthase (iNOS) immunosignals and significantly attenuated the damage in chronic experimental colitis [73]. In a randomized controlled trial, it was detected that the addition of curcumin to mesalamine therapy was superior to only mesalamine in inducing clinical and endoscopic remission in UC patients [74]. Curcumin has shown ameliorative effect by downregulating the various pro-inflammatory cytokines (IFN-γ, TNF-α, IL-1β, IL-12, IL-17 and IL-23) and by affecting some signalling pathways and enzymes (Janus kinase/signal transducer and cyclooxygenase-2) in the chronic inflammation associated with IBS [67, 75 - 79].

Catechins

Further clinical trials should be done to confirm the beneficial effects of popular natural polyphenols in IBD. Among them, catechins, including some types of polyphenols, have also beenmore focused over the last decade [80 - 82]. Thanks to its high potential for anti-inflammation, anti-oxidant, and anti-bacterial effects, catechins contribute to the remission of IBD. The main underlying mechanisms responsible for the effects of catechins in IBD are oxidative stress, cell filtration, cell signaling pathways (NF-κB associated anti-inflammation), and interactions with intestinal microbiota [80, 81, 83, 84]. Catechins and their metabolites in the acidic environment of the stomach, can be easily absorbed from the gastrointestinal tract [85]. Catechins that exist in green tea (*Camelia sinensis*) and some foods exhibit significant efficacy in murine colitis and clinical trials [80, 85]. The oxiradical overload is considered to aggravate the pathogenesis of IBD. Although the occurence of reactive oxygen species (ROS) is necessary and normal for the function of the pathways that provide signal transmission in the body, they can be effective in the deterioration of the intestinal mucosa [81, 86]. Hence, the antioxidant defense against reactive oxygen radicals and oxidative stress may be useful in IBD patients. The catechins can scavenge free radicals directly chelating with redox-active metals, or they can regulate protein synthesis and signaling mechanisms indirectly to reduce the oxidative stress [87 - 89]. Najafzadeh *et al.* reported that epicathecin (EC) demonstrated a protective activity for *in vitro* lymphocytes of IBD patients [90]. Renato *et al.* have proved that the antioxidant capacity of (+)-catechin is dose-dependent (10-100μM) [91].

Catechins have several forms of diastereoisomers: Epicatechin (EC), epicatechin gallate (ECG), epigallocatechin (EGC), and epigallocatechine gallate (EGCG) [92]. Epigallocatechin-3-gallate (EGCG), one of the major polyphenols in green tea, has an inhibitory effect on TNF-α activity [64, 93]. In the study with murine colitis model, it was determined that EGCG exerts an anti-inflammatory effect by suppressing mast cell and macrophage function [81]. Peracetylated EGCG, with similar anti-inflammatory activity as EGCG, was found to be more effective than EGCG in DSS-induced colitis [94]. It was also indicated that EGCG inhibited colon inflammation, when applied intraperitoneally in colitis in rat models, causing a decline in weight loss [95]. The inflammatory damages due to IBD pathonegenesis have been primarily related to large amount of infiltration of the immune system components (T helper cells, neutrophils, leukocytes) and extention of the damage that depends on the production of pro-inflammatory cytokines, chemokines, and reactive oxygen species [80, 81, 84, 86, 90, 95]. The results of studies investigating the effect of catechins on cell filtration are remarkable with their effects on neutrophil infiltration. It was reported that EGCG showed a reductive effect on MPO activity that resulted in the reduction of neutrophil infiltration [95, 96]. Brückner *et al.* observed that the piperine and ECGC combination exhibit an inhibitory effect on MPO, in the colon tissue of murine colitis model. Interestingly, it was also indicated that ECGC alone could not eliminate MPO and piperine also failed to inhibit the neutrophil infiltration in the same study [95].

The relationship between the human gut microbiota and its composition and the pathogenesis of IBD has been further understood in recent studies. It has been noticed in several clinical trials that flavonoids (which include catechins) are beneficial for improving IBS sypmtoms as they cause the suppression of the bacterial growth (particularly pathogenic gut bacteria) and the regulation of imbalanced intestinal microbiota [97, 98]. Human studies have also pointed out the lethal effects of catechins, whose antimicrobial activities have been determined by many *in vitro* studies, especially on pathogenic bacterial species [99, 100]. It was demonstrated that catechins have antimicrobial activity against Staphylococcus spp., Pseudomonas spp., and *Clostridium perfringens,* which are pathogenic bacterial species. Xue *et al.* reported that catechins have a less promoter effect on the growth of Bacteroidetes, an Furmucites species dominating the gut microbiota [100]. In contrast, Rastmanesh *et al.* suggested that polyphenols may have a stimulating effect on Bacteroidetes, but not on *Firmicutes* [101]. The research also highlights that the antimicrobial effect of catechin against Gram-positive bacteria (B. subtilis) was more obvious than the Gram-negative bacteria (*E. coli*) [92]. Hence, catechins may be helpful for stabilizing intestinal flora to the recovery of IBD. Even though the mechanisms are not fully understood, it is revealed that catechins (with their anti-inflammatory, antioxidative, and antibacterial activity) and microorganisms in the gut interact and these interactions may have the potential to ameliorate IBD and related GIS conditions [80].

Andrographis paniculata

Andrographis paniculata (A. paniculata) which is known as the 'king of bitters' is an herbaceous plant belonging to the Acanthaceae family. The leaves and roots of this plant have been used for various medicinal purposes in Southern Asia and Europe for centuries [102]. The main pharmacological uses of *A. paniculata* include stimulating the components of the immune system and the treatment of respiratory tract infections. Numerous different studies on *Andrographis paniculata* have also reported its antioxidant, antimicrobial, antimalarial and anti-inflammatory effects [102 - 104]. It has been determined that *A. paniculata* contains different phytochemicals, in leaves and stem parts, responsible for its pharmacological activities such as andrographolide, neoandrographolide, isoandrographolide and andrographolide derivatives [105]. Andrographolide, a diterpenoid molecule, is the major phytochemical of *A. paniculata*. It has demonstrated benefical effects on the diseases associated with inflammation, bacterial and viral infections, dysentery, malaria, *etc* [106 - 110]. Pre-clinical and clinical trial results indicating the anti-inflammatory effect of *A.paniculata* have been reported in the literature [67]. It has been understood that *A. paniculata* exerts its anti-inflammatory effect by inhibiting T cells, macrophages, dendritic cells, cytokines and cell signaling pathways [111]. The anti-inflammatory activity of a herbal medicinal product named HMPL-004 made from the ethanol extract of *A.paniculata* has been investigated in various *in vitro* studies. In the studies on *Andrographis paniculata* extracts, it was reported that this plant inhibits the proliferation and differentiation of CD4+ T cells and Th1/Th17 cell responses in colitis models [112, 113]. Michelsen *et al.* detected a significant reduction in expression levels of the genes associated with TNF-α, IL-1β, IL-22, and IFN-γ [112]. Andrographolide exhibited a reduction effect on the protein levels of pro-inflammatory cytokines, and COX-2 and iNOS related gene expression was examined in a colitis mouse model [108]. With a limited number of randomized clinical trials, the efficacy of this plant extract alone and in combination with mesalamine was evaluated [113, 114]. Tang *et al.* investigated the HPML-004 and mesalamine combination in 108 active UC patients for 8 weeks, and they reported a similar effect of HPML-004 to mesalamine [114]. Another clinical study conducted in UC patients receiving a specific dose of mesalamine examined the effect of different doses of HPML-004. The primary endpoint of this study was the clinical response, defined as a decrease in the rectal bleeding subscore and no significant differences were detected for tested doses (1.2 or 1.8 g/day of HMPL-004) in terms of clinical remission [113]. More randomized controlled clinical trials and molecular level studies are needed to elucidate the chemical components and mechanisms responsible for the anti-inflammatory effect of *A.paniculata* [102].

Boswellia serrata

Boswellia species has been used as a medicinal herb for the treatment of inflammatory diseases in India, Africa and Middle East for years [115]. *Boswellia serrata* and the resin (called Frankincense) obtained from this plant have demonstrated antioxidant and anti-inflammatory properties in arthritis, asthma, colitis and cancer, which are associated with chronic inflammation [116, 117]. The resin of *B.serrata* includes terpenoids (monoterpenes, diterpenes), especially tetracyclic triterpenic acids. β-boswellic acid (β-BA), 11-keto-β-boswellic acid (KBA), and acetyl-11-keto-β-boswellic acid (AKBA) are active derivates that are considered responsible for the anti-inflammotory effect [118, 119]. *In vitro* experimental studies and preclinical trials revealed that *Boswellia serrata* can decrease TNF-α, IFN-γ, IL-6, and IL-12 and increase IL-4, and IL-10 [120 - 123].

The mechanisms underlying these effects are indicated as the inhibition of lipid peroxidation, P-selectin expression, iNOS expression, and leukocyte adhesion [67]. Gerhardt *et al.* stated that *B. serrata* extract was applied for 8 weeks and it provided a significant reduction in DAI in 102 Crohn's patients [124]. On the other hand, no beneficial clinical effect of *B. serrata* extract (Boswelan 800 mg tid orally) was observed at a randomised controlled trial of 82 patients [125].

Aloe vera

Aloe vera is a medicinal plant that has been used medicinally for over 5000 years by Egyptians, Indians, and Europeans. Its biological acitivity profile has been widely investigated for years and proved that it has antiinflammatory, immunmodulating, wound healing, and antidiabetic properties [126, 127]. *Aloe vera* gel has been used for the treatment of various gastrointestinal disorders and skin diseases associated with inflammation. It is known that IBD patients commonly use *Aloe vera* gel orally as a complement to medicines [128]. Even though there is limited scientific evidence about the effect of *A.vera* in IBD, randomized trials have shown that *Aloe vera* gel might be beneficial for improving IBD symptoms thanks to the mechanisms associated with TNF-α and several interleukins [67]. The major active phytochemicals of *A.vera* are polymannans, anthraquinones (aloe-emodin) anthrones, chromones, and lectins [69]. Experiments with mouse models indicate a reduction in inflammation in the intestinal mucosa following oral administration of *A. vera* gel. It has been determined that this effect occurs as a result of a decrease in myeloperoxidase activity and a decrease in the expression of TNF-α and IL-1β-related genes [129, 130]. In a placebo-controlled randomised trial including 44 patients, Langmead *et al.* investigated the effect of *A. vera* gel (taken orally, twice daily) for 4 weeks. They reported that clinical remission, improvement and response occurred in 30%, 37% and 47%, in 30 patients given *Aloe vera* gel, respectively. It has also been highlighted that clinical trials with a larger patient groups are needed to reach a certain point with respect to the clinical efficacy of *A.vera* in IBD [131].

CONCLUDING REMARKS

Side effects of conventional pharmacological therapies and the lack of a definitive treatment for some diseases such as IBD increase the interest in herbal treatments. Herbal remedies and natural products are some of the alternative treatments commonly preferred by IBD patients. However, it should not be forgotten that herbal medicines can directly or indirectly affect various signal transmission pathways and the immune system, and also interfere with different drugs. Hence, herbal medicines should be used by patients in consultation with physicians every time. In addition, there should be sufficient evidence-based data on the herbal product to be used. Intensive research based on preclinical and clinical trials of IBD, is the gold standard for evaluating the efficacy of herbal medicines and their active compounds. Various randomized controlled studies on herbs showing potential for use in IBD were attempted that are summarized in this study. Among herbal medicines used for IBS, *A. paniculata* and *B. serrata* are prominent plant species, catechins and curcumin are the most commonly investigated phytochemicals. Randomised controlled trials showed that *B. serrata* resin extract in high dose showed therapeutic efficacy in CD patients. *A. paniculata* extract, curcumin and catechins have significant anti-inflammatory effects. However, the most important disadvantage of animal models and clinical studies on herbal medicines in IBD treatment is the low sample size. The superiority of these studies, which mostly compare herbal therapy with placebo, over conventional therapy in IBD should be evaluated separately.

LIST OF ABBREVIATIONS

CD	Crohn's Disease
COX-2	Cyclooxygenase 2
DSS	Dextran Sulfate Sodium
EC	Epicatechin
ECG	Epicatechin Gallate
EGC	Epigallocatechin
EGCG	Epigallocatechine Gallate
GIS	Gastrointestinal System
GWAS	Genome-wide Association Atudies
IBD	Inflammatory Bowel Disease
IFN-γ	Interferon- γ
iNOS	Inducible Nitric Oxide Synthase
MDP	Muramyl Dipeptide in Peptidoglycan
MPO	Myeloperoxidase
NF-Kb	Nuclear Factor-kappa B
NOD	Nucleotide-binding Oligomerization Domain protein
NSAID	Nonsteroidal Anti-inflammatory Drug
PAMP	Pathogen-associated Molecular Patterns
PRR	Pattern Recognition Receptors
ROS	Reactive Oxygen Species
TLR	Toll-like Receptor
TNF	Tumor Necrosis Factor
UC	Ulcerative Colitis

REFERENCES

[1]   Rosen MJ, Dhawan A, Saeed SA. Inflammatory Bowel Disease in Children and Adolescents. JAMA Pediatr 2015; 169(11): 1053-60.
        [PMID: 26414706]

[2]   Seyedian SS, Nokhostin F, Malamir MD. A review of the diagnosis, prevention, and treatment methods of inflammatory bowel disease. J Med Life 2019; 12(2): 113-22.
        [PMID: 31406511]

[3]   Baldassano RN, Piccoli DA. Inflammatory bowel disease in pediatric and adolescent patients. Gastroenterol Clin North Am 1999; 28(2): 445-58.
        [PMID: 10372276]

[4]   Guan Q. A Comprehensive Review and Update on the Pathogenesis of Inflammatory Bowel Disease. J Immunol Res 2019; 2019: 7247238.
        [PMID: 31886308]

[5]   Ng SC, Shi HY, Hamidi N, *et al.* Worldwide incidence and prevalence of inflammatory bowel disease in the 21st century: a systematic review of population-based studies. Lancet 2017; 390(10114): 2769-78.
        [PMID: 29050646]

[6]   M'Koma AE. Inflammatory Bowel Disease: Clinical Diagnosis and Surgical Treatment-Overview. Medicina (Kaunas) 2022; 58(5): 567.
        [PMID: 35629984]

[7]   Sciberras M, Karmiris K, Nascimento C, *et al.* Mental Health, Work Presenteeism, and Exercise in Inflammatory Bowel Disease. J Crohn's Colitis 2022; 16(8): 1197-201.
        [PMID: 35239962]

[8]   Parra RS, Chebli JMF, Amarante HMBS, *et al.* Quality of life, work productivity impairment and healthcare resources in inflammatory bowel diseases in Brazil. World J Gastroenterol 2019; 25(38): 5862-82.
        [PMID: 31636478]

[9]   Vadstrup K, Alulis S, Borsi A, *et al.* Societal costs attributable to Crohn's disease and ulcerative colitis within the first 5 years after diagnosis: a Danish nationwide cost-of-illness study 2002-2016. Scand J Gastroenterol 2020; 55(1): 41-6.
        [PMID: 31960726]

[10]   Khor B, Gardet A, Xavier RJ. Genetics and pathogenesis of inflammatory bowel disease. Nature 2011; 474(7351): 307-17.
        [PMID: 21677747]

[11]   Zhang YZ, Li YY. Inflammatory bowel disease: pathogenesis. World J Gastroenterol 2014; 20(1): 91-9.
        [PMID: 24415861]

[12]   Ott SJ, Musfeldt M, Wenderoth DF, *et al.* Reduction in diversity of the colonic mucosa associated bacterial microflora in patients with active inflammatory bowel disease. Gut 2004; 53(5): 685-93.
        [PMID: 15082587]

[13]   Johansson ME, Phillipson M, Petersson J, Velcich A, Holm L, Hansson GC. The inner of the two Muc2 mucin-dependent mucus layers in colon is devoid of bacteria. Proc Natl Acad Sci USA 2008; 105(39): 15064-9.
        [PMID: 18806221]

[14]   Szigethy E, McLafferty L, Goyal A. Inflammatory bowel disease. Child Adolesc Psychiatr Clin N Am 2010; 19(2): 301-318, ix. [ix.].
        [PMID: 20478501]

[15]   Stokkers PC, Hommes DW. New cytokine therapeutics for inflammatory bowel disease. Cytokine 2004; 28(4-5): 167-73.
[PMID: 15588691]

[16]   Farmer RG, Hawk WA, Turnbull RB Jr. Clinical patterns in Crohn's disease: a statistical study of 615 cases. Gastroenterology 1975; 68(4 Pt 1): 627-35.
[PMID: 1123132]

[17]   Mehdizadeh S, Chen G, Enayati PJ, *et al.* Diagnostic yield of capsule endoscopy in ulcerative colitis and inflammatory bowel disease of unclassified type (IBDU). Endoscopy 2008; 40(1): 30-5.
[PMID: 18058654]

[18]   Duerr RH. Genome-wide association studies herald a new era of rapid discoveries in inflammatory bowel disease research. Gastroenterology 2007; 132(5): 2045-9.
[PMID: 17484895]

[19]   Mak WY, Zhao M, Ng SC, Burisch J. The epidemiology of inflammatory bowel disease: East meets west. J Gastroenterol Hepatol 2020; 35(3): 380-9.
[PMID: 31596960]

[20]   Jostins L, Ripke S, Weersma RK, *et al.* Host-microbe interactions have shaped the genetic architecture of inflammatory bowel disease. Nature 2012; 491(7422): 119-24.
[PMID: 23128233]

[21]   Ogura Y, Bonen DK, Inohara N, *et al.* A frameshift mutation in NOD2 associated with susceptibility to Crohn's disease. Nature 2001; 411(6837): 603-6.
[PMID: 11385577]

[22]   Inohara N, Ogura Y, Fontalba A, *et al.* Host recognition of bacterial muramyl dipeptide mediated through NOD2. Implications for Crohn's disease. J Biol Chem 2003; 278(8): 5509-12.
[PMID: 12514169]

[23]   Travassos LH, Carneiro LA, Ramjeet M, *et al.* Nod1 and Nod2 direct autophagy by recruiting ATG16L1 to the plasma membrane at the site of bacterial entry. Nat Immunol 2010; 11(1): 55-62.
[PMID: 19898471]

[24]   Kuballa P, Huett A, Rioux JD, Daly MJ, Xavier RJ. Impaired autophagy of an intracellular pathogen induced by a Crohn's disease associated ATG16L1 variant. PLoS One 2008; 3(10): e3391.
[PMID: 18852889]

[25]   Duerr RH, Taylor KD, Brant SR, *et al.* A genome-wide association study identifies IL23R as an inflammatory bowel disease gene. Science 2006; 314(5804): 1461-3.
[PMID: 17068223]

[26]   Anderson CA, Boucher G, Lees CW, *et al.* Meta-analysis identifies 29 additional ulcerative colitis risk loci, increasing the number of confirmed associations to 47. Nat Genet 2011; 43(3): 246-52.
[PMID: 21297633]

[27]   Brand S. Crohn's disease: Th1, Th17 or both? The change of a paradigm: new immunological and genetic insights implicate Th17 cells in the pathogenesis of Crohn's disease. Gut 2009; 58(8): 1152-67.
[PMID: 19592695]

[28]   Liu JZ, van Sommeren S, Huang H, *et al.* Association analyses identify 38 susceptibility loci for inflammatory bowel disease and highlight shared genetic risk across populations. Nat Genet 2015; 47(9): 979-86.
[PMID: 26192919]

[29]   Loftus EV Jr. Clinical epidemiology of inflammatory bowel disease: Incidence, prevalence, and environmental influences. Gastroenterology 2004; 126(6): 1504-17.
[PMID: 15168363]

[30]   Maunder RG. Evidence that stress contributes to inflammatory bowel disease: evaluation, synthesis, and future directions. Inflamm Bowel Dis 2005; 11(6): 600-8.
[PMID: 15905709]

[31]   Mawdsley JE, Rampton DS. The role of psychological stress in inflammatory bowel disease. Neuroimmunomodulation 2006; 13(5-6): 327-36.
[PMID: 17709955]

[32]   Bitton A, Dobkin PL, Edwardes MD, *et al.* Predicting relapse in Crohn's disease: a biopsychosocial model. Gut 2008; 57(10): 1386-92.
[PMID: 18390994]

[33]   Cámara RJ, Schoepfer AM, Pittet V, Begré S, von Känel R. Mood and nonmood components of perceived stress and exacerbation of Crohn's disease. Inflamm Bowel Dis 2011; 17(11): 2358-65.
[PMID: 21287671]

[34]   Ananthakrishnan AN, Higuchi LM, Huang ES, *et al.* Aspirin, nonsteroidal anti-inflammatory drug use, and risk for Crohn disease and ulcerative colitis: a cohort study. Ann Intern Med 2012; 156(5): 350-9.
[PMID: 22393130]

[35]   Shaw SY, Blanchard JF, Bernstein CN. Association between the use of antibiotics in the first year of life and pediatric inflammatory bowel disease. Am J Gastroenterol 2010; 105(12): 2687-92.
[PMID: 20940708]

[36]   Hviid A, Svanström H, Frisch M. Antibiotic use and inflammatory bowel diseases in childhood. Gut 2011; 60(1): 49-54.
[PMID: 20966024]

[37]   Ng SC, Tang W, Leong RW, *et al.* Environmental risk factors in inflammatory bowel disease: a population-based case-control study in Asia-Pacific. Gut 2015; 64(7): 1063-71.
[PMID: 25217388]

[38]   Aksoyalp ZS, Temel A, Erdogan BR. Iron in infectious diseases friend or foe?: The role of gut microbiota. J Trace Elem Med Biol 2023; 75: 127093.
[PMID: 36240616]

[39]   Saleh M, Elson CO. Experimental inflammatory bowel disease: insights into the host-microbiota dialog. Immunity 2011; 34(3): 293-302.
[PMID: 21435584]

[40]   Nell S, Suerbaum S, Josenhans C. The impact of the microbiota on the pathogenesis of IBD: lessons from mouse infection models. Nat Rev Microbiol 2010; 8(8): 564-77.
[PMID: 20622892]

[41]   Nishida A, Inoue R, Inatomi O, Bamba S, Naito Y, Andoh A. Gut microbiota in the pathogenesis of inflammatory bowel disease. Clin J Gastroenterol 2018; 11(1): 1-10.
[PMID: 29285689]

[42]   Kamada N, Seo SU, Chen GY, Núñez G. Role of the gut microbiota in immunity and inflammatory disease. Nat Rev Immunol 2013; 13(5): 321-35.
[PMID: 23618829]

[43]   Devi TB, Devadas K, George M, *et al.* Low *Bifidobacterium* Abundance in the Lower Gut Microbiota Is Associated With *Helicobacter pylori*-Related Gastric Ulcer and Gastric Cancer. Front Microbiol 2021; 12: 631140.
[PMID: 33717022]

[44]   Socała K, Doboszewska U, Szopa A, *et al.* The role of microbiota-gut-brain axis in neuropsychiatric and neurological disorders. Pharmacol Res 2021; 172: 105840.
[PMID: 34450312]

[45]   Richard ML, Sokol H. The gut mycobiota: insights into analysis, environmental interactions and role

in gastrointestinal diseases. Nat Rev Gastroenterol Hepatol 2019; 16(6): 331-45.
[PMID: 30824884]

[46]   Ni J, Wu GD, Albenberg L, Tomov VT. Gut microbiota and IBD: causation or correlation? Nat Rev Gastroenterol Hepatol 2017; 14(10): 573-84.
[PMID: 28743984]

[47]   Melgar S, Shanahan F. Inflammatory bowel disease—from mechanisms to treatment strategies. Autoimmunity 2010; 43(7): 463-77.
[PMID: 20388058]

[48]   Medzhitov R, Janeway C Jr. Innate immunity. N Engl J Med 2000; 343(5): 338-44.
[PMID: 10922424]

[49]   Abreu MT, Fukata M, Arditi M. TLR signaling in the gut in health and disease. J Immunol 2005; 174(8): 4453-60.
[PMID: 15814663]

[50]   Marks DJ, Harbord MW, MacAllister R, *et al.* Defective acute inflammation in Crohn's disease: a clinical investigation. Lancet 2006; 367(9511): 668-78.
[PMID: 16503465]

[51]   Takatori H, Kanno Y, Watford WT, *et al.* Lymphoid tissue inducer-like cells are an innate source of IL-17 and IL-22. J Exp Med 2009; 206(1): 35-41.
[PMID: 19114665]

[52]   Bonen DK, Ogura Y, Nicolae DL, *et al.* Crohn's disease-associated NOD2 variants share a signaling defect in response to lipopolysaccharide and peptidoglycan. Gastroenterology 2003; 124(1): 140-6.
[PMID: 12512038]

[53]   Wehkamp J, Harder J, Weichenthal M, *et al.* NOD2 (CARD15) mutations in Crohn's disease are associated with diminished mucosal alpha-defensin expression. Gut 2004; 53(11): 1658-64.
[PMID: 15479689]

[54]   Watanabe T, Kitani A, Murray PJ, Strober W. NOD2 is a negative regulator of Toll-like receptor 2-mediated T helper type 1 responses. Nat Immunol 2004; 5(8): 800-8.
[PMID: 15220916]

[55]   Korn T, Bettelli E, Oukka M, Kuchroo VK. IL-17 and Th17 Cells. Annu Rev Immunol 2009; 27: 485-517.
[PMID: 19132915]

[56]   Breese E, Braegger CP, Corrigan CJ, Walker-Smith JA, MacDonald TT. Interleukin-2- and interferon-gamma-secreting T cells in normal and diseased human intestinal mucosa. Immunology 1993; 78(1): 127-31.
[PMID: 8436398]

[57]   Di Sabatino A, Biancheri P, Rovedatti L, MacDonald TT, Corazza GR. New pathogenic paradigms in inflammatory bowel disease. Inflamm Bowel Dis 2012; 18(2): 368-71.
[PMID: 21538717]

[58]   Rovedatti L, Kudo T, Biancheri P, *et al.* Differential regulation of interleukin 17 and interferon gamma production in inflammatory bowel disease. Gut 2009; 58(12): 1629-36.
[PMID: 19740775]

[59]   Wilson MS, Ramalingam TR, Rivollier A, *et al.* Colitis and intestinal inflammation in IL10-/- mice results from IL-13Rα2-mediated attenuation of IL-13 activity. Gastroenterology 2011; 140(1): 254-64.
[PMID: 20951137]

[60]   Hou JK, Abraham B, El-Serag H. Dietary intake and risk of developing inflammatory bowel disease: a systematic review of the literature. Am J Gastroenterol 2011; 106(4): 563-73.
[PMID: 21468064]

[61]   Sairenji T, Collins KL, Evans DV. An Update on Inflammatory Bowel Disease. Prim Care 2017; 44(4): 673-92.
[PMID: 29132528]

[62]   Grundmann O, Yoon SL. Complementary and alternative medicines in irritable bowel syndrome: an integrative view. World J Gastroenterol 2014; 20(2): 346-62.
[PMID: 24574705]

[63]   Hussain Z, Quigley EM. Systematic review: Complementary and alternative medicine in the irritable bowel syndrome. Aliment Pharmacol Ther 2006; 23(4): 465-71.
[PMID: 16441466]

[64]   Guo BJ, Bian ZX, Qiu HC, Wang YT, Wang Y. Biological and clinical implications of herbal medicine and natural products for the treatment of inflammatory bowel disease. Ann N Y Acad Sci 2017; 1401(1): 37-48.
[PMID: 28891095]

[65]   Akter J, Hossain MA, Takara K, Islam MZ, Hou DX. Antioxidant activity of different species and varieties of turmeric (Curcuma spp): Isolation of active compounds. Comp Biochem Physiol C Toxicol Pharmacol 2019; 215: 9-17.
[PMID: 30266519]

[66]   Ayati Z, Ramezani M, Amiri MS, *et al.* Ethnobotany, Phytochemistry and Traditional Uses of Curcuma spp. and Pharmacological Profile of Two Important Species (C. longa and C. zedoaria): A Review. Curr Pharm Des 2019; 25(8): 871-935.
[PMID: 30947655]

[67]   Holleran G, Scaldaferri F, Gasbarrini A, Currò D. Herbal medicinal products for inflammatory bowel disease: A focus on those assessed in double-blind randomised controlled trials. Phytother Res 2020; 34(1): 77-93.
[PMID: 31701598]

[68]   Pagano E, Romano B, Izzo AA, Borrelli F. The clinical efficacy of curcumin-containing nutraceuticals: An overview of systematic reviews. Pharmacol Res 2018; 134: 79-91.
[PMID: 29890252]

[69]   Ganji-Arjenaki M, Rafieian-Kopaei M. Phytotherapies in inflammatory bowel disease. J Res Med Sci 2019; 24: 42.
[PMID: 31160909]

[70]   Zhang M, Deng CS, Zheng JJ, Xia J. Curcumin regulated shift from Th1 to Th2 in trinitrobenzene sulphonic acid-induced chronic colitis. Acta Pharmacol Sin 2006; 27(8): 1071-7.
[PMID: 16867261]

[71]   Jiang H, Deng CS, Zhang M, Xia J. Curcumin-attenuated trinitrobenzene sulphonic acid induces chronic colitis by inhibiting expression of cyclooxygenase-2. World J Gastroenterol 2006; 12(24): 3848-53.
[PMID: 16804969]

[72]   Deguchi Y, Andoh A, Inatomi O, *et al.* Curcumin prevents the development of dextran sulfate Sodium (DSS)-induced experimental colitis. Dig Dis Sci 2007; 52(11): 2993-8.
[PMID: 17429738]

[73]   Camacho-Barquero L, Villegas I, Sánchez-Calvo JM, *et al.* Curcumin, a Curcuma longa constituent, acts on MAPK p38 pathway modulating COX-2 and iNOS expression in chronic experimental colitis. Int Immunopharmacol 2007; 7(3): 333-42.
[PMID: 17276891]

[74]   Lang A, Salomon N, Wu JC, *et al.* Curcumin in Combination With Mesalamine Induces Remission in Patients With Mild-to-Moderate Ulcerative Colitis in a Randomized Controlled Trial. Clin Gastroenterol Hepatol 2015; 13(8): 1444-9.e1.

[PMID: 25724700]

[75]   Sugimoto K, Hanai H, Tozawa K, *et al.* Curcumin prevents and ameliorates trinitrobenzene sulfonic acid-induced colitis in mice. Gastroenterology 2002; 123(6): 1912-22.
[PMID: 12454848]

[76]   Salh B, Assi K, Templeman V, *et al.* Curcumin attenuates DNB-induced murine colitis. Am J Physiol Gastrointest Liver Physiol 2003; 285(1): G235-43.
[PMID: 12637253]

[77]   Ukil A, Maity S, Karmakar S, Datta N, Vedasiromoni JR, Das PK. Curcumin, the major component of food flavour turmeric, reduces mucosal injury in trinitrobenzene sulphonic acid-induced colitis. Br J Pharmacol 2003; 139(2): 209-18.
[PMID: 12770926]

[78]   Larmonier CB, Uno JK, Lee KM, *et al.* Limited effects of dietary curcumin on Th-1 driven colitis in IL-10 deficient mice suggest an IL-10-dependent mechanism of protection. Am J Physiol Gastrointest Liver Physiol 2008; 295(5): G1079-91.
[PMID: 18818316]

[79]   Ung VY, Foshaug RR, MacFarlane SM, *et al.* Oral administration of curcumin emulsified in carboxymethyl cellulose has a potent anti-inflammatory effect in the IL-10 gene-deficient mouse model of IBD. Dig Dis Sci 2010; 55(5): 1272-7.
[PMID: 19513843]

[80]   Fan FY, Sang LX, Jiang M. Catechins and Their Therapeutic Benefits to Inflammatory Bowel Disease. Molecules 2017; 22(3): 484.
[PMID: 28335502]

[81]   Mochizuki M, Hasegawa N. (-)-Epigallocatechin-3-gallate reduces experimental colon injury in rats by regulating macrophage and mast cell. Phytother Res 2010; 24 (Suppl. 1): S120-2.
[PMID: 19548282]

[82]   Melgarejo E, Medina MA, Sánchez-Jiménez F, Urdiales JL. Targeting of histamine producing cells by EGCG: a green dart against inflammation? J Physiol Biochem 2010; 66(3): 265-70.
[PMID: 20652470]

[83]   Dryden GW, Lam A, Beatty K, Qazzaz HH, McClain CJ. A pilot study to evaluate the safety and efficacy of an oral dose of (-)-epigallocatechin-3-gallate-rich polyphenon E in patients with mild to moderate ulcerative colitis. Inflamm Bowel Dis 2013; 19(9): 1904-12.
[PMID: 23846486]

[84]   Rosillo MA, Sanchez-Hidalgo M, Cárdeno A, de la Lastra CA. Protective effect of ellagic acid, a natural polyphenolic compound, in a murine model of Crohn's disease. Biochem Pharmacol 2011; 82(7): 737-45.
[PMID: 21763290]

[85]   Stevens JF, Maier CS. The Chemistry of Gut Microbial Metabolism of Polyphenols. Phytochem Rev 2016; 15(3): 425-44.
[PMID: 27274718]

[86]   Biasi F, Astegiano M, Maina M, Leonarduzzi G, Poli G. Polyphenol supplementation as a complementary medicinal approach to treating inflammatory bowel disease. Curr Med Chem 2011; 18(31): 4851-65.
[PMID: 21919842]

[87]   Fraga CG, Oteiza PI. Dietary flavonoids: Role of (-)-epicatechin and related procyanidins in cell signaling. Free Radic Biol Med 2011; 51(4): 813-23.
[PMID: 21699974]

[88]   Fraga CG, Galleano M, Verstraeten SV, Oteiza PI. Basic biochemical mechanisms behind the health benefits of polyphenols. Mol Aspects Med 2010; 31(6): 435-45.

[PMID: 20854840]

[89]   Dryden GW, Song M, McClain C. Polyphenols and gastrointestinal diseases. Curr Opin Gastroenterol 2006; 22(2): 165-70.
[PMID: 16462174]

[90]   Najafzadeh M, Reynolds PD, Baumgartner A, Anderson D. Flavonoids inhibit the genotoxicity of hydrogen peroxide (H_2O_2) and of the food mutagen 2-amino-3-methylimadazo[4,5-f]-quinoline (IQ) in lymphocytes from patients with inflammatory bowel disease (IBD). Mutagenesis 2009; 24(5): 405-11.
[PMID: 19553277]

[91]   Pereira RB, Sousa C, Costa A, Andrade PB, Valentão P. Glutathione and the antioxidant potential of binary mixtures with flavonoids: synergisms and antagonisms. Molecules 2013; 18(8): 8858-72.
[PMID: 23892632]

[92]   Fathima A, Rao JR. Selective toxicity of Catechin-a natural flavonoid towards bacteria. Appl Microbiol Biotechnol 2016; 100(14): 6395-402.
[PMID: 27052380]

[93]   Yanofsky VR, Patel RV, Goldenberg G. Genital warts: a comprehensive review. J Clin Aesthet Dermatol 2012; 5(6): 25-36.
[PMID: 22768354]

[94]   Chiou YS, Ma NJ, Sang S, Ho CT, Wang YJ, Pan MH. Peracetylated (-)-epigallocatechin-3-gallate (AcEGCG) potently suppresses dextran sulfate sodium-induced colitis and colon tumorigenesis in mice. J Agric Food Chem 2012; 60(13): 3441-51.
[PMID: 22409325]

[95]   Brückner M, Westphal S, Domschke W, Kucharzik T, Lügering A. Green tea polyphenol epigallocatechin-3-gallate shows therapeutic antioxidative effects in a murine model of colitis. J Crohn's Colitis 2012; 6(2): 226-35.
[PMID: 22325177]

[96]   Abboud PA, Hake PW, Burroughs TJ, *et al.* Therapeutic effect of epigallocatechin-3-gallate in a mouse model of colitis. Eur J Pharmacol 2008; 579(1-3): 411-7.
[PMID: 18022615]

[97]   Kaulmann A, Bohn T. Bioactivity of Polyphenols: Preventive and Adjuvant Strategies toward Reducing Inflammatory Bowel Diseases-Promises, Perspectives, and Pitfalls. Oxid Med Cell Longev 2016; 2016: 9346470.
[PMID: 27478535]

[98]   Hold GL, Smith M, Grange C, Watt ER, El-Omar EM, Mukhopadhya I. Role of the gut microbiota in inflammatory bowel disease pathogenesis: what have we learnt in the past 10 years? World J Gastroenterol 2014; 20(5): 1192-210.
[PMID: 24574795]

[99]   Kawai K, Tsuno NH, Kitayama J, *et al.* Epigallocatechin gallate induces apoptosis of monocytes. J Allergy Clin Immunol 2005; 115(1): 186-91.
[PMID: 15637567]

[100]   Xue B, Xie J, Huang J, *et al.* Plant polyphenols alter a pathway of energy metabolism by inhibiting fecal Bacteroidetes and Firmicutes *in vitro*. Food Funct 2016; 7(3): 1501-7.
[PMID: 26882962]

[101]   Rastmanesh R. High polyphenol, low probiotic diet for weight loss because of intestinal microbiota interaction. Chem Biol Interact 2011; 189(1-2): 1-8.
[PMID: 20955691]

[102]   Dai Y, Chen SR, Chai L, Zhao J, Wang Y, Wang Y. Overview of pharmacological activities of Andrographis paniculata and its major compound andrographolide. Crit Rev Food Sci Nutr 2019; 59(1): S17-29.

[103] Chao WW, Lin BF. Isolation and identification of bioactive compounds in Andrographis paniculata (Chuanxinlian). Chin Med 2010; 5: 17.
[PMID: 20465823]

[104] Suebsasana S, Pongnaratorn P, Sattayasai J, Arkaravichien T, Tiamkao S, Aromdee C. Analgesic, antipyretic, anti-inflammatory and toxic effects of andrographolide derivatives in experimental animals. Arch Pharm Res 2009; 32(9): 1191-200.
[PMID: 19784573]

[105] Chao WW, Kuo YH, Lin BF. Isolation and Identification of *Andrographis paniculata* (*Chuanxinlian*) and Its Biologically Active Constituents Inhibited Enterovirus 71-Induced Cell Apoptosis. Front Pharmacol 2021; 12: 762285.
[PMID: 34955832]

[106] Gupta S, Mishra KP, Ganju L. Broad-spectrum antiviral properties of andrographolide. Arch Virol 2017; 162(3): 611-23.
[PMID: 27896563]

[107] Li ZZ, Tan JP, Wang LL, Li QH. Andrographolide Benefits Rheumatoid Arthritis *via* Inhibiting MAPK Pathways. Inflammation 2017; 40(5): 1599-605.
[PMID: 28584977]

[108] Liu Y, Liang RM, Ma QP, *et al.* Synthesis of thioether andrographolide derivatives and their inhibitory effect against cancer cells. MedChemComm 2017; 8(6): 1268-74.
[PMID: 30108837]

[109] Wen L, Xia N, Chen X, *et al.* Activity of antibacterial, antiviral, anti-inflammatory in compounds andrographolide salt. Eur J Pharmacol 2014; 740: 421-7.
[PMID: 24998876]

[110] Zhu T, Wang DX, Zhang W, *et al.* Andrographolide protects against LPS-induced acute lung injury by inactivation of NF-κB. PLoS One 2013; 8(2): e56407.
[PMID: 23437127]

[111] Tan WSD, Liao W, Zhou S, Wong WSF. Is there a future for andrographolide to be an anti-inflammatory drug? Deciphering its major mechanisms of action. Biochem Pharmacol 2017; 139: 71-81.
[PMID: 28377280]

[112] Michelsen KS, Wong MH, Ko B, Thomas LS, Dhall D, Targan SR. HMPL-004 (Andrographis paniculata extract) prevents development of murine colitis by inhibiting T-cell proliferation and TH1/TH17 responses. Inflamm Bowel Dis 2013; 19(1): 151-64.
[PMID: 23292349]

[113] Sandborn WJ, Targan SR, Byers VS, *et al.* Andrographis paniculata extract (HMPL-004) for active ulcerative colitis. Am J Gastroenterol 2013; 108(1): 90-8.
[PMID: 23044768]

[114] Tang T, Targan SR, Li ZS, Xu C, Byers VS, Sandborn WJ. Randomised clinical trial: herbal extract HMPL-004 in active ulcerative colitis - a double-blind comparison with sustained release mesalazine. Aliment Pharmacol Ther 2011; 33(2): 194-202.
[PMID: 21114791]

[115] Siddiqui MZ. Boswellia serrata, a potential antiinflammatory agent: an overview. Indian J Pharm Sci 2011; 73(3): 255-61.
[PMID: 22457547]

[116] Poeckel D, Werz O. Boswellic acids: biological actions and molecular targets. Curr Med Chem 2006; 13(28): 3359-69.
[PMID: 17168710]

[117] Sharma ML, Bani S, Singh GB. Anti-arthritic activity of boswellic acids in bovine serum albumin

(BSA)-induced arthritis. Int J Immunopharmacol 1989; 11(6): 647-52.
[PMID: 2807636]

[118] Abdel-Tawab M, Werz O, Schubert-Zsilavecz M. Boswellia serrata: an overall assessment of *in vitro*, preclinical, pharmacokinetic and clinical data. Clin Pharmacokinet 2011; 50(6): 349-69.
[PMID: 21553931]

[119] Ammon HP. Boswellic Acids and Their Role in Chronic Inflammatory Diseases. Adv Exp Med Biol 2016; 928: 291-327.
[PMID: 27671822]

[120] Krieglstein CF, Anthoni C, Rijcken EJ, *et al.* Acetyl-11-keto-beta-boswellic acid, a constituent of a herbal medicine from Boswellia serrata resin, attenuates experimental ileitis. Int J Colorectal Dis 2001; 16(2): 88-95.
[PMID: 11355324]

[121] Anthoni C, Laukoetter MG, Rijcken E, *et al.* Mechanisms underlying the anti-inflammatory actions of boswellic acid derivatives in experimental colitis. Am J Physiol Gastrointest Liver Physiol 2006; 290(6): G1131-7.
[PMID: 16423918]

[122] Gayathri B, Manjula N, Vinaykumar KS, Lakshmi BS, Balakrishnan A. Pure compound from Boswellia serrata extract exhibits anti-inflammatory property in human PBMCs and mouse macrophages through inhibition of TNFalpha, IL-1beta, NO and MAP kinases. Int Immunopharmacol 2007; 7(4): 473-82.
[PMID: 17321470]

[123] Hartmann RM, Fillmann HS, Martins MI, Meurer L, Marroni NP. Boswellia serrata has beneficial anti-inflammatory and anti-oxidant properties in a model of experimental colitis. Phytother Res 2014; 28(9): 1392-8.
[PMID: 24619538]

[124] Gerhardt H, Seifert F, Buvari P, Vogelsang H, Repges R. [Therapy of active Crohn disease with Boswellia serrata extract H 15]. Z Gastroenterol 2001; 39(1): 11-7. [Therapy of active Crohn disease with Boswellia serrata extract H 15].
[PMID: 11215357]

[125] Holtmeier W, Zeuzem S, Preiss J, *et al.* Randomized, placebo-controlled, double-blind trial of Boswellia serrata in maintaining remission of Crohn's disease: good safety profile but lack of efficacy. Inflamm Bowel Dis 2011; 17(2): 573-82.
[PMID: 20848527]

[126] Langmead L, Makins RJ, Rampton DS. Anti-inflammatory effects of aloe vera gel in human colorectal mucosa *in vitro*. Aliment Pharmacol Ther 2004; 19(5): 521-7.
[PMID: 14987320]

[127] Grindlay D, Reynolds T. The Aloe vera phenomenon: a review of the properties and modern uses of the leaf parenchyma gel. J Ethnopharmacol 1986; 16(2-3): 117-51.
[PMID: 3528673]

[128] Langmead L, Chitnis M, Rampton DS. Use of complementary therapies by patients with IBD may indicate psychosocial distress. Inflamm Bowel Dis 2002; 8(3): 174-9.
[PMID: 11979137]

[129] Korkina L, Suprun M, Petrova A, Mikhal'chik E, Luci A, De Luca C. The protective and healing effects of a natural antioxidant formulation based on ubiquinol and Aloe vera against dextran sulfate-induced ulcerative colitis in rats. Biofactors 2003; 18(1-4): 255-64.
[PMID: 14695941]

[130] Park MY, Kwon HJ, Sung MK. Dietary aloin, aloesin, or aloe-gel exerts anti-inflammatory activity in a rat colitis model. Life Sci 2011; 88(11-12): 486-92.
[PMID: 21277867]

[131]　Langmead L, Feakins RM, Goldthorpe S, *et al.* Randomized, double-blind, placebo-controlled trial of oral aloe vera gel for active ulcerative colitis. Aliment Pharmacol Ther 2004; 19(7): 739-47.
[PMID: 15043514]

CHAPTER 6

Multiple Sclerosis (MS) and its Treatment with Natural Products

Ceylan Dönmez[1,*], **Fatma Ayaz**[1] and **Nuraniye Eruygur**[1]

[1] Department of Pharmacognosy, Faculty of Pharmacy, Selçuk University, Konya, Türkiye

Abstract: Multiple sclerosis (MS) is an autoimmune disease that causes myelination defects and axonal impairment in the central nervous (CNS) system, causing inhibition of electrical transmission. The disease's typical symptoms include stiffness, persistent discomfort, exhaustion, motor and mobility problems, and cognitive deficits. Although immunosuppressive and immune-modulating medications have been the fundamental basis of MS treatment, there is currently no known treatment for the disease. Herbal-originated therapies are now being considered a possible therapeutic option for MS by using medicinal plant extracts or phytochemicals. Numerous research works have emphasized the medicinal herbs' anti-inflammatory and antioxidant properties, which make them a natural treatment for MS. According to the literature, several plants, such as hemp, turmeric, ginkgo, St. John's wort, black cumin, ginseng, and ginger have been reported to have various therapeutic effects in MS patients. Otherwise, the most promising substances that have been suggested to treat MS symptoms include curcumin, resveratrol, cannabinoids, apigenin, omega 3, and vitamin D. In this chapter, we compiled medicinal plants, and phytochemicals that have potential effects on MS. It is suggested that clinical trials were conducted on MS patients with medicinal plants, which were prominent *in vivo* findings. We also advise further research in this field to identify the precise active ingredients present in these extracts for the best composition necessary for the intended therapeutic effect.

Keywords: Herbal remedy, Multiple sclerosis (MS), Natural product, Neurodegenerative diseases.

INTRODUCTION

Multiple sclerosis (MS) is a central nervous system (CNS) problem related to autoreactive T cells and inflammation. It is characterized by the immune system mistakenly attacking the protective covering of nerve fibers called myelin. This leads to inflammation, demyelination (loss of myelin), and disruption of nerve signals [1].

---

* **Corresponding author Ceylan Dönmez:** Department of Pharmacognosy, Faculty of Pharmacy, Selçuk University, Konya, Türkiye; E-mail: ceylan.donmez@sulcuk.edu.tr

Cennet Ozay & Gokhan Zengin (Eds.)
All rights reserved-© 2024 Bentham Science Publishers

The symptoms of MS can vary widely and may include fatigue, muscle weakness, coordination and balance problems, numbness or tingling, cognitive impairment, and visual disturbances. The course of the disease can also vary, with some individuals experiencing relapses and remissions (RMS). In contrast, others may have a progressive decline in function without remission (primary progressive MS-PPMS) [2].

The exact reason for MS is not fully understood, but it is believed to involve a combination of genetic and environmental factors. There is currently no cure for MS, but various treatment options are available to manage symptoms, slow down disease progression, and improve the quality of life. These may include disease-modifying therapies, symptom management medications, physical and occupational therapy, and lifestyle modifications. Ongoing research in the field of MS aims to better understand the underlying mechanisms of the disease, identify new therapeutic targets, and develop more effective treatments. Advances in imaging techniques, such as magnetic resonance imaging (MRI), have provided valuable insights into the progression and pathology of MS. Moreover, patient advocacy groups and organizations play a crucial role in raising awareness, providing support, and advocating for better access to care and research funding for individuals with MS. Individuals with MS need to work closely with healthcare professionals to develop a personalized treatment plan and to actively manage their condition through regular monitoring, lifestyle modifications, and adherence to prescribed medications [3].

Natural products, especially medicinal plants, are the new leading therapeutic targets. Studies conducted to date have revealed that herbs play a complementary role in the treatment of MS disease by relieving symptoms or preventing the progression of the disease. Recently, in newly published articles, it has been seen that drug discovery studies based on phytochemical compounds responsible for the effect and different formulations and different techniques have gained importance [4].

Pathophysiology of MS

The pathophysiology of MS involves a complex interplay of immune system dysfunction, inflammation, demyelination, and neurodegeneration [5]. While the exact cause of MS remains unknown, several key mechanisms contribute to the development and progression of the disease.

Autoimmune Response

MS is considered an autoimmune disease, meaning the immune system mistakenly attacks the body's tissues. In MS, immune cells, particularly T cells, become activated and cross the blood-brain barrier into the CNS. This immune system malfunction leads to chronic inflammation within the CNS [6].

Inflammation and Blood-Brain Barrier Dysfunction

Inflammatory immune cells, such as T cells and macrophages, release cytokines and other pro-inflammatory molecules within the CNS. This inflammatory response causes damage to the blood-brain barrier, which normally protects the brain and spinal cord from harmful substances. The compromised blood-brain barrier allows immune cells to infiltrate the CNS, leading to further inflammation and tissue damage [7].

Demyelination

Myelin, the protective covering around nerve fibers, is a primary target in MS. Inflammatory processes in the CNS cause immune cells to attack and damage the myelin sheath. Demyelination disrupts the conduction of nerve impulses, resulting in impaired nerve signaling and the characteristic symptoms of MS [8].

Reactive Gliosis and Neurodegeneration

In response to demyelination and inflammation, supportive cells in the CNS called glial cells [astrocytes and microglia] become activated. This activation, known as reactive gliosis, leads to the release of inflammatory molecules and contributes to further damage to myelin and nerve fibers. Over time, neurodegeneration can occur, leading to an irreversible loss of neuronal tissue [9].

Remyelination and Repair

In some cases, the CNS can initiate a process called remyelination, in which oligodendrocytes [cells responsible for myelin production] attempt to repair damaged myelin. However, the effectiveness of remyelination can vary among individuals and may become less efficient as the disease progresses [10].

The interplay between immune dysregulation, inflammation, demyelination, and neurodegeneration results in the clinical manifestations and progression of MS. The heterogeneity of MS, with various disease courses and clinical phenotypes, further reflects the complex pathophysiology of the condition.

Understanding these underlying mechanisms is crucial for developing targeted therapies that modulate the immune response, reduce inflammation, promote remyelination, and protect against neurodegeneration. Ongoing research aims to unravel the precise factors that trigger MS and develop more effective treatments to halt or slow down disease progression.

Diagnosis of MS

In recent years, a newer classification system known as the McDonald criteria has been widely used for the diagnosis of MS. The McDonald criteria consider a combination of clinical presentation, magnetic resonance imaging (MRI) findings, and cerebrospinal fluid analysis to support the diagnosis and classification of MS [11].

Classifying MS helps healthcare professionals understand disease patterns, determine treatment approaches, and monitor disease progression. However, it is important to consult with a healthcare professional who specializes in MS for an accurate diagnosis and appropriate management of the disease.

Classification of MS

In 1996, the International Advisory Committee on Clinical Trials of MS originally identified four disease courses of MS based on the clinical course and characteristics of the disease (Fig. **1**). The most recognized classifications include [12]:

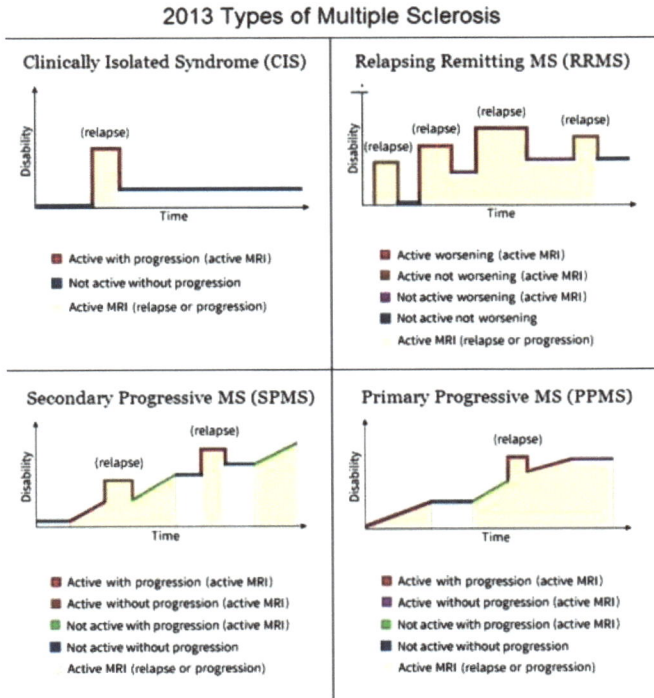

Fig. (1). New types of multiple sclerosis after 2013 [12].

- Relapsing-Remitting Multiple Sclerosis (RRMS): It is the most common form of MS, characterized by clearly defined relapses or flare-ups of symptoms followed by periods of partial or complete recovery (remission). In between relapses, there may be no disease progression or accumulation of disability.
- Primary Progressive Multiple Sclerosis (PPMS): This is characterized by a gradual and steady progression of symptoms from the onset, without distinct relapses or remissions. Individuals with PPMS experience a continuous accumulation of disability over time, which may vary in rate and severity.
- Secondary Progressive Multiple Sclerosis (SPMS): This form of MS typically follows an initial relapsing-remitting course. Over time, individuals with SPMS experience a gradual worsening of symptoms and disability, with or without superimposed relapses and remissions. In this stage, there may be a progression of disability even without relapses.
- Progressive-Relapsing Multiple Sclerosis (PRMS): PRMS is a relatively rare form of MS in which there is a steady progression of symptoms from the onset, with occasional superimposed relapses. Unlike RRMS, there is no remission between relapses, and disability continues to accumulate over time.

Although these four types matched the clinical types based on data and consensus at the time, imaging and biological correlations were found to be lacking over time. With the increase in data on MS and its pathology and the emergence of newer definitions, it has become necessary to reconsider the disease from a clinical point of view. The changes that were accepted in 2013 by the committee retained three of the disease course identifications first formed in 1996. They included the addition of clinically isolated syndrome (CIS) and eliminated progressive-relapsing MS (PRMS). Besides, modifiers have been added to promote more effective preservation of illness activity and progression and shared decision-making about therapy options [12].

It is important to note that these classifications serve as general descriptions and that MS can present with considerable variability from person to person. Additionally, other less common or atypical forms of MS may exhibit unique clinical features.

Prevalence of MS

The prevalence of MS varies geographically, with higher rates reported in certain regions. It is considered a relatively common neurological disease, particularly in temperate climates. Here are some estimates of MS prevalence:

Global Prevalence: The global prevalence of MS is estimated to be around 33 cases /100,000 people. However, prevalence rates can vary significantly between countries and regions [13].

North America and Europe: MS is more prevalent in North America and Europe compared to other parts of the world. In these regions, prevalence rates range from approximately 80 to 180 cases per 100,000 people. Some northern European countries, such as Norway and Sweden, have even higher prevalence rates, exceeding 200 cases per 100,000 people [14].

Asia, Africa, and South America: MS prevalence is generally lower in Asian, African, and South American countries compared to Europe and North America. Prevalence rates in these regions typically range from approximately 1 to 10 cases per 100,000 people. However, it is worth noting that prevalence rates may vary within specific populations and regions [15].

Gender and Ethnicity: MS is more commonly diagnosed in women than men, with a male-to-female ratio of approximately 1:2 [16]. It predominantly affects individuals of European descent, but the disease is also found in other ethnic groups [17].

It is important to keep in mind that these figures are approximate and can vary based on the methodology and data sources used in different studies. Additionally, the prevalence of MS may change over time due to factors such as improved diagnostic techniques, changes in disease awareness, and environmental influences. MS is a chronic condition that can have a significant impact on the quality of life of affected individuals. Understanding the prevalence of MS is crucial for healthcare planning, resource allocation, and raising awareness about the disease.

Research on MS

In MS research, various methods are employed to study the disease and evaluate potential treatments. These methods include *in vitro* [cell-based], *in vivo* [animal-based], and clinical approaches. One commonly used animal model for MS research is experimental autoimmune encephalomyelitis. Here is an overview of these research methods:

In Vitro Methods

Cell Cultures

Immune cells, such as T cells and macrophages, can be isolated from MS patients or animal models and cultured in the laboratory. These cultures can be used to investigate immune responses, cellular interactions, and the effects of potential therapies. Using single cells or mixed cell cultures, the complexity of the CNS, interactions of CNS cells with each other, and immune-neurological interactions may be simplified [18].

Cell-Based Assays

Researchers use various assays to examine cellular and molecular processes related to MS. Examples include measuring cytokine production, immune cell activation, cell migration, and myelin protein expression in response to different stimuli [18].

In Vivo Methods

Experimental Autoimmune Encephalomyelitis (EAE)

EAE is an animal model that mimics some aspects of MS. It involves inducing an autoimmune response against myelin components, typically by injecting myelin proteins or peptides combined with an adjuvant. EAE allows researchers to study the immune mechanisms, pathogenesis, and potential therapeutic interventions in a controlled experimental setting [19].

Transgenic Mice

Genetically modified mice can be used to study specific aspects of MS, such as the role of certain genes or immune cell populations in disease development or progression. These mice may express human genes or lack specific genes to mimic particular aspects of MS [20].

Clinical Methods

Observational Studies

Researchers conduct observational studies on individuals with MS to understand disease progression, risk factors, and potential associations between various factors and outcomes. These studies often involve collecting clinical data, conducting surveys, and analyzing medical records to identify patterns and correlations [21].

Clinical Trials

Clinical trials evaluate the safety and effectiveness of potential treatments for MS. These trials involve administering experimental therapies to human participants and monitoring their outcomes. They are typically performed in multiple phases, starting with small-scale studies to assess safety and dosage, followed by larger trials to evaluate efficacy and side effects [22].

It is important to note that while *in vitro* and *in vivo* methods provide valuable insights into MS pathophysiology and potential treatments, findings from animal models do not always directly translate to humans. Clinical studies, including randomized controlled trials, provide the most relevant and reliable evidence for the efficacy and safety of interventions in MS. The combination of *in vitro*, *in vivo*, and clinical methods allows researchers to gain a comprehensive understanding of MS, explore potential mechanisms, identify therapeutic targets, and develop new treatments [23].

Treatment of MS

Conventional Therapy

There is no cure for MS. Therapy typically focuses on speeding recovery from attacks, decreasing new radiographic and clinical relapses, decelerating the advance of the disease, and managing MS symptoms. Some people have such mild symptoms that no treatment is necessary [24]. The treatment of MS aims to manage symptoms, slow down disease progression, and improve the quality of life for individuals living with the condition. The approach to treatment may vary depending on the type and stage of MS, as well as the specific needs of each patient. Here are some common treatment options:

Conventional medicine plays a central role in the management of MS. The primary goals of conventional treatment for MS are to reduce relapse frequency, slow disease progression, manage symptoms, and improve the quality of life. Here are some commonly used conventional treatment approaches for MS:

Disease-Modifying Therapies (DMTs)

DMTs are a key component of MS treatment. These medications can help reduce the frequency and severity of relapses, slow down disease progression, and decrease the accumulation of new lesions in the central nervous system [25]. DMTs include various options such as injectable drugs [interferons, glatiramer acetate], oral medications (fingolimod, dimethyl fumarate) [26], and infused therapies (natalizumab, ocrelizumab) [27].

Symptom Management

MS symptoms can vary widely and may include fatigue, muscle weakness, spasticity, pain, bladder and bowel dysfunction, cognitive impairment, and depression. Symptom management strategies involve the use of medications, physical therapy, occupational therapy, speech therapy, and assistive devices to address specific symptoms and improve daily functioning [28].

Relapse Treatment

Relapses in multiple sclerosis (MS) are disruptive and usually devastating for patients, and therapy is frequently difficult. Despite advances in understanding the pathogenesis of MS and the development of novel medicines for the long-term management of MS, therapy choices for relapses have not altered significantly over the last several decades. During relapses or exacerbations of MS symptoms, corticosteroids such as intravenous methylprednisolone are often prescribed to reduce inflammation and shorten the duration of the relapse. These treatments help individuals recover from acute symptoms and return to their baseline functioning [29].

Rehabilitation Therapies

Rehabilitation plays an important role in MS management. Physical therapy, occupational therapy, and speech therapy can help individuals improve mobility, strengthen muscles, manage fatigue, enhance coordination, and address difficulties with activities of daily living. Rehabilitation programs may also include assistive devices, such as mobility aids or adaptive equipment, to maximize independence and quality of life [30].

Supportive Care

Comprehensive care for individuals with MS involves a multidisciplinary approach. This may include regular monitoring of disease progression, psychological support, counseling, and lifestyle modifications such as maintaining a healthy diet, smoking cessation, regular exercise, and stress management. Support groups and patient advocacy organizations can provide valuable resources, education, and emotional support for individuals with MS and their families [31].

Individuals with MS must work closely with a healthcare team, including neurologists, specialized MS nurses, and other healthcare professionals, to develop an individualized treatment plan based on their specific needs and disease course. Regular monitoring, adherence to prescribed treatments, and open communication with the healthcare team are key factors in effectively managing MS.

Natural Remedies

While conventional medicine is the primary approach for managing MS, some individuals may be interested in exploring complementary and alternative therapies, including natural remedies and herbal treatments [32]. It is important to note that the effectiveness and safety of these interventions for MS have not been extensively studied, and their use should always be discussed with a healthcare professional. Natural products have been extensively studied for their potential therapeutic benefits in the management of MS. While they should not be considered as a replacement for conventional medical treatments, some natural products have shown promise in alleviating symptoms and modulating the immune response in MS. It is important to note that further research is needed to establish their efficacy and safety.

MS is a central nervous system problem related to autoreactive T cells and chronic inflammatory and demyelinating disorders of the central nervous system. In the treatment of MS, which may cause instability, and sensorial and cognition degradations, natural remedies, especially plants, are often used symptomatically. Many medicinal plants with anti-inflammatory, antioxidant, and immuno-modulatory effects are used for this purpose [33]. Certain herbs possess anti-inflammatory properties that may help reduce inflammation associated with MS. Hemp, turmeric, ginkgo, St. John's wort, black cumin, ginseng, ginger, olive, grape, green tea, milk thistle, boswellia, and rue are the most known plant examples used in the treatment of MS [33]. These herbs can be consumed as part of a balanced diet or taken as supplements, but their use should be discussed with a healthcare professional to ensure safety and proper dosage. Antioxidant-rich foods, such as colorful fruits, and vegetables, can help combat oxidative stress in the body. This oxidative stress is thought to contribute to MS progression. Including a variety of antioxidant-rich foods in the diet can provide overall health benefits and support the body's natural defense mechanisms [34]. Stress reduction techniques are also thought to have an important place in the treatment of MS. Stress can exacerbate MS symptoms, so incorporating stress reduction techniques is essential [35]. Natural products such as chamomile tea, lavender oil, and adaptogenic herbs like ashwagandha and rhodiola may help promote relaxation and reduce stress levels [36]. However, it is important to consult with a healthcare professional before using herbal supplements.

Some studies have shown that oils, vitamins, and minerals are also effective in the treatment of MS. Omega-3 fatty acids, found in fatty fish [such as salmon and mackerel], flaxseed, and chia seeds, have anti-inflammatory properties. Some studies suggest that omega-3 supplementation may help reduce inflammation and potentially improve symptoms in MS. They have been studied for their potential to improve symptoms and slow disease progression. However, more research is needed to establish their efficacy [37, 38]. Low levels of vitamin D have been associated with an increased risk of developing MS and may contribute to disease progression. Ensuring adequate vitamin D levels through safe sun exposure, fortified foods, or dietary sources like fatty fish and fortified dairy products may have a beneficial impact on the immune system and disease activity in MS. However, the optimal dosage and long-term effects are still being investigated [39].

It is essential to approach natural remedies and herbal treatments for MS with caution. Some of these remedies may interact with medications or have side effects. It is always recommended to consult with a healthcare professional before starting any new treatments or supplements, especially if you are already on prescribed medications as they can interact with medications or have potential side effects. Additionally, natural products should be used in conjunction with conventional medical treatments under proper supervision. While natural remedies and herbal treatments may provide some symptom relief, they are not a substitute for conventional MS management strategies. It is crucial to continue working closely with your healthcare team to ensure comprehensive care and effective disease management.

Medicinal Plants used in MS Treatment

Plants have been used for the treatment of many diseases besides their nutritional benefits on human health for many years. Based on traditional use, many natural-origin drug discoveries have been and continue to be made. The effects of such valuable plants against many diseases are being studied on the scientific platform. In recent years, many new methods have been used, and applications for the treatment of diseases with natural substances of which relatively little work has been done and emphasized. One of these diseases is MS. MS, which appears between twenty-forty years of age, is an autoimmune disease affecting the central nervous system. Scientific studies have focused on the healing role of herbs in MS symptoms such as involuntary changes in muscle ton (spasticity), pain, tremors, ataxia, bladder dysfunction, sleep problems, and disability [40]. Though studies show that the therapeutic effects of many medicinal plants on MS, both *in vivo* and clinical human research are limited, information on seven plants on which extensive studies have been carried out is given in detail below:

Cannabis sativa L.

Cannabis sativa L. (Hemp) belongs to the Cannabaceae family and is grown in Asia and Europe besides being native to Central and Western Asia [41]. Hemp has been used traditionally for over 5000 years. Seeds of hemp, which are used for feeding animals and the production of industrial material, have anti-inflammatory, anti-lipogenic, neuroprotective, analgesic, and anti-microbial effects [42, 43]. Hemp is one of the most studied plants related to MS, with both its seeds, oil, and phytochemical compounds. About one hundred different cannabinoids have been isolated from *C. sativa* [44]. 9-tetrahydrocannabinol

(THC) and cannabidiol are major cannabinoid derivatives thought to be responsible for the neuroprotective effect. The most important reason for this is the presence of cannabinoid receptors known as CB1 and CB2. These receptors are present in the central and peripheral nervous and immune systems and are linked to adenylyl cyclase (-) and mitogen-activated protein kinase (+) by the Gi/o protein [45 - 47]. The effect of the ethanolic extract of *C. sativa*, which was standardized on cannabidiol (range 0.8-1.8 mg) and 2.5 mg Λ9-tetrahydrocannabinol, on parameters such as body pain, spasms, sleep quality, spasticity, and physical and psychological condition, in MS patients was evaluated in a placebo-controlled clinical study. According to the results of the evaluations made with an interval of four weeks, it was revealed that the recovery rate in the muscles of the extract group was two times higher than the placebo group [48]. In the treatment of neuropathic pain associated with multiple sclerosis, preclinical and clinical studies have been conducted and are being carried out with many extract formulations standardized on tetrahydrocannabinol and cannabidiol phytochemicals [49]. Considering many studies, possible mechanisms by which hemp may be effective in the treatment of MS include rising 5' adenosine monophosphate-activated protein kinase (AMPK) expression, suppressing the nuclear factor- kappa B (NF-κB), anti-oxidant and anti-neuroinflammatory effects, blocking pain pathways and improvement in the expanded disability status scale (EDSS) [50 - 52]. Cannabis-based products (CBD) may help alleviate pain, spasticity, and sleep disturbances. However, the use of cannabis-based products for MS should be discussed with a healthcare professional due to potential side effects and legal considerations. CBD-based medications have been approved for the treatment of spasticity in MS in some countries [53].

Curcuma longa L.

Curcuma longa L. (turmeric) belongs to the Zingiberaceae family and is known as turmeric, Indian saffron. The dried rhizome of turmeric has been used for the treatment of skin problems, colic, chest pains, and fractures for thousands of years in traditional Indian and Chinese medicine [54]. Scientific studies have also shown that turmeric has significant activities against cancer, inflammation, growth retardation, arthritis, atherosclerosis, depression, diabetes, skin illnesses, and memorial impairment [55]. Many activity studies have been carried out on MS disease, which is related to inflammation and memorial defect, of both turmeric and its effective compound curcumin (isolated from nonpolar turmeric rhizome extract) [56]. The most likely mechanism of action of the turmeric extract/curcumin is thought to be due to the inhibition of pro-inflammatory cytokine release. Experimental studies focus on curcumin rather than the extract. *In vitro* and *in vivo* studies have shown that curcumin inhibits Th17-induced blood-brain barrier disruption, and the severity of experimental autoimmune encephalomyelitis caused by inflammation is reduced or even improved [57]. In a placebo-controlled clinical study examining the effect of curcumin, the main component of turmeric, on MS, FoxP3, IL-10 mRNA, TGF-b, and Treg cells increased while EDSS decreased in blood peripheral mononuclear cells in patients [58]. According to the results of the studies, it is an undeniable fact that both turmeric and curcumin are beneficial in the treatment of neurological illnesses.

Ginkgo biloba L.

Ginkgo biloba L. (ginkgo) belongs to the Ginkgoaceae family. Its extracts have neuroprotective effects against Alzheimer's disease (AD), anxiety, and ischemia thanks to its antioxidant and anti-inflammatory properties [59]. Ginkgolide K, which is a diterpene lactone compound extracted from the leaves and roots of ginkgo, improved demyelination and behavioral dysfunction in the cuprizone-induced MS animal model. The nuclear factor Nrf2, which has been approved for clinical treatment of MS, ameliorates endogenous cellular antioxidant response by ginkgolide K [60]. In a double-blind and placebo-controlled pilot trial, the ginkgo special extract (EGb 761) treated group's parameters such as depression-anxiety, fatigue symptom severity, and functional performance were improved compared with the placebo group [61]. In another study, in which the same extract was applied twice a day, it was revealed that there was an increase in cognitive performance. It has been suggested to potentially improve cognitive function in individuals with MS, although scientific evidence is limited [62].

Hypericum perforatum L.

Hypericum perforatum L. (St John's wort) belongs to the Hypericaceae family and has been traditionally used for healing neurological diseases [63]. St John's wort extract has anti-inflammatory, antiapoptotic, and antioxidant activities and contains hyperforin, phloroglucinols, naphthodiathrones, hypericin, pseudo-hypericin, flavonoids, and other phenolic compounds [64]. According to the clinical study's results, dried ethanolic St John's wort extract showed modulation of oxidative stress, apoptosis, and calcium entry in leukocytes of nine newly diagnosed MS patients [65]. The *in vivo* study showed that clinical and pathological complications decreased in the experimental autoimmune encephalomyelitis-induced animal group administered with the nanoparticle formulation of hydro-alcoholic St John's wort extract [66]. *In vivo,* another study demonstrated that St John's wort oil improved the brain tissue myelin oligodendrocyte glycoprotein and myelin basic protein levels in animals with MS [67]. In a clinical study comparing the anti-inflammatory and proliferative effects of callus with field-growing plant extracts of St John's wort on mesenchymal stem cells-derived adipose tissue (AT-MSC) derived from MS patients; both extracts demonstrated effectiveness on AT-MSC proliferation and immunomodulatory properties at high concentrations [68, 69].

Nigella sativa L.

Nigella sativa L. (black cumin) belongs to the Ranunculaceae family and its seed oil is often used for medicinal purposes such as liver tonics for digestion, as an appetite stimulant, anti-diarrheal analgesics, for healing skin disorders, as diuretics and as an antihypertensive drug in Unani, Ayurveda, and Siddha system of medicine. It is a plant that has been studied in terms of many of its activities on the scientific platform [70]. It was thought that the preventive and therapeutic effect mechanisms of black cumin were as follows: suppressing inflammation, enhancing remyelination, and reducing the expression of transforming growth factor $\beta1$ by *in vivo* study on MS disorder. It has been demonstrated that thymoquinone in black cumin oil can be effective on MS; thanks to its antioxidant effect and upregulation of the Nrf2/HO-1 pathway [43]. In an *in silico* study examining the effects of black cumin seed, chemical compounds on MS, based on black cumin oil, which has an anti-inflammatory effect, phytochemicals of black cumin seed showed promising results as the therapeutic substance against target MS genes (such as FAU, RPL27, RPS14) for treatment of MS [71].

Panax ginseng L.

Panax ginseng L. (Korean red ginseng) belongs to the Araliaceae family and is widely used for healing fatigue as a tonic, and aging signs in traditional Chinese medicine [72]. A randomized, placebo-controlled, double-blind pilot study showed that the fatigue of the 3-month ginseng administrated group decreased and the group's quality of life improved [73]. Korean ginseng is probably a good candidate for the relief of MS-related fatigue. While the curative effect of Korean ginseng against MS-induced fatigue is quite high, it was revealed in a clinical study that the patients treated with American ginseng did not show any significant difference from the placebo control group [74]. In an *in vivo* study in adult male mice to determine the effective mechanism of ginseng in the treatment of MS, downregulation of proinflammatory mediators, and amelioration of demyelination and oligodendrocyte degeneration were observed. The possible mechanism was thought to be inhibition of immune cell activation and infiltration [75]. Considering the mechanism of action of Korean ginseng on inflammation, studies have shown that Korean ginseng has a high potential in the treatment of neurological problems related to COVID-19 [76]. In another clinical study, in which the meta-analysis method was applied, in which the effect of Korean ginseng herbal formulas on chronic fatigue was investigated, it was concluded that there was a significant improvement compared to the control group, although it was not big size [77].

Zingiber officinalis Roscoe

Zingiber officinalis Roscoe (ginger) belongs to the Zingiberaceae family and is widely used as a spice and medicine for the treatment of numerous diseases including vomiting, pain, and inflammation [78]. Especially the rhizomes of this plant, which is native to Southeastern Asia, continue to gain increasing importance in traditional treatment. Scientific studies showed that gingerols, shogaols, and phenolic ketone derivatives are important phytochemical compounds responsible for many biological activities [79 - 81]. A study examining a hydro-alcoholic ginger extract by constructing an animal [female mice] model of MS for 21 days found that interleukin-17 and interferon-γ were reduced and symptom strength relieved in the extract-treated group [82]. In the double-blind randomized controlled clinical trial, the effect of ginger supplementation on patients with MS was examined based on the following parameters body mass index, neurofilament light chain (NfL), interleukin-17, neutrophil/lymphocyte ratio, and matrix metalloproteinase-9. With respect to life quality such as any disability, it was revealed that there was a significant decrease in EDSS and the Multiple Sclerosis Impact Scale (MSIS) [83]. It is thought that inflammatory, oxidative, and immunopathological parameters are associated with Multiple sclerosis, which is featured by demyelination of nerve cells and degeneration of the nervous system. Ginger and its bioactive compounds could be taken into consideration as potential agents to treat MS due to their anti-inflammatory, antioxidant, and immunomodulatory properties. Ginger is on the Food and Drug Administration (FDA) list of herbs that are generally considered safe and can be used up to 4 mg per day [84].

Natural Compounds used in MS Treatment

Curcumin

A naturally occurring compound in the rhizome of turmeric, polyphenolic phytochemical called curcumin is known as an analgesic, wound healing, and anti-inflammatory agent. Curcumin has recently been found to be effective in treating autoimmune disorders such as rheumatoid arthritis, multiple sclerosis, psoriasis, and inflammatory bowel disease, according to studies conducted on both humans and lab animals. The preventive effects of curcumin in various disorders appear to result from the regulation of inflammatory cytokines and related signaling pathways in the immune systems [85].

Curcumin, dimethoxy curcumin, and bis dimethoxy curcumin are polyphenols from turmeric that, as antioxidants, save the brain against a variety of oxidative stresses. They also have neuroprotective and anti-aging properties by scavenging down superoxide anions [86]. Numerous genes that are connected to the induction of inflammatory, acute, and immunological responses are controlled at the rate of nuclear factor-kB (NF-kB) expression. Curcumin suppresses the stimulation of the NF-kB, which results in the down-regulation of particular inflammatory genes and has attractive therapeutic potential for MS [87]. The effects of curcumin on mitochondrial damage and apoptosis in the experimental autoimmune encephalomyelitis model were assessed. The numbers of TUNEL (+) cells were dramatically decreased by curcumin in both the acute and chronic stages. In addition, curcumin dramatically reduced the expression of caspase-3, cleaved caspase-9, and cytochrome complex while considerably increasing the expression of myelin basic protein [88].

Curcumin can be a great choice for use in the management of MS and other neurological illnesses, due to its capacity to enhance myelinogenesis, reduce astrocyte growth, and boost oligodendrocyte activity and differentiation [89]. Curcumin prevented lysine acetyltransferase enzyme function. By inhibiting the invasion of inflammatory cells into the nervous system, curcumin reduced the intensity of experimental autoimmune encephalomyelitis, the animal model of MS, in rats. Curcumin therapy also suppressed the expression of interleukins, transcription factors, and growth factors in animal models, which suggested that curcumin inhibits the differentiation of CD4+ helper T cells into T helper 17 cells, a key role in MS [90 - 92]. Studies demonstrate that curcumin can reduce the secretion of metalloproteinase-9, which is involved in the enhancement of blood-brain barrier permeability, in lipo-polysaccharide-induced human astrocyte cells [93]. Curcumin can prevent axon degeneration, a final destructive stage in the pathogenesis of MS, in the primary microglia of rats or mice [86].

A polymerized form of nano-curcumin was utilized in an investigation to treat the experimental autoimmune encephalomyelitis model of MS, which exhibited antioxidant and anti-inflammatory capabilities as well as a rise in remyelination and a decline in model score. However, more research is needed to establish its effectiveness and optimal dosage [94]. According to another study, curcumin supplementation may reduce inflammation and potentially alleviate symptoms through neuroprotective effects and by modulating immune responses in MS [95]. High doses of curcumin can have negative side effects, including nausea and diarrhea. Although curcumin has been shown to have therapeutic effects in several investigations, randomized controlled clinical trials are undoubtedly required to support the use of curcumin in MS patients [32, 56]. Curcumin, the active compound in turmeric, has anti-inflammatory and antioxidant properties.

Resveratrol

A phenolic molecule called resveratrol (trans-3, 4, 5-trihydroxystilbene) is formed in grapes because of fungal pathogenic damage. According to the reports, resveratrol has many therapeutic deeds, including neuroprotective, anti-inflammatory, anti-cancer, antioxidant, and antiviral characteristics [32]. Resveratrol demonstrated important neuroprotective benefits by blocking the stimulation of primary immune cells of the central nervous system and reducing the generation of inflammatory mediators [96, 97]. The blood-brain barrier is permeable to resveratrol, making it an optimal alternative for the treatment of neuroinflammatory and neurodegenerative disorders [32]. In experimental autoimmune encephalomyelitis models of MS in mice, oral treatment of resveratrol activated Sirt1 (deacetylase enzyme), resulting in low neurological degeneration [97]. Regular grape consumption within overeating results in intestinal discomfort and unpleasant symptoms, such as nausea, pain in the abdomen, flatulence, and diarrhea. Although grape was discovered to possess neuroprotective properties in a variety of neurodegenerative disorders, further research on their therapeutic potential for MS is required [32].

Epigallocatechin gallate

Numerous different plants with anti-inflammatory and antioxidant characteristics could treat MS, lowering the severity of the disease and its neuropathological alterations. The primary chemical constituents of green tea are phenolic compounds, including epigallo-catechin-3-gallate (EGCG), epicatechin-3-gallate, epigallocatechin, and epicatechin, which have antioxidant and anti-inflammatory properties [86].

One of the most significant active constituents of green tea, EGCG, is responsible for the anti-inflammatory and neuroprotective features of the plant by reducing the formation of inflammatory mediators, and stimulation of the microglia associated with lipopolysaccharide, as well as defending against damage to dopaminergic neurons. Green tea can be consumed routinely and without harm, but excessive quantities can be harmful to the liver [32, 98]. Because of the anti-inflammatory properties, it can defend the central nervous system from one of the neurodegenerative conditions, MS. By lowering inflammatory infiltration, proliferation, and differentiation of auto-reactive T cells in the central nervous system, EGCG treatment to experimental autoimmune encephalomyelitis mice reduced brain inflammation and neuronal damage [86]. In the clinical trial, EGCG also improved muscle metabolism and managed how much energy the body uses, which may help with exhaustion caused by MS [99].

Cannabinoids

The most prominent and widely utilized plant for treating MS is marijuana. Several studies presented that marijuana could help MS patients fall asleep better and decrease muscle rigidity, bladder problems, spasms, and neurological pain. Recent research on the endocannabinoid system has made it possible to explore potential targets for the curative purposes of several conditions, including MS [32, 86].

The main content of the plant is THC, which exhibits anti-inflammatory and neuroprotective effects by attaching to cannabinoid receptors [32]. Cannabinoid receptor 1, the most prevalent G protein-coupled receptor in the brain, has been linked to the neuroprotective effects of cannabis in MS, whereas cannabinoid receptor 2 has been linked to immunomodulatory effects. THC showed activity as a partial agonist to the cannabinoid receptors and exhibited anti-inflammatory and neuroprotective properties by inhibiting the synthesis of interferon-gamma, interleukins, and tumor necrosis factor-alpha in the brain and preventing immune cells from penetrating the CNS [86]. THC and cannabinoids taken orally can lessen the severity of many MS symptoms, including rigidity, strictness, and tremor, and it also can increase walking skills, handwriting capacity, and management of the bladder [100, 101]. In animal models of MS, cannabinoids and related synthetic analogs showed promising anti-inflammatory benefits [102]. Oral usage of cannabidiol decreased experimental autoimmune encephalomyelitis intensity by inhibiting interferon-gamma, chemokine ligands, interleukins, and generation of CD8+ helper T cells, as well as enhancing myeloid-derived suppressor cells [86]. By blocking immune cells from penetrating the CNS and reducing the release of pro-inflammatory cytokines, synthetic cannabinoids can reduce inflammation, and enhance motor performance. THC and cannabidiol are combined with oral spray to treat MS symptoms, such as neuropathic pain, stiffness, trouble falling asleep, and urinary disorders. The combination was more successful at treating MS patients' moderate to serious resistant rigidity [103]. In another clinical trial, cannabinoids reduced urinary symptoms, such as nocturia, frequency of urinary, incontinence events, and urine urgency, as well as advanced in spasticity and sleep quality in MS patients [104].

Although there are conflicting data on inadequate therapeutic practices as a result of many studies performed on MS patients, it is known that several cannabis-derived substances have been tested and approved for medical use and are legalized in some countries as a therapeutic option for MS-related spasticity and pain [86].

Vitamin D

According to the Scientific Advisory Committee on Nutrition study, there is strong proof that vitamin D supplementation can improve musculoskeletal health, including lowering the risk of rickets and osteomalacia, decreasing falls, and enhancing muscle strength and function. Numerous benefits of adequate vitamin D status have been reported, including decreased total mortality, lowered risk of autoimmune diseases like type 1 diabetes and multiple sclerosis, decreased risk of osteoporosis fractures in the elderly, and decreased risk of cancer, hypertension, arthritis, Parkinson's disease, and asthma. According to the conclusion of the European Food Standards Agency, "a cause-effect relationship has been established between the normal function of the immune system, contribution to healthy inflammatory response as well as maintenance of normal muscle function and dietary intake of vitamin D." [105].

Omega-3

The role and underlying mechanisms of omega-3 polyunsaturated fatty acids and their metabolites in the prevention and treatment of autoimmune pathologies like rheumatoid arthritis, systemic lupus erythematosus, type 1 diabetes, and multiple sclerosis have come to light in recent years thanks to growing evidence from genetic mouse models and clinical studies [106]. Unquestionably, a large portion of the advantageous benefits of omega-3 polyunsaturated fatty acids (PUFAs) can be attributed to their anti-inflammatory properties; nevertheless, additional mechanisms, such as the control of mTOR activity, may also be at work. The use of high doses of eicosapentaenoic acid / docosahexaenoic acid or fat-1 gene therapy to produce endogenous omega-3 PUFAs has significant promise in the clinical treatment of these crippling disorders, even still having certain technical challenges, particularly clinical evaluation of efficacy and safety [85, 106].

Apigenin

Natural flavonoid apigenin is often present in a wide range of plants, fruits, vegetables, herbs, and spices. Parsley and dried chamomile flowers are the primary sources of apigenin. Apigenin's anticancer, anti-inflammatory, and antioxidant properties have all been thoroughly investigated. It works well to treat conditions like shingles, Parkinson's disease, neuralgia, and asthma. The modulation of the immune system by Apigenin prevented the progression and relapse of two MS mice models. Apigenin was administered orally and intraperitoneally. Apigenin has been shown to have anti-inflammatory and antioxidant properties, however, no clinical trials have been performed on MS patients [107, 108].

Berberine

Berberine is one of the isoquinoline alkaloid. It is isolated from several herbs, including Rhizoma coptidis (Huanglian), Cortex phellodendri (Huang bai), and *Hydrastis canadensis* (goldenseal). It is thought to have a variety of pharmacological activities, including anti-inflammatory and neuroprotective behaviors. Berberine was found to alleviate behavioral impairments, pathological indices, and blood-brain barrier permeability in rats with EAE when given orally. Additionally, oral berberine therapy in rats with an experimental autoimmune neuritis model improved the condition. The peripheral nerve system therefore may benefit from its therapeutic benefits for various autoimmune illnesses [109]. There has not been a clinical study on how berberine affects MS patients. However, to date, more than 90 clinical trials including this substance have been reported. These investigations mainly concentrated on its antidyslipidemic effects [110].

β-Elemene

The primary chemical component of the Chinese and Brazilian medicinal plants *Curcuma zedoaria* (Christm.) Roscoe and *Pterodon emarginatus* Vogel, respectively, is elemene. This substance can penetrate the blood-brain barrier and exhibits anti-inflammatory and anticancer effects. According to the literature, β-elemene improved motor impairment and decreased inflammation of the optic nerve in mice with experimental autoimmune encephalomyelitis. Additionally, it was shown that reduction of the differentiation and growth of Th17 cells mediate inflammation. Furthermore, a recent study showed that giving mice with experimental autoimmune encephalomyelitis the essential oil from *P. emarginatus* orally reduced neurological symptoms and demyelination. The positive impact of β-elemene on lung cancer has been examined in a small number of clinical trials. No clinical research has been conducted to assess its impact on MS [108].

Chrysin and caffeic acid

According to reports, propolis and honey are rich sources of the flavonoids chrysin and caffeic acid. They are beneficial against neurodegenerative disorders including Alzheimer's and Parkinson's disorders, improve cognitive decline, and have neuroprotective properties. Caffeic acid therapy improved behavioral impairments in experimental allergic encephalomyelitis rats by reducing reactive oxygen species generation brought on by the disease [111]. Additionally, oral chrysin administration for three days before the induction of experimental autoimmune encephalomyelitis reduced behavioral impairments and inhibited dendritic and Th1 cells [112]. Chrysin and caffeine have not been tested in any clinical studies on MS patients. On the other hand, prior clinical research showed that caffeic acid was useful in treating various types of cancer [108].

Genistein

Numerous plants, particularly soybeans, contain genistein, a typical form of phytoestrogen. A class of plant chemicals known as phytoestrogens, which possess a chemical similarity with estrogen, has estrogen-like and antiestrogenic properties. In mice with experimental autoimmune encephalomyelitis, genistein treatment improved the behavioral problems and regulated the amounts of cytokines that were pro-inflammatory and anti-inflammatory. Recent research has shown that if symptoms begin in the early stages of the disease, oral genistein administration lowers the intensity of experimental allergic encephalomyelitis. Although genistein is the subject of numerous clinical trials for meta-bolicdisorders, prostate ailments osteoporosis, and breast cancer, there has not been any clinical study carried out on MS patients yet [108].

Hesperidin

A widespread natural flavonoid found in citrus species like lemon and orange is called hesperidin. Hesperidin has been found to have many biological abilities, such as anticancer, antiviral, and anti-inflammatory effects. Hesperidin was recently used to treat experimental autoimmune encephalomyelitis mice, by reducing behavioral deficiencies in these mice and preventing oxidative stress. Although hesperidin has been thoroughly examined for medicinal effects in various disorders, no clinical trial on MS sufferers has yet been carried out [113].

Huperzine A

A sesquiterpene alkaloid known as huperzine A is obtained from the Indian and Southeast Asian natural plant *Huperzia serrata*, often known as club moss. Huperzine A might have anti-inflammatory and anticholinesterase activities; therefore, AD and other neurodegenerative disorders have been treated with huperzine A. According to the literature, huperzine A treatment reduced the symptoms of experimental autoimmune encephalomyelitis in mice by reducing demyelination and axonal damage in the neural pathway as well as autoimmune and inflammatory reactions. Although huperzine A has undergone a small number of clinical trials, the majority of which were individuals with AD, and the outcomes showed that huperzine A enhanced both cognitive capabilities and overall quality of life, there has not been a single clinical trial conducted on MS yet [108].

Lipoic Acid

A natural antioxidant called lipoic acid can be found in a variety of foods, such as liver, kidney, heart, spinach, broccoli, and yeast extract. Investigations have shown that lipoic acid can help treat diabetes, neurodegeneration, and injuries caused by ischemia-reperfusion. In numerous investigations, the impact of lipoic acid on experimental autoimmune encephalomyelitis has been assessed. The outcomes showed that lipoic acid decreased the model, perhaps by modifying inflammatory and immunological responses. The substance has been tested in clinical studies on MS patients. It was found that giving lipoic acid to MS patients decreased the frequency of relapses and the need for corticosteroids. Additionally, treating a mix of antioxidants in MS patients was more successful than giving lipoic acid alone. According to other studies, MS patients who consumed lipoic acid daily had lower levels of inflammatory cytokines. The effectiveness of lipoic acid in MS patients has been the subject of even more clinical trials. To evaluate the effects of lipoic acid on MS patients more clearly, more research with larger sample sizes is necessary [114].

Luteolin

Luteolin is a typical flavonoid that is widely distributed in a variety of plant items, such as celery, broccoli, spice, and pepper. Luteolin has been demonstrated to have advantageous neuroprotective properties both *in vitro* and *in vivo* by studies on immunomodulatory and antioxidant effects. It was claimed that luteolin, administered either orally or intraperitoneally, inhibited behavioral impairments, avoided relapse, and decreased inflammation and axonal damage in rats with experimental allergic encephalitis. Additionally, it was recently discovered that oligodendrocyte precursor cells, which create the layer of myelin around neurons, become more mature after being exposed to a specific palmitoylethanolamide/luteolin mixture. Instead of lessening the severity of the condition, it was also reported that taking oral supplements of luteolin prolonged the healing of behavioral defects. Clinical studies have demonstrated the usefulness of luteolin in treating cancer, type 2 diabetes, and autism, however, clinical trials on MS sufferers have not existed [108].

Matrine

Two naturally occurring alkaloid substances, matrine, and oxymatrine, were isolated from the herb Radix Sophorae flavescentis. Matrine has been linked to a few therapeutic actions, such as anti-inflammatory, anti-allergic, and cardiovascular protective properties. Matrine was found to improve behavioral impairments, inflammatory cells, and blood-brain barrier permeability in rats with experimental autoimmune encephalomyelitis, according to an increasing number of studies. Furthermore, matrine has long been used without any known negative side effects to treat cardiac arrhythmia, skin irritation, and viral hepatitis. Therefore, participating MS patients in clinical studies can be advised [115].

N-Acetylglucosamine

A simple sugar [monosaccharide derivative of glucose] is *N*-acetylglucosamine, which primarily comes from the chitin that fungi produce in large quantities. It is used as a nutritional supplement administered orally to people due to several biological functions, including immune system modification. *N*-acetylglucosamine was given orally to mice with experimental autoimmune encephalomyelitis, as a result, it increased *N*-glycosylation, decreased inflammatory T-cell reactions, and prevented behavioral symptoms. Patients with MS have not been the subject of clinical studies [108].

CONCLUDING REMARKS

AD, dementia, MS, and Parkinson's disease are CNS problems related to oxidative stress. The oxidative stress has caused the loss the myelination, disruption of remyelination, and triggering the inflammation in the CNS cells [116]. MS is the first thing that comes to mind when it comes to an autoimmune disease characterized by myelination defect and axonal impairment. So far, a treatment method that completely cures this disease has not been found yet. Improvement methods are mostly applied for symptoms such as pain, stiffness, persistent discomfort, exhaustion, and motor and mobility problems, and patients try to maintain a more comfortable life by managing the disease process well. Rather than conventional treatment, the tendency of patients to natural resources, which are thought to be more reliable and have fewer side effects, is increasing day by day, and in parallel, there is an increase in scientific studies in this field. The natural sources on which many *in vivo* and clinical studies have been conducted are asfollows: hemp and its main components cannabinoids; turmeric and its main component curcumin; standardized ginkgo extract; ginger extract; Korean red ginseng extract; St. John's wort oil; phytochemical compounds such as apigenin, epigallocatechin gallate, resveratrol, omega-3 and vitamin D. As a result, it is thought that more studies are needed both to develop the mechanisms and formulations of these sources and to determine the effects and mechanisms of phytochemicals such as *β*-elemene, berberine, chrysin, caffeic acid, genistein, hesperidin, huperzine A, lipoic acid, luteolin, matrine, *N*-acetylglucosamine, *etc.* *in vivo* and clinical studies.

REFERENCES

[1]   Ghasemi N, Razavi S, Nikzad E. Multiple sclerosis: pathogenesis, symptoms, diagnoses and cell-based therapy. Cell J 2017; 19(1): 1-10. [Yakhteh].
[PMID: 28367411]

[2]   Hauser SL, Cree BA. Treatment of multiple sclerosis: a review. The American Journal of Medicine. 2020; 133(12): 1380-90.
[http://dx.doi.org/10.1016/j.amjmed.2020.05.049]

[3]   Robertson D, Moreo N. Disease-modifying therapies in multiple sclerosis: overview and treatment considerations. Fed Pract 2016; 33(6): 28-34.
[PMID: 30766181]

[4]   Alam MZ. A review on plant-based remedies for the treatment of multiple sclerosis. Ann Pharm Fr 2023; 81(5): 775-89.
[http://dx.doi.org/10.1016/j.pharma.2023.03.005] [PMID: 36963654]

[5]   Korn T. Pathophysiology of multiple sclerosis. J Neurol 2008; 255(S6) (Suppl. 6): 2-6.
[http://dx.doi.org/10.1007/s00415-008-6001-2] [PMID: 19300953]

[6]   Gold R, Linington C, Lassmann H. Understanding pathogenesis and therapy of multiple sclerosis *via* animal models: 70 years of merits and culprits in experimental autoimmune encephalomyelitis research. Brain 2006; 129(8): 1953-71.
[http://dx.doi.org/10.1093/brain/awl075] [PMID: 16632554]

[7]   Smith KJ, McDonald WI. The pathophysiology of multiple sclerosis: the mechanisms underlying the production of symptoms and the natural history of the disease. Philos Trans R Soc Lond B Biol Sci 1999; 354(1390): 1649-73.
[http://dx.doi.org/10.1098/rstb.1999.0510] [PMID: 10603618]

[8]   Lubetzki C, Stankoff B. Demyelination in multiple sclerosis. Handb Clin Neurol 2014; 122: 89-99.
[http://dx.doi.org/10.1016/B978-0-444-52001-2.00004-2] [PMID: 24507514]

[9]   Reynolds R, Roncaroli F, Nicholas R, Radotra B, Gveric D, Howell O. The neuropathological basis of clinical progression in multiple sclerosis. Acta Neuropathol 2011; 122(2): 155-70.
[http://dx.doi.org/10.1007/s00401-011-0840-0] [PMID: 21626034]

[10]   Miller A, Korem M, Almog R, Galboiz Y. Vitamin B12, demyelination, remyelination and repair in multiple sclerosis. J Neurol Sci 2005; 233(1-2): 93-7.
[http://dx.doi.org/10.1016/j.jns.2005.03.009] [PMID: 15896807]

[11]   McDonald WI, Compston A, Edan G, *et al.* Recommended diagnostic criteria for multiple sclerosis: Guidelines from the international panel on the diagnosis of multiple sclerosis. Ann Neurol 2001; 50(1): 121-7.
[http://dx.doi.org/10.1002/ana.1032] [PMID: 11456302]

[12]   org M-M. Types of Multiple Sclerosis My-MS.org for information on Multiple Sclerosis. Available from: https://my-ms.org/ms_types.htm

[13]   Rosati G. The prevalence of multiple sclerosis in the world: an update. Neurol Sci 2001; 22(2): 117-39.
[http://dx.doi.org/10.1007/s100720170011] [PMID: 11603614]

[14]   Kingwell E, Marriott JJ, Jetté N, *et al.* Incidence and prevalence of multiple sclerosis in Europe: a systematic review. BMC Neurol 2013; 13(1): 128.
[http://dx.doi.org/10.1186/1471-2377-13-128] [PMID: 24070256]

[15]   Wallin MT, Culpepper WJ, Nichols E, *et al.* Global, regional, and national burden of multiple sclerosis 1990–2016: a systematic analysis for the Global Burden of Disease Study 2016. Lancet Neurol 2019; 18(3): 269-85.
[http://dx.doi.org/10.1016/S1474-4422(18)30443-5] [PMID: 30679040]

[16]   Harbo HF, Gold R, Tintoré M. Sex and gender issues in multiple sclerosis. Ther Adv Neurol Disord 2013; 6(4): 237-48.
[http://dx.doi.org/10.1177/1756285613488434] [PMID: 23858327]

[17]   Bove RM, Healy B, Augustine A, Musallam A, Gholipour T, Chitnis T. Effect of gender on late-onset multiple sclerosis. Mult Scler 2012; 18(10): 1472-9.
[http://dx.doi.org/10.1177/1352458512438236] [PMID: 22383227]

[18]   J van der Star B, YS Vogel D, Kipp M, Puentes F, Baker D, Amor S. *In vitro* and *in vivo* models of

multiple sclerosis. CNS & Neurological Disorders-Drug Targets. Formerly Current Drug Targets-CNS & Neurological Disorders. 2012; 11(5): 570-88.

[19]   Baker D, Amor S. Publication guidelines for refereeing and reporting on animal use in experimental autoimmune encephalomyelitis. J Neuroimmunol 2012; 242(1-2): 78-83.
[http://dx.doi.org/10.1016/j.jneuroim.2011.11.003] [PMID: 22119102]

[20]   Scheikl T, Pignolet B, Mars LT, Liblau RS. Transgenic mouse models of multiple sclerosis. Cell Mol Life Sci 2010; 67(23): 4011-34.
[http://dx.doi.org/10.1007/s00018-010-0481-9] [PMID: 20714779]

[21]   Trojano M, Tintore M, Montalban X, *et al.* Treatment decisions in multiple sclerosis — insights from real-world observational studies. Nat Rev Neurol 2017; 13(2): 105-18.
[http://dx.doi.org/10.1038/nrneurol.2016.188] [PMID: 28084327]

[22]   van Munster CEP, Uitdehaag BMJ. Outcome measures in clinical trials for multiple sclerosis. CNS Drugs 2017; 31(3): 217-36.
[http://dx.doi.org/10.1007/s40263-017-0412-5] [PMID: 28185158]

[23]   Kipp M, van der Star B, Vogel DYS, *et al.* Experimental *in vivo* and *in vitro* models of multiple sclerosis: EAE and beyond. Mult Scler Relat Disord 2012; 1(1): 15-28.
[http://dx.doi.org/10.1016/j.msard.2011.09.002] [PMID: 25876447]

[24]   Clinic   M.   2022.   https://www.mayoclinic.org/diseases-conditions/multiple-sclerosis/diagnos-s-treatment/ drc-20350274

[25]   Goodin DS, Frohman EM, Garmany GP Jr, *et al.* Disease modifying therapies in multiple sclerosis. Neurology 2002; 58(2): 169-78.
[http://dx.doi.org/10.1212/WNL.58.2.169] [PMID: 11805241]

[26]   Faissner S, Gold R. Oral therapies for multiple sclerosis. Cold Spring Harb Perspect Med 2019; 9(1): a032011.
[http://dx.doi.org/10.1101/cshperspect.a032011] [PMID: 29500302]

[27]   Rath L, Bui MV, Ellis J, *et al.* Fast and safe: Optimising multiple sclerosis infusions during COVID-19 pandemic. Mult Scler Relat Disord 2021; 47: 102642.
[http://dx.doi.org/10.1016/j.msard.2020.102642] [PMID: 33321356]

[28]   Amatya B, Khan F, Galea M. Rehabilitation for people with multiple sclerosis: an overview of Cochrane Reviews. Cochrane Libr 2019; 2019(1): CD012732.
[http://dx.doi.org/10.1002/14651858.CD012732.pub2] [PMID: 30637728]

[29]   Ross AP, Ben-Zacharia A, Harris C, Smrtka J. Multiple sclerosis, relapses, and the mechanism of action of adrenocorticotropic hormone. Front Neurol 2013; 4: 21.
[http://dx.doi.org/10.3389/fneur.2013.00021] [PMID: 23482896]

[30]   Stevenson VL, Playford ED. Rehabilitation and MS. Int MS J 2007; 14(3): 85-92.
[PMID: 18028832]

[31]   Neate SL, Taylor KL, Jelinek GA, De Livera AM, Brown CR, Weiland TJ. Taking active steps: Changes made by partners of people with multiple sclerosis who undertake lifestyle modification. PLoS One 2019; 14(2): e0212422.
[http://dx.doi.org/10.1371/journal.pone.0212422] [PMID: 30817765]

[32]   Mojaverrostami S, Bojnordi MN, Ghasemi-Kasman M, Ebrahimzadeh MA, Hamidabadi HG. A review of herbal therapy in multiple sclerosis. Adv Pharm Bull 2018; 8(4): 575-90.
[http://dx.doi.org/10.15171/apb.2018.066] [PMID: 30607330]

[33]   Bahrami M, Mosayebi G, Ghazavi A, Ganji A. Immunomodulation in Multiple Sclerosis by Phytotherapy. Curr Immunol Rev 2020; 16(1): 28-36.
[http://dx.doi.org/10.2174/1573395516999200930122850]

[34]   Mirshafiey A, Mohsenzadegan M. Antioxidant therapy in multiple sclerosis. Immunopharmacol

Immunotoxicol 2009; 31(1): 13-29.
[http://dx.doi.org/10.1080/08923970802331943] [PMID: 18763202]

[35]   Crawford JD, McIvor GP. Stress management for multiple sclerosis patients. Psychol Rep 1987; 61(2): 423-9.
[http://dx.doi.org/10.2466/pr0.1987.61.2.423] [PMID: 3324144]

[36]   Sinha AK, Dilnashin H, Birla H, Kumar G. Role of Withania somnifera [Ashwagandha] in Neuronal Health. Indopathy for Neuroprotection: Recent Advances. 2022: 281.

[37]   AlAmmar WA, Albeesh FH, Ibrahim LM, Algindan YY, Yamani LZ, Khattab RY. Effect of omega-3 fatty acids and fish oil supplementation on multiple sclerosis: a systematic review. Nutr Neurosci 2021; 24(7): 569-79.
[http://dx.doi.org/10.1080/1028415X.2019.1659560] [PMID: 31462182]

[38]   Shinto L, Marracci G, Baldauf-Wagner S, *et al.* Omega-3 fatty acid supplementation decreases matrix metalloproteinase-9 production in relapsing-remitting multiple sclerosis. Prostaglandins Leukot Essent Fatty Acids 2009; 80(2-3): 131-6.
[http://dx.doi.org/10.1016/j.plefa.2008.12.001] [PMID: 19171471]

[39]   Pierrot-Deseilligny C, Souberbielle JC. Vitamin D and multiple sclerosis: An update. Mult Scler Relat Disord 2017; 14: 35-45.
[http://dx.doi.org/10.1016/j.msard.2017.03.014] [PMID: 28619429]

[40]   Haddad F, Dokmak G, Karaman R. The Efficacy of Cannabis on Multiple Sclerosis-Related Symptoms. Life (Basel) 2022; 12(5): 682.
[http://dx.doi.org/10.3390/life12050682] [PMID: 35629350]

[41]   Kuddus M, Ginawi I, AlHazimi A. Cannabis sativa: An ancient wild edible plant of India. Emir J Food Agric 2013; 25(10): 736-45.
[http://dx.doi.org/10.9755/ejfa.v25i10.16400]

[42]   Jin S, Lee MY. The ameliorative effect of hemp seed hexane extracts on the Propionibacterium acnes-induced inflammation and lipogenesis in sebocytes. PLoS One 2018; 13(8): e0202933.
[http://dx.doi.org/10.1371/journal.pone.0202933] [PMID: 30148860]

[43]   S A, J S-G, H J, Sr F. Therapeutic Effects of *Nigella Sativa* and *Cannabis Sativa* Seeds On Multiple Sclerosis. Clinics of Surgery 2021; 05(04): 1-5.

[44]   Rudroff T, Honce JM. Cannabis and Multiple Sclerosis—The Way Forward. Front Neurol 2017; 8: 299.
[http://dx.doi.org/10.3389/fneur.2017.00299] [PMID: 28690588]

[45]   Breijyeh Z, Jubeh B, Bufo SA, Karaman R, Scrano L. Cannabis: A Toxin-Producing Plant with Potential Therapeutic Uses. Toxins (Basel) 2021; 13(2): 117.
[http://dx.doi.org/10.3390/toxins13020117] [PMID: 33562446]

[46]   Howlett AC, Barth F, Bonner TI, *et al.* International Union of Pharmacology. XXVII. Classification of cannabinoid receptors. Pharmacol Rev 2002; 54(2): 161-202.
[http://dx.doi.org/10.1124/pr.54.2.161] [PMID: 12037135]

[47]   Pertwee RG. Pharmacology of cannabinoid CB1 and CB2 receptors. Pharmacol Ther 1997; 74(2): 129-80.
[http://dx.doi.org/10.1016/S0163-7258(97)82001-3] [PMID: 9336020]

[48]   Zajicek JP, Hobart JC, Slade A, Barnes D, Mattison PG. Multiple sclerosis and extract of cannabis: results of the MUSEC trial. J Neurol Neurosurg Psychiatry 2012; 83(11): 1125-32.
[http://dx.doi.org/10.1136/jnnp-2012-302468] [PMID: 22791906]

[49]   Maayah ZH, Takahara S, Ferdaoussi M, Dyck JRB. The anti-inflammatory and analgesic effects of formulated full-spectrum cannabis extract in the treatment of neuropathic pain associated with multiple sclerosis. Inflamm Res 2020; 69(6): 549-58.
[http://dx.doi.org/10.1007/s00011-020-01341-1] [PMID: 32239248]

[50] Rezapour-Firouzi S, Arefhosseini SR, Mehdi F, *et al.* Immunomodulatory and therapeutic effects of Hot-nature diet and co-supplemented hemp seed, evening primrose oils intervention in multiple sclerosis patients. Complement Ther Med 2013; 21(5): 473-80.
[http://dx.doi.org/10.1016/j.ctim.2013.06.006] [PMID: 24050582]

[51] Rodriguez-Martin NM, Toscano R, Villanueva A, *et al.* Neuroprotective protein hydrolysates from hemp (*Cannabis sativa* L.) seeds. Food Funct 2019; 10(10): 6732-9.
[http://dx.doi.org/10.1039/C9FO01904A] [PMID: 31576391]

[52] Wang S, Luo Q, Zhou Y, Fan P. CLG from Hemp Seed Inhibits LPS-Stimulated Neuroinflammation in BV2 Microglia by Regulating NF-κB and Nrf-2 Pathways. ACS Omega 2019; 4(15): 16517-23.
[http://dx.doi.org/10.1021/acsomega.9b02168] [PMID: 31616830]

[53] Schabas AJ, Vukojevic V, Taylor C, *et al.* Cannabis-based product use in a multiple sclerosis cohort. Mult Scler J Exp Transl Clin 2019; 5(3).
[http://dx.doi.org/10.1177/2055217319869360] [PMID: 31598330]

[54] Kocaadam B, Şanlier N. Curcumin, an active component of turmeric (*Curcuma longa*), and its effects on health. Crit Rev Food Sci Nutr 2017; 57(13): 2889-95.
[http://dx.doi.org/10.1080/10408398.2015.1077195] [PMID: 26528921]

[55] Aggarwal BB, Yuan W, Li S, Gupta SC. Curcumin-free turmeric exhibits anti-inflammatory and anticancer activities: Identification of novel components of turmeric. Mol Nutr Food Res 2013; 57(9): 1529-42.
[http://dx.doi.org/10.1002/mnfr.201200838] [PMID: 23847105]

[56] Ghanaatian N, Lashgari NA, Abdolghaffari AH, *et al.* Curcumin as a therapeutic candidate for multiple sclerosis: Molecular mechanisms and targets. J Cell Physiol 2019; 234(8): 12237-48.
[http://dx.doi.org/10.1002/jcp.27965] [PMID: 30536381]

[57] Kimura K, Teranishi S, Fukuda K, Kawamoto K, Nishida T. Delayed disruption of barrier function in cultured human corneal epithelial cells induced by tumor necrosis factor-α in a manner dependent on NF-kappaB. Invest Ophthalmol Vis Sci 2008; 49(2): 565-71.
[http://dx.doi.org/10.1167/iovs.07-0419] [PMID: 18235000]

[58] Dolati S, Babaloo Z, Ayromlou H, *et al.* Nanocurcumin improves regulatory T-cell frequency and function in patients with multiple sclerosis. J Neuroimmunol 2019; 327: 15-21.
[http://dx.doi.org/10.1016/j.jneuroim.2019.01.007] [PMID: 30683426]

[59] Singh SK, Srivastav S, Castellani RJ, Plascencia-Villa G, Perry G. Neuroprotective and Antioxidant Effect of Ginkgo biloba Extract Against AD and Other Neurological Disorders. Neurotherapeutics 2019; 16(3): 666-74.
[http://dx.doi.org/10.1007/s13311-019-00767-8] [PMID: 31376068]

[60] Li QY, Miao Q, Sui RX, *et al.* Ginkgolide K supports remyelination *via* induction of astrocytic IGF/PI3K/Nrf2 axis. Int Immunopharmacol 2019; 75: 105819.
[http://dx.doi.org/10.1016/j.intimp.2019.105819] [PMID: 31421546]

[61] Johnson SK, Diamond BJ, Rausch S, Kaufman M, Shiflett SC, Graves L. The effect of *Ginkgo biloba* on functional measures in multiple sclerosis: a pilot randomized controlled trial. Explore (NY) 2006; 2(1): 19-24.
[http://dx.doi.org/10.1016/j.explore.2005.10.007] [PMID: 16781604]

[62] Lovera J, Bagert B, Smoot K, *et al.* Ginkgo biloba for the improvement of cognitive performance in multiple sclerosis. Mult Scler 2007; 13(3): 376-85.
[http://dx.doi.org/10.1177/1352458506071213] [PMID: 17439907]

[63] Zou YP, Lu YH, Wei DZ. Protective effects of a flavonoid-rich extract of *Hypericum perforatum* L. against hydrogen peroxide-induced apoptosis in PC12 cells. Phytother Res 2010; 24(S1) (Suppl. 1): S6-S10.
[http://dx.doi.org/10.1002/ptr.2852] [PMID: 19548287]

[64]   Kasper S. Hypericum perforatum--a review of clinical studies. Pharmacopsychiatry 2001; 34 (Suppl. 1): 51-5.
[http://dx.doi.org/10.1055/s-2001-15467] [PMID: 11518077]

[65]   Naziroglu M, Kutluhan S, Övey İS, Aykur M, Yurekli VA. Modulation of oxidative stress, apoptosis, and calcium entry in leukocytes of patients with multiple sclerosis by *Hypericum perforatum*. Nutr Neurosci 2014; 17(5): 214-21.
[http://dx.doi.org/10.1179/1476830513Y.0000000083] [PMID: 24075078]

[66]   Mahmoudi M, Rastin M, Kazemi Arababadi M, Anaeigoudari A, Nosratabadi R. Enhancing the efficacy of *Hypericum perforatum* in the treatment of an experimental model of multiple sclerosis using gold nanoparticles: an *in vivo* study. Avicenna J Phytomed 2022; 12(3): 325-36.
[PMID: 36186934]

[67]   Selek S, Esrefoglu M, Meral I, *et al.* Effects of *Oenothera biennis* L. and *Hypericum perforatum* L. extracts on some central nervous system myelin proteins, brain histopathology and oxidative stress in mice with experimental autoimmune encephalomyelitis. Biotech Histochem 2019; 94(2): 75-83.
[http://dx.doi.org/10.1080/10520295.2018.1482001] [PMID: 30957550]

[68]   Afsharzadeh N, Lavi Arab F, Sankian M, *et al.* Comparative assessment of proliferation and immunomodulatory potential of *Hypericum perforatum* plant and callus extracts on mesenchymal stem cells derived adipose tissue from multiple sclerosis patients. Inflammopharmacology 2021; 29(5): 1399-412.
[http://dx.doi.org/10.1007/s10787-021-00838-3] [PMID: 34510276]

[69]   Zha Z, Liu S, Liu Y, Li C, Wang L. Potential Utility of Natural Products against Oxidative Stress in Animal Models of Multiple Sclerosis. Antioxidants 2022; 11(8): 1495.
[http://dx.doi.org/10.3390/antiox11081495] [PMID: 36009214]

[70]   Ahmad A, Husain A, Mujeeb M, *et al.* A review on therapeutic potential of *Nigella sativa*: A miracle herb. Asian Pac J Trop Biomed 2013; 3(5): 337-52.
[http://dx.doi.org/10.1016/S2221-1691(13)60075-1] [PMID: 23646296]

[71]   Kapadia H, Vora DS, Manjegowda D, Nair A, Sharma S, Dinesh S. Integrating network pharmacology and molecular docking for the identification of key genes and therapeutic targets of *Nigella sativa* in multiple sclerosis treatment. Biomedicine (Taipei) 2023; 43(3): 936-44.
[http://dx.doi.org/10.51248/.v43i3.2867]

[72]   Kim YK, Guo Q, Packer L. Free radical scavenging activity of red ginseng aqueous extracts. Toxicology 2002; 172(2): 149-56.
[http://dx.doi.org/10.1016/S0300-483X(01)00585-6] [PMID: 11882354]

[73]   Etemadifar M, Sayahi F, Abtahi SH, *et al.* Ginseng in the treatment of fatigue in multiple sclerosis: a randomized, placebo-controlled, double-blind pilot study. Int J Neurosci 2013; 123(7): 480-6.
[http://dx.doi.org/10.3109/00207454.2013.764499] [PMID: 23301896]

[74]   Kim E, Cameron M, Lovera J, Schaben L, Bourdette D, Whitham R. American ginseng does not improve fatigue in multiple sclerosis: a single center randomized double-blind placebo-controlled crossover pilot study. Mult Scler 2011; 17(12): 1523-6.
[http://dx.doi.org/10.1177/1352458511412062] [PMID: 21803872]

[75]   Lee MJ, Choi JH, Kwon TW, *et al.* Korean Red Ginseng extract ameliorates demyelination by inhibiting infiltration and activation of immune cells in cuprizone-administrated mice. J Ginseng Res 2023; 47(5): 672-80.
[http://dx.doi.org/10.1016/j.jgr.2023.05.001] [PMID: 37720568]

[76]   Shin SW, Cho IH. *Panax ginseng* as a potential therapeutic for neurological disorders associated with COVID-19; Toward targeting inflammasome. J Ginseng Res 2023; 47(1): 23-32.
[http://dx.doi.org/10.1016/j.jgr.2022.09.004] [PMID: 36213093]

[77]   Li X, Yang M, Zhang YL, *et al.* Ginseng and Ginseng Herbal Formulas for Symptomatic Management

of Fatigue: A Systematic Review and Meta-Analysis. Journal of Integrative and Complementary Medicine 2023; 29(8): 468-82.
[http://dx.doi.org/10.1089/jicm.2022.0532] [PMID: 36730693]

[78]   Bitari A, Oualdi I, Touzani R, Elachouri M, Legssyer A. *Zingiber officinale* Roscoe: A comprehensive review of clinical properties. Mater Today Proc 2023; 72: 3757-67.
[http://dx.doi.org/10.1016/j.matpr.2022.09.316]

[79]   Young HY, Luo YL, Cheng HY, Hsieh WC, Liao JC, Peng WH. Analgesic and anti-inflammatory activities of [6]-gingerol. J Ethnopharmacol 2005; 96(1-2): 207-10.
[http://dx.doi.org/10.1016/j.jep.2004.09.009] [PMID: 15588672]

[80]   Han JJ, Li X, Ye ZQ, *et al.* Treatment with 6-Gingerol Regulates Dendritic Cell Activity and Ameliorates the Severity of Experimental Autoimmune Encephalomyelitis. Mol Nutr Food Res 2019; 63(18): 1801356.
[http://dx.doi.org/10.1002/mnfr.201801356] [PMID: 31313461]

[81]   Sapkota A, Park SJ, Choi JW. Neuroprotective Effects of 6-Shogaol and Its Metabolite, 6-Paradol, in a Mouse Model of Multiple Sclerosis. Biomol Ther (Seoul) 2019; 27(2): 152-9.
[http://dx.doi.org/10.4062/biomolther.2018.089] [PMID: 30001610]

[82]   Kamankesh F, Ganji A, Ghazavi A, Mosayebi G. The Anti-inflammatory Effect of Ginger Extract on the Animal Model of Multiple Sclerosis. Iran J Immunol 2023; 20(2): 211-8.
[PMID: 37246522]

[83]   Foshati S, Poursadeghfard M, Heidari Z, Amani R. The effect of ginger (*Zingiber officinale*) supplementation on clinical, biochemical, and anthropometric parameters in patients with multiple sclerosis: a double-blind randomized controlled trial. Food Funct 2023; 14(8): 3701-11.
[http://dx.doi.org/10.1039/D3FO00167A] [PMID: 36974730]

[84]   Jafarzadeh A, Nemati M. Therapeutic potentials of ginger for treatment of Multiple sclerosis: A review with emphasis on its immunomodulatory, anti-inflammatory and anti-oxidative properties. J Neuroimmunol 2018; 324: 54-75.
[http://dx.doi.org/10.1016/j.jneuroim.2018.09.003] [PMID: 30243185]

[85]   Mannucci C, Casciaro M, Sorbara EE, *et al.* Nutraceuticals against oxidative stress in autoimmune disorders. Antioxidants 2021; 10(2): 261.
[http://dx.doi.org/10.3390/antiox10020261] [PMID: 33567628]

[86]   Costantini E, Masciarelli E, Casorri L, Di Luigi M, Reale M. Medicinal herbs and multiple sclerosis: Overview on the hard balance between new therapeutic strategy and occupational health risk. Front Cell Neurosci 2022; 16: 985943.
[http://dx.doi.org/10.3389/fncel.2022.985943] [PMID: 36439198]

[87]   Gachpazan M, Habbibirad S, Kashani H, Jamialahmadi T, Rahimi HR, Sahebkar A. Targeting nuclear factor-Kappa B signaling pathway by curcumin: implications for the treatment of multiple sclerosis. Studies on Biomarkers and New Targets in Aging Research in Iran: Focus on Turmeric and Curcumin. 2021: 41-53.

[88]   Feng J, Tao T, Yan W, Chen CS, Qin X. Curcumin inhibits mitochondrial injury and apoptosis from the early stage in EAE mice. Oxid Med Cell Longev 2014; 2014: 1-10.
[http://dx.doi.org/10.1155/2014/728751] [PMID: 24868317]

[89]   Mohammadi A, Hosseinzadeh Colagar A, Khorshidian A, Amini SM. The functional roles of curcumin on astrocytes in neurodegenerative diseases. Neuroimmunomodulation 2022; 29(1): 4-14.
[http://dx.doi.org/10.1159/000517901] [PMID: 34496365]

[90]   Fujino M, Funeshima N, Kitazawa Y, *et al.* Amelioration of experimental autoimmune encephalomyelitis in Lewis rats by FTY720 treatment. J Pharmacol Exp Ther 2003; 305(1): 70-7.
[http://dx.doi.org/10.1124/jpet.102.045658] [PMID: 12649354]

[91]   Xie L, Li XK, Funeshima-Fuji N, *et al.* Amelioration of experimental autoimmune encephalomyelitis

by curcumin treatment through inhibition of IL-17 production. Int Immunopharmacol 2009; 9(5): 575-81.
[http://dx.doi.org/10.1016/j.intimp.2009.01.025] [PMID: 19539560]

[92]   Kanakasabai S, Casalini E, Walline CC, Mo C, Chearwae W, Bright JJ. Differential regulation of CD4+ T helper cell responses by curcumin in experimental autoimmune encephalomyelitis. J Nutr Biochem 2012; 23(11): 1498-507.
[http://dx.doi.org/10.1016/j.jnutbio.2011.10.002] [PMID: 22402368]

[93]   Eghbaliferiz S, Farhadi F, Barreto GE, Majeed M, Sahebkar A. Effects of curcumin on neurological diseases: focus on astrocytes. Pharmacol Rep 2020; 72(4): 769-82.
[http://dx.doi.org/10.1007/s43440-020-00112-3] [PMID: 32458309]

[94]   Qureshi M, Al-Suhaimi EA, Wahid F, Shehzad O, Shehzad A. Therapeutic potential of curcumin for multiple sclerosis. Neurol Sci 2018; 39(2): 207-14.
[http://dx.doi.org/10.1007/s10072-017-3149-5] [PMID: 29079885]

[95]   Mohajeri M, Sadeghizadeh M, Najafi F, Javan M. Polymerized nano-curcumin attenuates neurological symptoms in EAE model of multiple sclerosis through down regulation of inflammatory and oxidative processes and enhancing neuroprotection and myelin repair. Neuropharmacology 2015; 99: 156-67.
[http://dx.doi.org/10.1016/j.neuropharm.2015.07.013] [PMID: 26211978]

[96]   Fonseca-Kelly Z, Nassrallah M, Uribe J, *et al.* Resveratrol neuroprotection in a chronic mouse model of multiple sclerosis. Front Neurol 2012; 3: 84.
[http://dx.doi.org/10.3389/fneur.2012.00084] [PMID: 22654783]

[97]   Shindler KS, Ventura E, Dutt M, Elliott P, Fitzgerald DC, Rostami A. Oral resveratrol reduces neuronal damage in a model of multiple sclerosis. J Neuroophthalmol 2010; 30(4): 328-39.
[http://dx.doi.org/10.1097/WNO.0b013e3181f7f833] [PMID: 21107122]

[98]   Li R, Huang YG, Fang D, Le WD. (−)□Epigallocatechin gallate inhibits lipopolysaccharide□induced microglial activation and protects against inflammation□mediated dopaminergic neuronal injury. J Neurosci Res 2004; 78(5): 723-31.
[http://dx.doi.org/10.1002/jnr.20315] [PMID: 15478178]

[99]   Mähler A, Steiniger J, Bock M, *et al.* Metabolic response to epigallocatechin-3-gallate in relapsing-remitting multiple sclerosis: a randomized clinical trial. Am J Clin Nutr 2015; 101(3): 487-95.
[http://dx.doi.org/10.3945/ajcn.113.075309] [PMID: 25733633]

[100] Zajicek JP, Sanders HP, Wright DE, *et al.* Cannabinoids in multiple sclerosis (CAMS) study: safety and efficacy data for 12 months follow up. J Neurol Neurosurg Psychiatry 2005; 76(12): 1664-9.
[http://dx.doi.org/10.1136/jnnp.2005.070136] [PMID: 16291891]

[101] Wade DT, Makela P, Robson P, House H, Bateman C. Do cannabis-based medicinal extracts have general or specific effects on symptoms in multiple sclerosis? A double-blind, randomized, placebo-controlled study on 160 patients. Mult Scler 2004; 10(4): 434-41.
[http://dx.doi.org/10.1191/1352458504ms1082oa] [PMID: 15327042]

[102] Saito VM, Rezende RM, Teixeira AL. Cannabinoid modulation of neuroinflammatory disorders. Curr Neuropharmacol 2012; 10(2): 159-66.
[http://dx.doi.org/10.2174/157015912800604515] [PMID: 23204985]

[103] Kmietowicz Z. Cannabis based drug is licensed for spasticity in patients with MS. BMJ 2010; 340(jun22 2): c3363.
[http://dx.doi.org/10.1136/bmj.c3363] [PMID: 20570870]

[104] Brady CM, DasGupta R, Dalton C, Wiseman OJ, Berkley KJ, Fowler CJ. An open-label pilot study of cannabis-based extracts for bladder dysfunction in advanced multiple sclerosis. Mult Scler 2004; 10(4): 425-33.
[http://dx.doi.org/10.1191/1352458504ms1063oa] [PMID: 15327041]

[105] Allergies. Scientific Opinion on the substantiation of health claims related to vitamin D and normal

function of the immune system and inflammatory response [ID 154, 159], maintenance of normal muscle function [ID 155] and maintenance of normal cardiovascular function [ID 159] pursuant to Article 13 [1] of Regulation [EC] No 1924/2006. EFSA J 2010; 8(2): 1468.

[106] Li X, Bi X, Wang S, Zhang Z, Li F, Zhao AZ. Therapeutic potential of ω-3 polyunsaturated fatty acids in human autoimmune diseases. Front Immunol 2019; 10: 2241.
[http://dx.doi.org/10.3389/fimmu.2019.02241] [PMID: 31611873]

[107] Ginwala R, McTish E, Raman C, *et al.* Apigenin, a natural flavonoid, attenuates EAE severity through the modulation of dendritic cell and other immune cell functions. J Neuroimmune Pharmacol 2016; 11(1): 36-47.
[http://dx.doi.org/10.1007/s11481-015-9617-x] [PMID: 26040501]

[108] Watson RR, Killgore WD. Nutrition and lifestyle in neurological autoimmune diseases: multiple sclerosis. Academic Press 2016.

[109] Li H, Li XL, Zhang M, *et al.* Berberine ameliorates experimental autoimmune neuritis by suppressing both cellular and humoral immunity. Scand J Immunol 2014; 79(1): 12-9.
[http://dx.doi.org/10.1111/sji.12123] [PMID: 24354407]

[110] Jiang Y, Wu A, Zhu C, *et al.* The protective effect of berberine against neuronal damage by inhibiting matrix metalloproteinase-9 and laminin degradation in experimental autoimmune encephalomyelitis. Neurol Res 2013; 35(4): 360-8.
[http://dx.doi.org/10.1179/1743132812Y.0000000156] [PMID: 23540404]

[111] Ilhan A, Akyol O, Gurel A, Armutcu F, Iraz M, Oztas E. Protective effects of caffeic acid phenethyl ester against experimental allergic encephalomyelitis-induced oxidative stress in rats. Free Radic Biol Med 2004; 37(3): 386-94.
[http://dx.doi.org/10.1016/j.freeradbiomed.2004.04.022] [PMID: 15223072]

[112] Zhang K, Ge Z, Xue Z, *et al.* Chrysin suppresses human CD14+ monocyte-derived dendritic cells and ameliorates experimental autoimmune encephalomyelitis. J Neuroimmunol 2015; 288: 13-20.
[http://dx.doi.org/10.1016/j.jneuroim.2015.08.017] [PMID: 26531689]

[113] Ciftci O, Ozcan C, Kamisli O, Cetin A, Basak N, Aytac B. Hesperidin, a citrus flavonoid, has the ameliorative effects against experimental autoimmune encephalomyelitis [EAE] in a C57BL/J6 mouse model. Neurochem Res 2015; 40(6): 1111-20.
[http://dx.doi.org/10.1007/s11064-015-1571-8] [PMID: 25859982]

[114] Chaudhary P, Marracci G, Galipeau D, Pocius E, Morris B, Bourdette D. Lipoic acid reduces inflammation in a mouse focal cortical experimental autoimmune encephalomyelitis model. J Neuroimmunol 2015; 289: 68-74.
[http://dx.doi.org/10.1016/j.jneuroim.2015.10.011] [PMID: 26616873]

[115] Zhu L, Pan Q, Zhang XJ, *et al.* Protective effects of matrine on experimental autoimmune encephalomyelitis *via* regulation of ProNGF and NGF signaling. Exp Mol Pathol 2016; 100(2): 337-43.
[http://dx.doi.org/10.1016/j.yexmp.2015.12.006] [PMID: 26681653]

[116] Asejeje FO, Asejeje GI. Plant-Based Antioxidants in the Prevention and Treatment of Neurodegenerative Diseases: Pros and Cons Curative and Preventive Properties of Medicinal Plants: Research on Disease Management and Animal Model Studies. Apple Academic Press 2023; pp. 81-104.

CHAPTER 7

Celiac Disease and Gut Microbiota: Herbal Treatment and Gluten-Free Diet

Ünkan Urganci[1,*]

[1] *Department of Food Engineering, Faculty of Engineering, Pamukkale University, Denizli 20160, Türkiye*

Abstract: Celiac disease (CD) manifests as a targeted autoimmune response that adversely affects the small intestine, primarily affecting individuals with a particular genetic predisposition. Diagnosis centers on identifying this gluten-sensitive enteropathy, which can be ameliorated through the implementation of a gluten-free diet (GFD), correlating with mucosal healing and symptom alleviation. The human microbiota, a vast symbiotic community within the gastrointestinal tract, profoundly impacts human health. Advances in genome sequencing have elucidated the intricate relationship between gut microbiota and autoimmune diseases, including CD, emphasizing the significant role of dietary patterns in shaping the gut microbiota. The influence of GFD on microbiota composition, the only clinically validated treatment for CD, leads to a nutritional shift and potential macronutrient imbalance. Emerging research also highlights the therapeutic potential of various herbs with antioxidant, anti-inflammatory, antimicrobial, gastroprotective, and immunomodulatory properties as complementary approaches to manage CD. This chapter synthesizes the complex interactions between genetics, diet, gut microbiota, and potential herbal interventions in CD, paving the way for more comprehensive understanding and management strategies.

Keywords: Autoimmune diseases, Antioxidant, Antimicrobial, Anti-inflammatory, Celiac disease, Gluten sensitivity, Gluten-free diet, Gut microbiota, Herbal treatment.

INTRODUCTION

Celiac disease (CD) is a complex autoimmune disorder characterized by an immune-mediated enteropathy that primarily inflicts damage upon the small intestine [1, 2]. This pathology is not arbitrary in its manifestation but is rather confined to individuals with a specific genetic predisposition, indicating the

---

* **Corresponding author Ünkan Urganci:** Department of Food Engineering, Faculty of Engineering, Pamukkale University, Denizli 20160, Türkiye; Tel: +90 2582962000; E-mail: uurganci11@posta.pau.edu.tr

Cennet Ozay & Gokhan Zengin (Eds.)

pivotal role of genetics in the onset of celiac disease [3]. These individuals demonstrate a detrimental reaction to the ingestion of gluten, a protein complex found in various grains.

The diagnosis of celiac disease hinges upon the identification of gluten-sensitive enteropathy, a damaging inflammation and structural deterioration of the small intestinal mucosa, culminating in malabsorption and diverse clinical symptoms [4]. This inflammation, triggered by an immune response specifically directed towards gluten, is notable for its amelioration through the implementation of a gluten-free diet (GFD), implying a direct correlation between gluten intake and intestinal damage [5]. Consequently, the exclusion of gluten leads to mucosal healing, alleviation of symptoms, and a reduced risk of associated complications, reaffirming the essential role of a GFD in the management of this autoimmune disorder [6].

Overview of Celiac Disease

CD is a multifaceted autoimmune disorder that exhibits variable global prevalence with estimates ranging from 0.3% to 1% [4]. Detailed regional analysis reveals a 1% prevalence in Europe and the United States, translating to a substantial affected population, considering the sizable demographics of these regions [7]. The CD also pervades the Middle East, North Africa, and India, although diagnostic limitations potentially lead to underdiagnosis or delayed diagnosis [8].

CD's prevalence shows a correlation with dietary habits; higher in countries where wheat, rich in gluten, is a dietary mainstay [9]. Conversely, in countries like China and Japan, where rice is a staple, CD incidence is low [10]. In Western Europe, CD prevalence exhibits age-related variations, with increasing incidence in adults and adolescents over 65 years of age [11].

A gender-related prevalence pattern also emerges, with women being more susceptible to CD than men, possibly pointing towards hormonal or genetic factors contributing to disease susceptibility [12, 13]. Genetic factors also play a vital role, evidenced by higher disease frequency among monozygotic twins and first-degree relatives, reinforcing genetic predisposition [14, 15].

Celiac patients and their first-degree relatives exhibit an elevated risk of other autoimmune diseases, suggesting a complex interplay of genetic and immune-related factors beyond CD [16]. Gluten absorption triggers a cascade of immune responses primarily involving T lymphocyte activation and the release of cytokines and surface antigens [17]. The intestinal epithelium's integrity, critical for gut health, deteriorates in CD, resulting in elevated gliadin levels, a key component of gluten implicated in CD [18]. Inflammatory response and immune reactions in CD prominently involve Immunoglobulin A (IgA) and a 33-mer peptide contained within gliadin [19].

Chronic inflammation in CD causes the destruction of intestinal villi, leading to malabsorption symptoms [15]. Clinical findings span a broad spectrum, dictated by disease duration, intestinal damage extent, patient age, and specific symptoms [20]. Given the significant number of undiagnosed patients vis-a-vis potential prevalence, the "Iceberg Model Theory" proposes a much higher number of undiagnosed CD patients in the community [21].

CD's complexity necessitates its categorization into five forms—classical, atypical, silent, or asymptomatic, latent, and refractory—each characterized by unique symptoms and disease progression, demanding a personalized approach to diagnosis and treatment [22 - 24].

Celiac Disease and Gut Microbiota

The human microbiota, a symbiotic community of approximately 10-100 trillion microbial cells, primarily resides within the gastrointestinal tract (GIS), skin, genitourinary system (GUS), and respiratory system [25]. The microbiome, encompassing the genes of these microbes, profoundly impacts human health and disease [26]. These co-inhabitants, estimated to be around 1014, are largely bacteria, supplemented by viruses and fungi [27]. The GIS is particularly hospitable due to its abundant nutritional supply, accounting for over 70% of the body's microorganisms [27]. Determining the number and diversity of intestinal bacteria is challenging; however, advances in high-throughput genome sequencing have yielded significant insights, suggesting the GIS hosts over 35,000 bacterial species [28, 29].

The GIS microbiota encompass aerobic, anaerobic, and facultative anaerobic bacteria. However, they predominantly consist of anaerobic bacteria, including Firmicutes, Bacteroides, Proteobacteria, and Actinobacteria [28]. A human GIS tract may host between 500-1000 distinct gut bacteria types, with Firmicutes and Bacteroidetes comprising over 60% and 20% of the microbiota, respectively [30]. Other substantial anaerobic bacteria include Fusobacteria, Verrucomicrobia, Spirochaet, Lentisphaerae, and Cyanobacteria [31]. Notably, obligate anaerobes are more prevalent than facultative anaerobes. The intestinal microbiota exhibits dynamic shifts over time, primarily influenced by diet, diseases, antibiotic use, and environmental changes [32, 33]. A study indicated that approximately 95% of the virome content in a healthy adult remained stable over a year, and attributed to dietary habits [34].

Dietary patterns significantly affect gut microbiota's composition and diversity [35]. High-carbohydrate and high-fat diets notably alter the microbiota profile. Consumption of prebiotics, especially those containing inulin, leads to a predominance of *Faecalibacterium prausnitzii* and Bifidobacterium [36]. High-fat diets coincide with increased Gram-negative bacteria in the gut microbiota, triggering lipopolysaccharides production. Studies in mice show that high-fat diets cause increased lipopolysaccharide production, leading to weight gain, hyperinsulinemia, and fasting hyperglycemia [37].

A comparative study of gut microbiota in African and European children accentuated diet's role in microbiota composition [38]. The study showed a protective effect of plant-based, high-fiber diets on the microbiota in African children, while high protein and fat diets in European children increased *Bacteroidetes* and decreased Firmicutes. Additionally, lower short-chain fatty acid quantities were found in African children's feces.

Another comprehensive study examined the short-term effects of animal-based (69% fat, 30% protein, and 0 g fiber) and plant-based diets (22% fat, 10% protein, and 25 g fiber) on intestinal microbiota [39]. Animal-based diet increased bile-acid-resistant *Alistipes putredinis*, Bacteroides, and *Bilophila wadsworthia*, while a plant-based diet amplified levels of plant polysaccharide metabolizers, including Prevotella, *Ruminococcus bromii*, Roseburia, *Eubacterium rectale*, and *Faecalibacterium prausnitzii*. These findings underscore dietary interventions' potential in modulating gut microbiota for health promotion and disease prevention.

The colon's microbiota, notably Lactobacilli and Bifidobacterium spp., have been associated with gluten metabolism, potentially influencing gluten and gluten peptide breakdown and modifying their immunogenic properties [40, 41]. Caminero *et al.* showed variations in gluten breakdown patterns as a function of different gut microorganisms, potentially impacting autoimmune disease risk [41].

Studies have shown Lactobacilli's ability to neutralize gliadin peptides' toxicity post partial digestion by human proteases, suggesting the potential usage of probiotics as an adjunct therapy for CD [42]. Alterations in gut microbiota composition can impact the intestinal barrier function and increase epithelial permeability [43]. Elevated intestinal permeability in CD patients is linked to zonulin degradation, a protein involved in the tight junction function. Certain studies associate dysbiosis with increased zonulin release, compromising tight junctions and allowing partially digested gliadin peptides into the lamina propria [44, 45].

The gut microbiota plays a critical role in modulating host metabolism and immune responses [46]. Recent research illuminates how gut microbiota, and their metabolic byproducts may enhance autoimmune disease risk *via* epigenetic mechanisms [47]. Bifidobacteria and Lactobacilli, recognized for potential immunomodulation in disease management, have been intensively studied; Bifidobacteria strains can mitigate gluten-induced epithelial permeability [48], downregulate the Th1 pathway of CD [49], and lessen damage to jejunal architecture [50].

Escherichia coli is proposed to have a protective effect on gut barrier function [51], while certain *Lactobacilli* strains possess immunomodulatory properties [52]. Cross-sectional studies examining fecal, salivary, and duodenal microbiota in CD have noted reduced beneficial species like Lactobacillus and Bifidobacterium, and an increase in potentially pathogenic species such as Bacteroides and *E. coli*, compared to healthy subjects [53].

Specifically, various studies have reported lower proportions of Bifidobacterium spp., *Bifidobacterium longum, Clostridium histolyticum, C. lituseburense*, and *Faecalibacterium prausnitzii* group in untreated CD patients than in healthy controls [54 - 56]. A study by Ou Gangwei *et al.* [57] found rod-shaped bacteria in the proximal small intestine microbiota in children with CD during the Swedish epidemics, absent in controls. Such findings emphasize that gut microbiota changes are particularly significant in the active CD phase, suggesting a critical role of host-microbiota interactions in CD's manifestation and progression.

Gluten-Free Diet and Gut Microbiota

GFD therapy, the only clinically validated treatment for CD, requires the exclusion of wheat (gliadin and glutenin), rye (secalin), and barley (hordein) derived products known to contain prolamins, causing high celiac reactivity. This diet excludes a wide array of items such as bread, pasta, bulgur, vermicelli, cakes, biscuits, cereal flakes, and various bakery products [58]. The gluten reactivity of oats (avenin) was previously controversial, but recent studies affirm their safety in CD [59, 60]. Systematic reviews and meta-analyses support these findings, suggesting that oats' inclusion in a GFD does not affect symptoms, histology, immunity, or serological outcomes negatively [61]. Still, potential oat contamination with wheat and geographic variability necessitate further investigation.

Upon adherence to a GFD, significant improvements can be observed in the clinical course of the disease. Immediate effects include rapid alleviation of gastrointestinal symptoms [62], while long-term benefits comprise correction of nutrient deficiencies, reduction of extraintestinal symptoms, malaise, oral ulcers, and weight loss, alongside improved bone health after one year. Concurrently, the diet decreases the risk of fractures, cancer, and lymphoma [63]. These improvements are paramount in reducing the overall morbidity and enhancing the quality of life of CD patients. Thus, persistent research and patient education are essential for effective GFD implementation and maintenance in CD individuals.

Maintaining a gluten-free lifestyle involves significant considerations. Among these, mitigating gluten cross-contamination in household settings is paramount. It necessitates the segregation of gluten-free products from those containing gluten to prevent inadvertent consumption [64]. Ensuring the cleanliness of all food-related kitchen utensils, appliances, and service wares is essential. Literature indicates that as long as cleanliness is rigorously maintained, no risk is posed [64]. Adhering to a GFD becomes markedly challenging during external food consumption due to a higher risk of gluten cross-contamination [65] and limited availability of gluten-free offerings. Studies emphasize the necessity of employee training and best manufacturing practices for standardization in establishments providing gluten-free services [66, 67]. Beyond food, gluten is present in numerous non-food items such as medications, oral care, and cosmetic products, and even children's items like playdough and finger paints, posing a potential ingestion risk [68]. Consequently, vigilant reading of product labels and manufacturer's consultation when necessary are vital for avoiding such sources of gluten consumption.

The myriad of challenges in gluten avoidance inevitably questions the potential intestinal damage from inadvertent gluten exposure and permissible gluten levels. Although no single threshold exists, it is proposed that daily gluten intake below 10 mg would not cause histopathological alterations [69]. Notably, the average daily gluten intake in a regular diet is substantial, approximately 10-20 g [70]. Even with strict precautions, individuals with CD on a GFD may unintentionally ingest gluten levels exceeding the tolerable amount (~150-400 mg, based on fecal tests) [71], partly due to gluten contamination in industrial gluten-free products [72]. This necessitates heightened awareness about potential gluten sources in CD patients.

Adopting a GFD prompts a dietary shift, particularly in food composition and nutritional value. Gluten-free products frequently use more carbohydrates and fats to maintain texture and structure [73, 74], generally containing lower protein levels than gluten counterparts [75 - 78]. Certain gluten-free products display elevated saturated fat content [76 - 78], while gluten-free biscuits and breads have diminished dietary fiber [75 - 77].

This substitution-induced nutritional shift can lead to diet macronutrient imbalance, posing challenges, especially among risk groups such as children and adolescents fond of packaged food items [75]. Although these products serve those with dietary restrictions like CD or gluten sensitivity, they could inadvertently result in a diet rich in carbohydrates and fats but poor in protein and fiber. Interestingly, the mere initiation of a GFD can trigger behavioral changes, potentially driving increased consumption of packaged food products [79]. Within GFDs, attention must be given to the intake of dietary fiber, saturated fats, B-group vitamins, minerals, sugar, and glycemic index [80, 81].

A systematic review by Di Nardo *et al.* [82] revealed that children, irrespective of adherence to a GFD, tend to consume excess fat and insufficient dietary fiber, iron, calcium, and vitamin D. GFDs particularly reduced folate, magnesium, and zinc intake while increasing high glycemic index food consumption. Yet, dietary patterns of children with CD resemble those of non-celiac peers, with dietary fiber, vitamin D, and magnesium intake below, and sucrose and saturated fat above the recommended values [83].

Cereal exclusion in a GFD necessitates viable substitutes, with pseudocereals, such as amaranth, quinoa, and buckwheat, gaining recognition as nutritionally sound gluten-free alternatives [84]. These grains, when utilized in gluten-free products or directly added to diets, bolster the intake of plant protein, dietary fiber, key vitamins and minerals, and bioactive compounds like polyphenols and phytosterols [85]. Use of low fiber, high carbohydrate gluten-free flours (e.g., rice flour, potato starch) in bread-making leads to high glycemic index products. Nonetheless, bread made with inulin-type fructans, or alternative cereal flours could aid in blood sugar regulation. Thus, thoughtfully planned GFDs with appropriate food choices can circumvent nutrient deficiencies and moderate dietary pattern shifts anticipated with GFD [86].

Drabinska *et al.* [87] investigated the efficacy of prebiotics in correcting nutrient imbalances in GFD, and their role in microbiota-targeted treatments for dysbiosis. Children on GFD were administered oligofructose-enriched inulin (10 g/day) for three months, resulting in significant increases in Bifidobacterium numbers and fecal acetate and butyrate levels. These findings were interpreted as evidence for prebiotic supplementation potentially reducing future complications related to CD, underscoring the potential of prebiotics and microbiota-targeted treatments in addressing nutritional imbalances associated with GFD.

The evaluation of the isolated impact of GFD on microbiota in CD presents a challenge due to the diets' therapeutic role in CD, resulting in the regression of intestinal atrophy concomitant with therapy [82]. The improvements in gastrointestinal health follow gluten removal, yet when considered as a dietary regimen alone, GFD exhibits notable variances in dietary patterns, quality, and nutrient content compared to gluten-inclusive diets [80].

Dietary constituents play an instrumental role in directly impacting the microbiota [88, 89]. Repeated research evidence substantiates the direct influence of dietary patterns (*e.g.*, Mediterranean, and Western diets) [88], specific foods (*e.g.*, fermented foods) [90], and certain nutrients (including dietary fiber, fats, and proteins) on gut microbiota regulation [91, 92]. Given these associations, the influence of GFD on the microbiota is an unavoidable consideration [93], underscoring the relevance of dietary patterns and constituents in microbiota research.

A short-term study involving healthy participants highlighted the transformative potential of GFD on microbiota, demonstrating significant alterations within a four-week adherence period, particularly within starch-metabolizing taxa [94]. In another study, GFD adoption led to reduced polysaccharide consumption and a decrease in Bifidobacterium, *Bifidobacterium longum*, and Lactobacillus species in healthy adults, while *Escherichia coli* and total Enterobacteriaceae populations increased [95]. Conversely, substituting alternative grains for gluten-containing foods—thus preserving dietary fiber intake—induced changes in adult microbiota and appeared to inhibit the production of pro-inflammatory cytokines by the immune system [96]. These results underscore the need for prudent dietary planning to optimize GFD's therapeutic efficacy for celiac patients. Missteps may negatively affect the microbiota and encourage pro-inflammatory processes [97], underlining the importance of careful dietary planning when adopting a gluten-free diet, particularly for therapeutic purposes, where the objective extends beyond symptom control to optimizing microbiota balance and overall health improvement.

The transformative potential of gluten detoxification has been investigated in a highly controlled *in vitro* environment that accurately mimics the digestive systems of both healthy individuals and those afflicted with CD. Bread undergoing this gluten detoxification process has displayed intriguing implications for the maintenance of the gut microbiota. Notably, this detoxified gluten product has been linked to the preservation of *Lactobacillus acidophilus*, a beneficial bacterium in the gut microbiota [98]. Moreover, the bread has also been reported to exert an antibacterial effect on potentially pathogenic species such as *Staphylococcus aureus* and *Salmonella typhimurium*. This effect is believed to be mediated through the continuous presence of *L. acidophilus*, as mentioned previously. This may pave the way for the exploitation of gluten-friendly foods not just for the management of CD but also for the broader context of gut health.

Furthermore, an increase in *Lactobacillus* due to this bread product also showed a favorable impact on the short-chain fatty acid profile, a critical aspect in maintaining gut health [99]. These *in vitro* findings, while intriguing and promising, are simply the first step in comprehensively understanding the full potential of that bread and its influence on the gut microbiota. The results must be substantiated by *in vivo* studies to ascertain the practicality of such an approach in a real-world context. It is crucial to remember that *in vitro* environments, while valuable for initial observations and hypotheses, may not fully encapsulate the complex interplays at work within a living organism. Thus, the translation of these findings to *in vivo* applications will provide the ultimate validation of their true significance.

Herbal Treatments for Celiac Disease

As a critical facet of the healthcare landscape, medical nutrition therapy has been firmly established as the sole effective method for the treatment of CD, as mentioned in detail above [100]. It is pertinent to note that this dietary strategy is not just another diet fed; rather, it is a stringent and mandatory recommendation for all individuals who have received a clinical diagnosis of CD. This therapeutic diet hinges on the fundamental understanding that the consumption of gluten by CD patients can result in severe intestinal inflammation and damage. Hence, the determination of safe gluten thresholds is crucial in managing this condition [101]. While the GFD necessitates the elimination of gluten-containing grains and their derivatives, it permits the consumption of an array of naturally gluten-free food categories. These include fish, lean cuts of meat, a diversity of fruits, and an assortment of vegetables. By focusing on these naturally gluten-free food groups, individuals with CD can maintain a balanced and nutrient-dense diet that supports overall health and disease management [102]. Moreover, it is vital for CD patients to be instructed about the importance of taking gluten-free multivitamins. As CD may impede the absorption of critical vitamins and minerals, supplementation can assist in averting deficiencies that could otherwise compromise the nutritional status and health of these patients [103].

An intriguing area of emerging research revolves around the therapeutic potential of various herbs for the management of CD. As delved deeper into this realm, it is crucial to note that this approach should always be explored under the guidance of healthcare professionals and should complement, rather than replace, the established GFD [104]. As research continues to unfold, the scientific community anticipates further insights into the benefits of these herbs, paving the way for more comprehensive and holistic approaches to managing CD.

Chamomile (*Matricaria chamomilla* L.), a member of the Asteraceae family, is a therapeutic plant that has a venerable tradition in herbal medicine, tracing its use back to thousands of years. Its diverse applications have established chamomile as a potent herbal remedy across cultures and throughout history. The efficacy of chamomile primarily manifests as an antiseptic, demonstrating profound capabilities in combating various microbial intrusions [105]. This characteristic extends its application to a range of conditions where microbial invasion is the root cause. In addition to its antiseptic properties, chamomile is also recognized for its potent anti-inflammatory effects. This feature underscores its significance in managing numerous conditions characterized by inflammation, ranging from minor irritations to severe systemic inflammation [106]. It has been instrumental in alleviating spasmodic conditions, most notably in the urinary tract, where it provides effective relief from associated swelling [107]. Simultaneously, it has been an essential aid for menstrual pain, providing comfort from cramps and other associated discomforts. Beyond its antiseptic, anti-inflammatory, and antispasmodic properties, chamomile also demonstrates other therapeutic potentials, including acting as a carminative, thereby aiding digestion and alleviating symptoms of gastrointestinal distress. Additionally, its healing properties have been leveraged in wound management, accelerating the process of recovery and tissue regeneration [108]. Lastly, the sedative qualities of chamomile provide a soothing effect, reducing anxiety, aiding sleep, and promoting overall relaxation. Thus, chamomile, with its rich range of therapeutic properties, continues to be a cornerstone in herbal treatments, as it has been for millennia.

Meadowsweet (*Filipendula ulmaria* L.) is a multifaceted herbal plant traditionally utilized for its diverse medicinal properties across several European countries. The comprehensive range of therapeutic uses of Meadowsweet spans a variety of health conditions, reflecting its broad spectrum of medicinal properties. In the capacity of a diuretic, meadowsweet plays an instrumental role in promoting renal health by facilitating the elimination of excess fluids and toxins from the body [109]. This attribute aids in the management of conditions related to fluid retention, further contributing to the regulation of blood pressure [109]. Concurrently, its utilization as an anti-hemorrhoidal agent underlines its effectiveness in managing the discomfort and complications associated with hemorrhoids. As a natural sedative, meadow sweet offers a holistic approach to managing anxiety and promoting sleep, thus playing a significant role in mental well-being. Its anti-inflammatory characteristics extend its applicability to numerous conditions characterized by inflammation, ranging from mild irritations to systemic inflammatory diseases [110]. Furthermore, the wound-healing properties of meadowsweet underline its utility in external applications, where it contributes to tissue regeneration and recovery. Additionally, it demonstrates analgesic properties, providing symptomatic relief from various forms of pain, further emphasizing its broad therapeutic scope [111]. Meadowsweet's antiulcerogenic attributes are particularly noteworthy, given the increasing prevalence of peptic ulcers. It helps prevent and manage peptic ulcers, providing a natural therapeutic option for mitigating this condition [112]. Moreover, it displays hypoglycemic properties, making it potentially beneficial for regulating blood sugar levels, a critical aspect of managing diabetes [113]. Finally, as an astringent, meadowsweet plays a crucial role in constricting tissues, thereby reducing secretions or discharges of bodily fluids.

Belonging to the illustrious mint family, lemon balm (*Melissa officinalis* L.), has established a considerable reputation in traditional medicinal practice owing to its extensive array of healing properties. Imbued with a delightful citrus fragrance and characterized by its distinctive leaves, lemon balm exemplifies the immense potential of medicinal plants in providing therapeutic benefits across a range of health conditions, primarily, lemon balm has been recognized for its carminative properties, efficiently relieving the discomfort caused by excess gas in the digestive system [114]. This alleviation of gastrointestinal distress is not limited merely to symptomatic relief but extends to the improvement of the overall digestive process. Indeed, lemon balm's ability to promote digestion underscores its role in enhancing gut health, thereby contributing to the body's overall nutritional uptake and energy production. The therapeutic potential of lemon balm is further amplified by its powerful antidepressant properties. In the face of the escalating incidence of mental health issues worldwide, lemon balm provides a holistic and natural approach to alleviating symptoms of depression, thereby offering a potential alternative or supplement to conventional pharmaceutical interventions [115]. Moreover, its strong antioxidant activities underscore lemon balm's contribution to cellular health by neutralizing harmful free radicals in the body [116]. This mechanism not only protects individual cells and tissues from oxidative damage but also contributes to the prevention of chronic diseases, including heart disease and cancer, that are closely linked to oxidative stress. Furthermore, lemon balm has been recognized for its notable antiviral properties, which equip it to combat various viral pathogens, thus bolstering the body's immune response [117]. This reinforces lemon balm's multi-faceted therapeutic potential, thereby broadening its utility in managing diverse health conditions. According to the authoritative German Commission E monograph, lemon balm is particularly recommended for alleviating gastrointestinal complaints, particularly cramps in the digestive tract and flatulent dyspepsia [117]. These therapeutic implications of lemon balm further affirm its enduring relevance in traditional medicinal practice, reinforcing its status as a versatile and efficacious medicinal plant.

Holding a distinguished position in traditional medicine systems worldwide, liquorice (*Glycyrrhiza glabra* L.), is a plant species recognized for its extensive ethnopharmacological value, predominantly found in subtropical and warm temperate regions; this plant species is distinguished by its sweet, anise-like flavor and a rich history of utilization in various therapeutic applications, each testifying to its comprehensive medicinal potential [118]. Foremost, liquorice has been lauded as a preventive agent for duodenal and gastric ulcers [118]. Ulcers, defined by the erosion of the stomach or duodenal lining, are a common health condition worldwide and can lead to severe complications if left untreated. In light of this, liquorice's anti-ulcerogenic properties can play a significant role in prophylaxis, reducing the risk and recurrence of such conditions and contributing to gastrointestinal health preservation. Beyond its anti-ulcerogenic properties, liquorice also comes into play in managing allergy-related conditions. Its use as an anti-inflammatory agent, particularly in cases of dyspepsia, underscores its versatility and potential to provide relief across a spectrum of allergic reactions [119]. Dyspepsia, characterized by chronic or recurrent discomfort in the upper abdomen, often presents with inflammation, and liquorice's ability to mitigate such inflammation points to its relevance in enhancing the quality of life for individuals affected by this condition. Its therapeutic scope further extends to include applications as an emmenagogue, a substance stimulating or increasing menstrual flow, thereby addressing issues of irregular menstrual cycles. Concurrently, it has been reported to possess contraceptive properties, illustrating its potential impact on reproductive health and family planning [118]. Moreover, its use as an anti-asthmatic, laxative, galactagogue, which promotes lactation in humans and other animals, and antiviral agent speaks to the multi-dimensional nature of its therapeutic value [120]. In essence, liquorice's role in folk therapy transcends merely symptomatic relief and delves into the broader realm of preventive and curative healthcare. It stands as a testament to the profound influence of traditional medicinal practices and the untapped potential of plant-derived therapies in today's modern medical landscape.

Peppermint (*Mentha piperita* L.), is an intriguing herbal specimen that belongs to the Lamiaceae (Labiatae) family, typified by an endless, lush green stem, and punctuated by vibrant purple flowers. An intriguing aspect of its botanical lineage is that it is essentially a hybrid plant, resulting from the intersection of two distinct species, namely spearmint (*Mentha spicata* L.) and water mint (*Mentha aquatica* L.) [121]. The amalgamation of these two species provides the potent medicinal properties and unique aromatic profile characteristic of peppermint. Held in high regard in numerous folk and traditional medicine systems around the world, peppermint has been utilized over centuries as a powerful tool in managing disorders related to the digestive and nervous systems. Its notable therapeutic repertoire is marked by its carminative and antispasmodic properties, which not only alleviate various gastrointestinal symptoms such as cramps and bloating but also effectively treat digestive complaints like anorexia, nausea, and diarrhea [122]. Interestingly, the benefits of this medicinal herb are not confined to the gastrointestinal tract; extending beyond digestive relief, peppermint also possesses remarkable antitumor properties, making it a potential natural alternative in cancer management strategies [121]. Its antimicrobial properties further underline its extensive therapeutic scope, offering an array of potential applications in treating various microbial infections. Additional beneficial attributes include its chemopreventive potential and renal actions. Chemoprevention refers to the use of natural or synthetic substances to prevent, suppress, or reverse the process of carcinogenesis, and peppermint's role in this is increasingly being recognized [123]. Meanwhile, its renal actions suggest potential beneficial effects on kidney health and function. Notably, it also boasts antiallergenic effects, making it an effective treatment for various allergy symptoms. This versatile herb's calming and soothing properties are beneficial to the nervous system, potentially helping to manage stress and anxiety, further illustrating the breadth of its medicinal properties [123]. Therefore, peppermint's diverse therapeutic capacities not only showcase its significant role in traditional medicine but also highlight the potential for its increased incorporation into modern medicinal practices. From digestive health to cancer prevention, peppermint stands as an emblem of nature's profound ability to heal and nurture health.

Fennel (*Foeniculum vulgare* Mill) belongs to the Umbelliferae (Apiaceae) family, a group of perennial herbs noted for their distinctive flower shape, reminiscent of an umbrella. Fennel has been steeped in medicinal usage for centuries and is renowned for its wide-ranging therapeutic properties, as evidenced by its incorporation into various traditional medicine systems [124]. One of the most widely recognized uses of fennel pertains to the realm of digestive health. It has long been used as an effective remedy for a plethora of gastrointestinal ailments, including stomach pain, constipation, and the condition known as irritable colon [124]. Furthermore, its carminative properties are highly sought after, particularly in the relief of flatulence. Some cultures also regard it as an appetite stimulant, which can be beneficial for individuals dealing with anorexia or other appetite disorders [125]. Beyond the digestive system, the utility of fennel extends to the respiratory, reproductive, and endocrine systems. In terms of respiratory health, its soothing properties have been employed for managing conditions such as asthma and bronchitis. In the domain of reproductive health, its emmenagogue function is widely recognized, facilitating, and regulating menstrual flow, and it has also been used as a treatment for leucorrhea, a vaginal discharge condition [126]. As a testament to its extensive medicinal potential, fennel has even been used in the management of fever, arthritis, and cancer, pointing to its potential anti-inflammatory and antitumor properties [127]. Moreover, fennel's role in addressing endocrine system disorders is of considerable interest, hinting at possible therapeutic potential in conditions such as diabetes or thyroid disorders. Other notable therapeutic uses of fennel include its application as a laxative, its purported benefits in liver health, evidenced by its use for liver pain, and its usage as a depurative, purifying and detoxifying the body [127]. Furthermore, it is worth noting that fennel has been utilized in mitigating symptoms of insomnia, suggesting potential sedative or relaxing properties. This provides a glimpse into the broad spectrum of ailments that this versatile plant can address, from digestive discomfort to sleep disorders, reflecting the impressive diversity of its therapeutic applications [127]. To conclude, fennel's myriad medicinal uses, as demonstrated in diverse traditional medicinal practices, underscore the vast potential of this therapeutic plant. Its comprehensive healing profile, spanning from digestive to endocrine health, underlines the immense promise of this humble herb in the arena of natural health and healing.

Slippery elm (*Ulmus rubra*) represents an intriguing instance of a medicinal plant whose therapeutic potential is obtained primarily from its inner bark. This plant, native to North America, is deeply rooted in the indigenous traditions of the region and has since permeated into a wider, global recognition within the herbal medicine sphere, as documented in the Natural Medicines Comprehensive Database and various scientific studies [128]. The applications of slippery elm in medicinal practice are impressively diverse, spanning a wide array of health issues and bodily systems [128]. Within the realm of upper respiratory ailments, slippery elm has long been favored as a potent remedy for sore throats. Its mucilaginous properties, yielding a gel-like substance when mixed with water, can coat the throat, thereby providing soothing relief from pain and irritation [129]. Furthermore, its beneficial effects extend to digestive health, an area where slippery elm is particularly known for its therapeutic contributions, including its use in the management of dyspepsia, colic, loose motions, and notably, irritable bowel syndrome, which has been substantiated by anecdotal reports and traditional medicinal practices [129]. These benefits can be ascribed in part to the mucilaginous substance it forms, which can create a protective barrier along the gastrointestinal tract. This coating action may alleviate various digestive issues by reducing inflammation, neutralizing acidity, and facilitating smoother digestion [129]. A particularly significant aspect of slippery elm's medicinal repertoire is its role in managing ulcers [130]. Evidence suggests that it may provide protection against stomach and duodenal ulcers, which can be attributed to its ability to produce a soothing, protective layer over these vulnerable areas, thereby reducing irritation and promoting healing. Similarly, it has also been used to ameliorate swelling of the colon, further highlighting its value in addressing gastrointestinal disorders [130]. Beyond its substantial applications in respiratory and digestive health, Slippy Elm's therapeutic scope embraces other areas of health as well.

Intriguingly, it has been enlisted in the fight against certain infectious diseases, such as septicemia of the urinary tract and syphilis, underscoring its potential antimicrobial properties. It has even been used in the expulsion of tapeworms, hinting at a possible role as an anthelmintic agent [130].

Green tea (*Camellia sinensis* L.), is an abundant source of numerous organic compounds, including a class of polyphenols that exert a myriad of biological effects [131]. A pivotal constituent amongst these compounds is Epigallocatechin-3-gallate (EGCG), which is primarily found in white and green tea varieties and demonstrates an interaction with the immunodominant peptide (32-mer gliadin), which plays a significant role in CD. This interaction between EGCG and gliadin not only illuminates new potential therapeutic avenues but also broadens the understanding of the mechanistic relationships at play within this complex condition [131, 132]. Furthermore, the evidence of green tea's protective role in chronic inflammatory ailments such as metabolic syndrome and inflammatory bowel disease has been reported across several research studies [133 - 135]. According to the results, green tea polyphenols were found to inhibit the digestion of gliadin proteins by obstructing the function of digestive proteases. This interaction results in the formation of a complex that diminishes the permeability-enhancing effect of gliadin on the intestinal wall, thus, compellingly pointing towards the promise of green tea polyphenols in the management of CD [135]. In addition, other studies have found that catechins found in green tea can inhibit gliadin digestion *in vitro*, leading to a reduction in gliadin-induced intestinal permeability and inflammation [136].

Echinacea, a genus belonging to the Asteraceae family, is noted for its potent immunostimulatory and anti-inflammatory effects [137]. This plant genus is rich in a variety of bioactive components, such as polysaccharides, caffeic acid derivatives, and alkyl amides, each contributing to its distinct therapeutic properties [138]. Medicinal preparations often favor three species of *Echinacea* for their notable properties: *E. angustifolia* DC., *E. pallida* Nutt., and *E. purpurea* L. These *Echinacea* species have been highlighted for their potential therapeutic role in addressing recurrent aphthous stomatitis, a clinical manifestation associated with CD [139]. However, it is important to note that *Echinacea* supplementation has been associated with alterations in the gastrointestinal microbiota, specifically an increase in the Bacteroides group. Considering the findings of previous studies, a role of *Bacteroides fragilis* in the pathogenesis of CD has been suggested, such alterations could potentially pose challenges for CD patients [140, 141]. Thus, while Echinacea offers promising therapeutic potential, its use must be guided by a comprehensive understanding of its effects on the complex ecosystem of the human gut.

An extensive body of scientific literature delineates the role of various plants, including cloves, cayenne pepper, and cinnamon, in modulating inflammatory responses, thus suggesting potential therapeutic benefits for conditions characterized by chronic inflammation [137, 142, 143]. Further extending the list of medicinal plants with notable gastrointestinal applications are species like coriander, ginger, and Ceylon leadwort that have demonstrated considerable efficacy in mitigating the symptoms associated with gastrointestinal disorders, thereby presenting intriguing possibilities for their incorporation into traditional and alternative treatment strategies [144]. The merit of certain herbal medicines in managing functional gastrointestinal disorders such as IBS is increasingly supported by robust evidence from randomized controlled trials. For instance, tormentil, carob bean juice, apple pectin, and peppermint oil have emerged as potential candidates for managing these complex gastrointestinal disorders [145]. These observations underscore the need for rigorous scientific investigation into the therapeutic potential, safety, and efficacy of these herbal supplements to guide their integration into standard clinical practice.

CONCLUSION

The only recognized treatment for CD is currently a strict GFD that requires significant dietary restrictions and presents numerous challenges due to the pervasive presence of gluten in many foods and beverages. As a consequence, recent research has been increasingly focused on identifying alternative treatments, particularly from medicinal herbs and other natural resources, to alleviate the burden of strict dietary adherence. This review has examined potential herbal treatments that could play a role in managing CD. A variety of plants with antioxidant, anti-inflammatory, antimicrobial, gastroprotective, and immunomodulatory properties have been discussed, which could potentially be utilized to control the gluten-mediated inflammation that characterizes CD. These natural remedies are characterized by their wide availability, low cost, and fewer side effects compared to conventional treatments, which might make them an attractive alternative for individuals contending with the demands of a strict GFD. Moreover, a significant role has been noted for gut microbiota in CD, adding an additional layer of complexity to the disease's management. The relationship between gut microbiota, CD, and dietary interventions has the potential to yield novel therapeutic strategies when fully understood. In conclusion, while a GFD remains the cornerstone of CD management, the potential of natural remedies such as herbal treatment and a comprehensive understanding of gut microbiota's role might pave the way for enhanced treatment strategies. Nevertheless, the validation of these potential alternative treatments and the complete understanding of the intricate interplay between diet, microbiota, and CD necessitates further rigorous research.

REFERENCES

[1]   Hill ID, Bhatnagar S, Cameron DJS, *et al.* Celiac Disease: Working Group Report of the First World Congress of Pediatric Gastroenterology, Hepatology, and Nutrition. J Pediatr Gastroenterol Nutr 2002; 35 (Suppl. 2): S78-88.
[http://dx.doi.org/10.1097/00005176-200208002-00004] [PMID: 12192175]

[2]   Cummins AG, Roberts-Thomson IC. Prevalence of celiac disease in the Asia–Pacific region. J Gastroenterol Hepatol 2009; 24(8): 1347-51.
[http://dx.doi.org/10.1111/j.1440-1746.2009.05932.x] [PMID: 19702902]

[3]   Casella G, Bordo BM, Schalling R, *et al.* Neurological disorders and celiac disease. Minerva Gastroenterol Dietol 2016; 62(2): 197-206.
[PMID: 26619901]

[4]   Catassi C, Gatti S, Lionetti E. World perspective and celiac disease epidemiology. Dig Dis 2015; 33(2): 141-6.
[http://dx.doi.org/10.1159/000369518] [PMID: 25925915]

[5]   Lebwohl B, Rubio-Tapia A. Epidemiology, presentation, and diagnosis of celiac disease. Gastroenterology 2021; 160(1): 63-75.
[http://dx.doi.org/10.1053/j.gastro.2020.06.098] [PMID: 32950520]

[6]   Iversen R, Sollid LM. The immunobiology and pathogenesis of celiac disease. Annu Rev Pathol 2023; 18(1): 47-70.
[http://dx.doi.org/10.1146/annurev-pathmechdis-031521-032634] [PMID: 36067801]

[7]   Raiteri A, Granito A, Giamperoli A, Catenaro T, Negrini G, Tovoli F. Current guidelines for the management of celiac disease: A systematic review with comparative analysis. World J Gastroenterol 2022; 28(1): 154-76.
[http://dx.doi.org/10.3748/wjg.v28.i1.154] [PMID: 35125825]

[8]   Poddighe D, Abdukhakimova D. Celiac Disease in Asia beyond the Middle East and Indian subcontinent: Epidemiological burden and diagnostic barriers. World J Gastroenterol 2021; 27(19): 2251-6.
[http://dx.doi.org/10.3748/wjg.v27.i19.2251] [PMID: 34040319]

[9]   Cataldo F, Montalto G. Celiac disease in the developing countries: A new and challenging public health problem. World J Gastroenterol 2007; 13(15): 2153-9.
[http://dx.doi.org/10.3748/wjg.v13.i15.2153] [PMID: 17465493]

[10]   Poddighe D, Rakhimzhanova M, Marchenko Y, Catassi C. Pediatric celiac disease in central and east Asia: current knowledge and prevalence. Medicina (Kaunas) 2019; 55(1): 11.
[http://dx.doi.org/10.3390/medicina55010011] [PMID: 30642036]

[11]   Elsurer R, Tatar G, Simsek H, Balaban YH, Aydinli M, Sokmensuer C. Celiac disease in the Turkish population. Dig Dis Sci 2005; 50(1): 136-42.
[http://dx.doi.org/10.1007/s10620-005-1291-z] [PMID: 15712651]

[12]   Lee SK, Lo W, Memeo L, Rotterdam H, Green PHR. Duodenal histology in patients with celiac disease after treatment with a gluten-free diet. Gastrointest Endosc 2003; 57(2): 187-91.
[http://dx.doi.org/10.1067/mge.2003.54] [PMID: 12556782]

[13]   Ivarsson A, Persson LÅ, Nyström L, Hernell O. The Swedish coeliac disease epidemic with a prevailing twofold higher risk in girls compared to boys may reflect gender specific risk factors. Eur J Epidemiol 2002; 18(7): 677-84.
[http://dx.doi.org/10.1023/A:1024873630588] [PMID: 12952142]

[14]   Fasano A. Clinical presentation of celiac disease in the pediatric population. Gastroenterology 2005; 128(4) (Suppl. 1): S68-73.
[http://dx.doi.org/10.1053/j.gastro.2005.02.015] [PMID: 15825129]

[15]   Mustalahti K. Unusual manifestations of celiac disease. Indian J Pediatr 2006; 73(8): 711-6.
       [http://dx.doi.org/10.1007/BF02898450] [PMID: 16936367]

[16]   Cataldo F, Marino V. Increased prevalence of autoimmune diseases in first-degree relatives of patients
       with celiac disease. J Pediatr Gastroenterol Nutr 2003; 36(4): 470-3.
       [PMID: 12658037]

[17]   Bajor J, Szakács Z, Farkas N, *et al.* Classical celiac disease is more frequent with a double dose of
       HLA-DQB1*02: A systematic review with meta-analysis. PLoS One 2019; 14(2): e0212329.
       [http://dx.doi.org/10.1371/journal.pone.0212329] [PMID: 30763397]

[18]   Di Sabatino A, Corazza GR. Coeliac disease. Lancet 2009; 373(9673): 1480-93.
       [http://dx.doi.org/10.1016/S0140-6736(09)60254-3] [PMID: 19394538]

[19]   Molberg Ø, McAdam S, Lundin KEA, *et al.* T cells from celiac disease lesions recognize gliadin
       epitopes deamidated in situ by endogenous tissue transglutaminase. Eur J Immunol 2001; 31(5): 1317-
       23.
       [http://dx.doi.org/10.1002/1521-4141(200105)31:5<1317::AID-IMMU1317>3.0.CO;2-I]   [PMID:
       11465088]

[20]   Catassi C, Verdu EF, Bai JC, Lionetti E. Coeliac disease. Lancet 2022; 399(10344): 2413-26.
       [http://dx.doi.org/10.1016/S0140-6736(22)00794-2] [PMID: 35691302]

[21]   Goddard CJR, Gillett HR. Complications of coeliac disease: are all patients at risk? Postgrad Med J
       2006; 82(973): 705-12.
       [http://dx.doi.org/10.1136/pgmj.2006.048876] [PMID: 17099088]

[22]   Green PHR, Krishnareddy S, Lebwohl B. Clinical manifestations of celiac disease. Dig Dis 2015;
       33(2): 137-40.
       [http://dx.doi.org/10.1159/000370204] [PMID: 25925914]

[23]   Rostom A, Murray JA, Kagnoff MF. American Gastroenterological Association (AGA) Institute
       technical review on the diagnosis and management of celiac disease. Gastroenterology 2006; 131(6):
       1981-2002.
       [http://dx.doi.org/10.1053/j.gastro.2006.10.004] [PMID: 17087937]

[24]   Wahab PJ, Meijer JWR, Goerres MS, Mulder CJJ. Coeliac disease: changing views on gluten-sensitive
       enteropathy. Scand J Gastroenterol 2002; 37(236): 60-5.
       [http://dx.doi.org/10.1080/003655202320621472] [PMID: 12408506]

[25]   Turnbaugh PJ, Ley RE, Hamady M, Fraser-Liggett CM, Knight R, Gordon JI. The human microbiome
       project. Nature 2007; 449(7164): 804-10.
       [http://dx.doi.org/10.1038/nature06244] [PMID: 17943116]

[26]   Thursby E, Juge N. Introduction to the human gut microbiota. Biochem J 2017; 474(11): 1823-36.
       [http://dx.doi.org/10.1042/BCJ20160510] [PMID: 28512250]

[27]   Miele L, Giorgio V, Alberelli MA, De Candia E, Gasbarrini A, Grieco A. Impact of gut microbiota on
       obesity, diabetes, and cardiovascular disease risk. Curr Cardiol Rep 2015; 17(12): 120.
       [http://dx.doi.org/10.1007/s11886-015-0671-z] [PMID: 26497040]

[28]   Belenguer A, Holtrop G, Duncan SH, *et al.* Rates of production and utilization of lactate by microbial
       communities from the human colon. FEMS Microbiol Ecol 2011; 77(1): 107-19.
       [http://dx.doi.org/10.1111/j.1574-6941.2011.01086.x] [PMID: 21395623]

[29]   Frank DN, St Amand AL, Feldman RA, Boedeker EC, Harpaz N, Pace NR. Molecular-phylogenetic
       characterization of microbial community imbalances in human inflammatory bowel diseases. Proc
       Natl Acad Sci USA 2007; 104(34): 13780-5.
       [http://dx.doi.org/10.1073/pnas.0706625104] [PMID: 17699621]

[30]   Eckburg PB, Relman DA. The role of microbes in Crohn's disease. Clin Infect Dis 2007; 44(2): 256-
       62.

[http://dx.doi.org/10.1086/510385] [PMID: 17173227]

[31]   Herrema H, IJzerman RG, Nieuwdorp M. Emerging role of intestinal microbiota and microbial metabolites in metabolic control. Diabetologia 2017; 60(4): 613-7.
[http://dx.doi.org/10.1007/s00125-016-4192-0] [PMID: 28013341]

[32]   Clemente JC, Ursell LK, Parfrey LW, Knight R. The impact of the gut microbiota on human health: an integrative view. Cell 2012; 148(6): 1258-70.
[http://dx.doi.org/10.1016/j.cell.2012.01.035] [PMID: 22424233]

[33]   Reyes A, Haynes M, Hanson N, *et al*. Viruses in the faecal microbiota of monozygotic twins and their mothers. Nature 2010; 466(7304): 334-8.
[http://dx.doi.org/10.1038/nature09199] [PMID: 20631792]

[34]   Turnbaugh PJ, Ridaura VK, Faith JJ, Rey FE, Knight R, Gordon JI. The effect of diet on the human gut microbiome: a metagenomic analysis in humanized gnotobiotic mice. Sci Transl Med 2009; 1(6): 6ra14-6ra14.
[http://dx.doi.org/10.1126/scitranslmed.3000322]

[35]   Ramirez-Farias C, Slezak K, Fuller Z, Duncan A, Holtrop G, Louis P. Effect of inulin on the human gut microbiota: stimulation of *Bifidobacterium adolescentis* and *Faecalibacterium prausnitzii*. Br J Nutr 2009; 101(4): 541-50.
[http://dx.doi.org/10.1017/S0007114508019880] [PMID: 18590586]

[36]   Shin NR, Whon TW, Bae JW. Proteobacteria: microbial signature of dysbiosis in gut microbiota. Trends Biotechnol 2015; 33(9): 496-503.
[http://dx.doi.org/10.1016/j.tibtech.2015.06.011] [PMID: 26210164]

[37]   Cani PD, Amar J, Iglesias MA, *et al*. Metabolic endotoxemia initiates obesity and insulin resistance. Diabetes 2007; 56(7): 1761-72.
[http://dx.doi.org/10.2337/db06-1491] [PMID: 17456850]

[38]   De Filippo C, Cavalieri D, Di Paola M, *et al*. Impact of diet in shaping gut microbiota revealed by a comparative study in children from Europe and rural Africa. Proc Natl Acad Sci USA 2010; 107(33): 14691-6.
[http://dx.doi.org/10.1073/pnas.1005963107] [PMID: 20679230]

[39]   David LA, Maurice CF, Carmody RN, *et al*. Diet rapidly and reproducibly alters the human gut microbiome. Nature 2014; 505(7484): 559-63.
[http://dx.doi.org/10.1038/nature12820] [PMID: 24336217]

[40]   Caminero A, Herrán AR, Nistal E, *et al*. Diversity of the cultivable human gut microbiome involved in gluten metabolism: isolation of microorganisms with potential interest for coeliac disease. FEMS Microbiol Ecol 2014; 88(2): 309-19.
[http://dx.doi.org/10.1111/1574-6941.12295] [PMID: 24499426]

[41]   Olivares M, Laparra M, Sanz Y. Influence of Bifidobacterium longum CECT 7347 and gliadin peptides on intestinal epithelial cell proteome. J Agric Food Chem 2011; 59(14): 7666-71.
[http://dx.doi.org/10.1021/jf201212m] [PMID: 21651295]

[42]   Caminero A, Galipeau HJ, McCarville JL, *et al*. Duodenal bacteria from patients with celiac disease and healthy subjects distinctly affect gluten breakdown and immunogenicity. Gastroenterology 2016; 151(4): 670-83.
[http://dx.doi.org/10.1053/j.gastro.2016.06.041] [PMID: 27373514]

[43]   Heyman M, Abed J, Lebreton C, Cerf-Bensussan N. Intestinal permeability in coeliac disease: insight into mechanisms and relevance to pathogenesis. Gut 2012; 61(9): 1355-64.
[http://dx.doi.org/10.1136/gutjnl-2011-300327] [PMID: 21890812]

[44]   Vorobjova T, Raikkerus H, Kadaja L, *et al*. Circulating zonulin correlates with density of enteroviruses and tolerogenic dendritic cells in the small bowel mucosa of celiac disease patients. Dig Dis Sci 2017; 62(2): 358-71.

[http://dx.doi.org/10.1007/s10620-016-4403-z] [PMID: 27995404]

[45] Lammers KM, Lu R, Brownley J, *et al.* Gliadin induces an increase in intestinal permeability and zonulin release by binding to the chemokine receptor CXCR3. Gastroenterology 2008; 135(1): 194-204.e3.
[http://dx.doi.org/10.1053/j.gastro.2008.03.023] [PMID: 18485912]

[46] Hooper LV, Littman DR, Macpherson AJ. Interactions between the microbiota and the immune system. Science 2012; 336(6086): 1268-73.
[http://dx.doi.org/10.1126/science.1223490] [PMID: 22674334]

[47] Serena G, Yan S, Camhi S, *et al.* Proinflammatory cytokine interferon-γ and microbiome-derived metabolites dictate epigenetic switch between forkhead box protein 3 isoforms in coeliac disease. Clin Exp Immunol 2017; 187(3): 490-506.
[http://dx.doi.org/10.1111/cei.12911] [PMID: 27936497]

[48] Lindfors K, Blomqvist T, Juuti-Uusitalo K, *et al.* Live probiotic *Bifidobacterium lactis* bacteria inhibit the toxic effects induced by wheat gliadin in epithelial cell culture. Clin Exp Immunol 2008; 152(3): 552-8.
[http://dx.doi.org/10.1111/j.1365-2249.2008.03635.x] [PMID: 18422736]

[49] Medina M, De Palma G, Ribes-Koninckx C, Calabuig M, Sanz Y. Bifidobacterium strains suppress *in vitro* the pro-inflammatory milieu triggered by the large intestinal microbiota of coeliac patients. J Inflamm (Lond) 2008; 5(1): 19.
[http://dx.doi.org/10.1186/1476-9255-5-19] [PMID: 18980693]

[50] Laparra JM, Olivares M, Gallina O, Sanz Y. Bifidobacterium longum CECT 7347 modulates immune responses in a gliadin-induced enteropathy animal model. PLoS One 2012; 7(2): e30744.
[http://dx.doi.org/10.1371/journal.pone.0030744] [PMID: 22348021]

[51] Zyrek AA, Cichon C, Helms S, Enders C, Sonnenborn U, Schmidt MA. Molecular mechanisms underlying the probiotic effects of *Escherichia coli* Nissle 1917 involve ZO-2 and PKC? redistribution resulting in tight junction and epithelial barrier repair. Cell Microbiol 2007; 9(3): 804-16.
[http://dx.doi.org/10.1111/j.1462-5822.2006.00836.x] [PMID: 17087734]

[52] D'Arienzo R, Stefanile R, Maurano F, *et al.* Immunomodulatory effects of Lactobacillus casei administration in a mouse model of gliadin-sensitive enteropathy. Scand J Immunol 2011; 74(4): 335-41.
[http://dx.doi.org/10.1111/j.1365-3083.2011.02582.x] [PMID: 21615450]

[53] Nadal I, Donant E, Ribes-Koninckx C, Calabuig M, Sanz Y, Sanz Y. Imbalance in the composition of the duodenal microbiota of children with coeliac disease. J Med Microbiol 2007; 56(12): 1669-74.
[http://dx.doi.org/10.1099/jmm.0.47410-0] [PMID: 18033837]

[54] De Palma G, Nadal I, Medina M, *et al.* Intestinal dysbiosis and reduced immunoglobulin-coated bacteria associated with coeliac disease in children. BMC Microbiol 2010; 10(1): 63.
[http://dx.doi.org/10.1186/1471-2180-10-63] [PMID: 20181275]

[55] Collado MC, Donat E, Ribes-Koninckx C, Calabuig M, Sanz Y. Imbalances in faecal and duodenal Bifidobacterium species composition in active and non-active coeliac disease. BMC Microbiol 2008; 8(1): 232.
[http://dx.doi.org/10.1186/1471-2180-8-232] [PMID: 19102766]

[56] Collado MC, Donat E, Ribes-Koninckx C, Calabuig M, Sanz Y. Specific duodenal and faecal bacterial groups associated with paediatric coeliac disease. J Clin Pathol 2009; 62(3): 264-9.
[http://dx.doi.org/10.1136/jcp.2008.061366] [PMID: 18996905]

[57] Ou G, Hedberg M, Hörstedt P, *et al.* Proximal small intestinal microbiota and identification of rod-shaped bacteria associated with childhood celiac disease. Am J Gastroenterol 2009; 104(12): 3058-67.
[http://dx.doi.org/10.1038/ajg.2009.524] [PMID: 19755974]

[58] Niewinski MM. Advances in celiac disease and gluten-free diet. J Am Diet Assoc 2008; 108(4): 661-

72.
[http://dx.doi.org/10.1016/j.jada.2008.01.011] [PMID: 18375224]

[59]   Lionetti E, Gatti S, Galeazzi T, *et al.* Safety of oats in children with celiac disease: a double-blind, randomized, placebo controlled trial. J Pediatr 2018; 194: 116-122.e2.
[http://dx.doi.org/10.1016/j.jpeds.2017.10.062] [PMID: 29478494]

[60]   Tapsas D, Fälth-Magnusson K, Högberg L, Hammersjö JÅ, Hollén E. Swedish children with celiac disease comply well with a gluten-free diet, and most include oats without reporting any adverse effects: a long-term follow-up study. Nutr Res 2014; 34(5): 436-41.
[http://dx.doi.org/10.1016/j.nutres.2014.04.006] [PMID: 24916557]

[61]   Pinto-Sánchez MI, Causada-Calo N, Bercik P, *et al.* Safety of adding oats to a gluten-free diet for patients with celiac disease: systematic review and meta-analysis of clinical and observational studies. Gastroenterology 2017; 153(2): 395-409.e3.
[http://dx.doi.org/10.1053/j.gastro.2017.04.009] [PMID: 28431885]

[62]   Murray JA, Watson T, Clearman B, Mitros F. Effect of a gluten-free diet on gastrointestinal symptoms in celiac disease. Am J Clin Nutr 2004; 79(4): 669-73.
[http://dx.doi.org/10.1093/ajcn/79.4.669] [PMID: 15051613]

[63]   See JA, Kaukinen K, Makharia GK, Gibson PR, Murray JA. Practical insights into gluten-free diets. Nat Rev Gastroenterol Hepatol 2015; 12(10): 580-91.
[http://dx.doi.org/10.1038/nrgastro.2015.156] [PMID: 26392070]

[64]   Studerus D, Hampe EI, Fahrer D, Wilhelmi M, Vavricka SR. Cross-contamination with gluten by using kitchen utensils: fact or fiction? J Food Prot 2018; 81(10): 1679-84.
[http://dx.doi.org/10.4315/0362-028X.JFP-17-383] [PMID: 30230372]

[65]   Verma A, Gatti S, Galeazzi T, *et al.* Gluten contamination in naturally or labeled gluten-free products marketed in Italy. Nutrients 2017; 9(2): 115-25.
[http://dx.doi.org/10.3390/nu9020115] [PMID: 28178205]

[66]   Oliveira OMV, Zandonadi RP, Gandolfi L, de Almeida RC, Almeida LM, Pratesi R. Evaluation of the presence of gluten in beans served at selfservice restaurants: a problem for celiac disease carriers. J Culin Sci Technol 2014; 12(1): 22-33.
[http://dx.doi.org/10.1080/15428052.2013.798606]

[67]   Farage P, Puppin Zandonadi R, Cortez Ginani V, Gandolfi L, Yoshio Nakano E, Pratesi R. Gluten-free diet: From development to assessment of a check-list designed for the prevention of gluten cross-contamination in food services. Nutrients 2018; 10(9): 1274-86.
[http://dx.doi.org/10.3390/nu10091274] [PMID: 30201860]

[68]   Hlywiak KH. Hidden sources of gluten. Pract Gastroenterol 2008; 32: 27-39.

[69]   Akobeng AK, Thomas AG. Systematic review: tolerable amount of gluten for people with coeliac disease. Aliment Pharmacol Ther 2008; 27(11): 1044-52.
[http://dx.doi.org/10.1111/j.1365-2036.2008.03669.x] [PMID: 18315587]

[70]   Theethira TG, Dennis M. Celiac disease and the gluten-free diet: consequences and recommendations for improvement. Dig Dis 2015; 33(2): 175-82.
[http://dx.doi.org/10.1159/000369504] [PMID: 25925920]

[71]   Syage JA, Kelly CP, Dickason MA, *et al.* Determination of gluten consumption in celiac disease patients on a gluten-free diet. Am J Clin Nutr 2018; 107(2): 201-7.
[http://dx.doi.org/10.1093/ajcn/nqx049] [PMID: 29529159]

[72]   Falcomer AL, Santos Araújo L, Farage P, Santos Monteiro J, Yoshio Nakano E, Puppin Zandonadi R. Gluten contamination in food services and industry: A systematic review. Crit Rev Food Sci Nutr 2018; 60(2): 1-15.
[PMID: 30582343]

[73]   Bascuñán KA, Vespa MC, Araya M. Celiac disease: understanding the gluten-free diet. Eur J Nutr

2017; 56(2): 449-59.
[http://dx.doi.org/10.1007/s00394-016-1238-5] [PMID: 27334430]

[74] Melini V, Melini F. Gluten-free diet: gaps and needs for a healthier diet. Nutrients 2019; 11(1): 170-91.
[http://dx.doi.org/10.3390/nu11010170] [PMID: 30650530]

[75] Cornicelli M, Saba M, Machello N, Silano M, Neuhold S. Nutritional composition of gluten-free food versus regular food sold in the Italian market. Dig Liver Dis 2018; 50(12): 1305-8.
[http://dx.doi.org/10.1016/j.dld.2018.04.028] [PMID: 29857960]

[76] Missbach B, Schwingshackl L, Billmann A, *et al.* Gluten-free food database: the nutritional quality and cost of packaged gluten-free foods. PeerJ 2015; 3: e1337.
[http://dx.doi.org/10.7717/peerj.1337] [PMID: 26528408]

[77] Bagolin do Nascimento A, Medeiros Rataichesck Fiates G, dos Anjos A, Teixeira E. Availability, cost and nutritional composition of gluten-free products. Br Food J 2014; 116(12): 1842-52.
[http://dx.doi.org/10.1108/BFJ-05-2013-0131]

[78] Calvo-Lerma J, Crespo-Escobar P, Martínez-Barona S, Fornés-Ferrer V, Donat E, Ribes-Koninckx C. Differences in the macronutrient and dietary fibre profile of gluten-free products as compared to their gluten-containing counterparts. Eur J Clin Nutr 2019; 73(6): 930-6.
[http://dx.doi.org/10.1038/s41430-018-0385-6] [PMID: 30647439]

[79] Levran N, Wilschanski M, Livovsky J, *et al.* Obesogenic habits among children and their families in response to initiation of gluten-free diet. Eur J Pediatr 2018; 177(6): 859-66.
[http://dx.doi.org/10.1007/s00431-018-3128-8] [PMID: 29594339]

[80] Vici G, Belli L, Biondi M, Polzonetti V. Gluten free diet and nutrient deficiencies: A review. Clin Nutr 2016; 35(6): 1236-41.
[http://dx.doi.org/10.1016/j.clnu.2016.05.002] [PMID: 27211234]

[81] Churruca I, Larretxi I, Lasa A. Gluten-free diet: nutritional status and dietary habits of celiac patients nutritional and analytical approaches of gluten-free diet in celiac disease. Springer 2017; pp. 79-94.
[http://dx.doi.org/10.1007/978-3-319-53342-1_6]

[82] Nardo GD, Villa MP, Conti L, *et al.* Nutritional deficiencies in children with celiac disease resulting from a gluten-free diet: a systematic review. Nutrients 2019; 11(7): 1588.
[http://dx.doi.org/10.3390/nu11071588] [PMID: 31337023]

[83] Öhlund K, Olsson C, Hernell O, Öhlund I. Dietary shortcomings in children on a gluten-free diet. J Hum Nutr Diet 2010; 23(3): 294-300.
[http://dx.doi.org/10.1111/j.1365-277X.2010.01060.x] [PMID: 20337845]

[84] Penagini F, Dilillo D, Meneghin F, Mameli C, Fabiano V, Zuccotti G. Gluten-free diet in children: an approach to a nutritionally adequate and balanced diet. Nutrients 2013; 5(11): 4553-65.
[http://dx.doi.org/10.3390/nu5114553] [PMID: 24253052]

[85] Alvarez-Jubete L, Arendt EK, Gallagher E. Nutritive value of pseudocereals and their increasing use as functional gluten-free ingredients. Trends Food Sci Technol 2010; 21(2): 106-13.
[http://dx.doi.org/10.1016/j.tifs.2009.10.014]

[86] Capriles VD, Arêas JAG. Approaches to reduce the glycemic response of gluten-free products: *in vivo* and *in vitro* studies. Food Funct 2016; 7(3): 1266-72.
[http://dx.doi.org/10.1039/C5FO01264C] [PMID: 26838096]

[87] Drabińska N, Jarocka-Cyrta E, Markiewicz L, Krupa-Kozak U. The effect of oligofructose-enriched inulin on faecal bacterial counts and microbiota-associated characteristics in celiac disease children following a gluten-free diet: results of a randomized, placebo-controlled trial. Nutrients 2018; 10(2): 201.
[http://dx.doi.org/10.3390/nu10020201] [PMID: 29439526]

[88] Gentile CL, Weir TL. The gut microbiota at the intersection of diet and human health. Science 2018;

362(6416): 776-80.
[http://dx.doi.org/10.1126/science.aau5812] [PMID: 30442802]

[89]   Kolodziejczyk AA, Zheng D, Elinav E. Diet–microbiota interactions and personalized nutrition. Nat Rev Microbiol 2019; 17(12): 742-53.
[http://dx.doi.org/10.1038/s41579-019-0256-8] [PMID: 31541197]

[90]   Marco ML, Heeney D, Binda S, *et al.* Health benefits of fermented foods: microbiota and beyond. Curr Opin Biotechnol 2017; 44: 94-102.
[http://dx.doi.org/10.1016/j.copbio.2016.11.010] [PMID: 27998788]

[91]   Simpson HL, Campbell BJ. Review article: dietary fibre-microbiota interactions. Aliment Pharmacol Ther 2015; 42(2): 158-79.
[http://dx.doi.org/10.1111/apt.13248] [PMID: 26011307]

[92]   Scott KP, Gratz SW, Sheridan PO, Flint HJ, Duncan SH. The influence of diet on the gut microbiota. Pharmacol Res 2013; 69(1): 52-60.
[http://dx.doi.org/10.1016/j.phrs.2012.10.020] [PMID: 23147033]

[93]   Sanz Y. Microbiome and Gluten. Ann Nutr Metab 2015; 67(2) (Suppl. 2): 28-41.
[PMID: 26605783]

[94]   Bonder MJ, Tigchelaar EF, Cai X, *et al.* The influence of a short-term gluten-free diet on the human gut microbiome. Genome Med 2016; 8(1): 45.
[http://dx.doi.org/10.1186/s13073-016-0295-y] [PMID: 27102333]

[95]   Sanz Y. Effects of a gluten-free diet on gut microbiota and immune function in healthy adult humans. Gut Microbes 2010; 1(3): 135-7.
[http://dx.doi.org/10.4161/gmic.1.3.11868] [PMID: 21327021]

[96]   Calabriso N, Scoditti E, Massaro M, *et al.* Non-celiac gluten sensitivity and protective role of dietary polyphenols. Nutrients 2022; 14(13): 2679.
[http://dx.doi.org/10.3390/nu14132679] [PMID: 35807860]

[97]   Hansen LBS, Roager HM, Søndertoft NB, *et al.* A low-gluten diet induces changes in the intestinal microbiome of healthy Danish adults. Nat Commun 2018; 9(1): 4630-43.
[http://dx.doi.org/10.1038/s41467-018-07019-x] [PMID: 30425247]

[98]   Caminero A, Meisel M, Jabri B, Verdu EF. Mechanisms by which gut microorganisms influence food sensitivities. Nat Rev Gastroenterol Hepatol 2019; 16(1): 7-18.
[http://dx.doi.org/10.1038/s41575-018-0064-z] [PMID: 30214038]

[99]   Bevilacqua A, Costabile A, Bergillos-Meca T, *et al.* Impact of gluten-friendly bread on the metabolism and function of *in vitro* gut microbiota in healthy human and coeliac subjects. PLoS One 2016; 11(9): e0162770.
[http://dx.doi.org/10.1371/journal.pone.0162770] [PMID: 27632361]

[100]   Mohn A, Cerruto M, Iafusco D, *et al.* Celiac disease in children and adolescents with type I diabetes: importance of hypoglycemia. J Pediatr Gastroenterol Nutr 2001; 32(1): 37-40.
[PMID: 11176322]

[101]   Stern M, Ciclitira PJ, van Eckert R, *et al.* Analysis and clinical effects of gluten in coeliac disease. Eur J Gastroenterol Hepatol 2001; 13(6): 741-7.
[http://dx.doi.org/10.1097/00042737-200106000-00023] [PMID: 11434606]

[102]   Tosun MS, Ertekin V, Selimoğlu MA. Autoimmune hepatitis associated with celiac disease in childhood. Eur J Gastroenterol Hepatol 2010; 22(7): 898-9.
[http://dx.doi.org/10.1097/MEG.0b013e32832faf09] [PMID: 20535074]

[103]   Dias R, Pereira CB, Pérez-Gregorio R, Mateus N, Freitas V. Recent advances on dietary polyphenol's potential roles in Celiac Disease. Trends Food Sci Technol 2021; 107: 213-25.
[http://dx.doi.org/10.1016/j.tifs.2020.10.033]

[104] Someya N, Endo MY, Fukuba Y, Hayashi N. Blood flow responses in celiac and superior mesenteric arteries in the initial phase of digestion. Am J Physiol Regul Integr Comp Physiol 2008; 294(6): R1790-6.
[http://dx.doi.org/10.1152/ajpregu.00553.2007] [PMID: 18385466]

[105] El Mihyaoui A, Esteves da Silva JCG, Charfi S, Candela Castillo ME, Lamarti A, Arnao MB. Chamomile (*Matricaria chamomilla* L.): A review of ethnomedicinal use, phytochemistry and pharmacological uses. Life (Basel) 2022; 12(4): 479.
[http://dx.doi.org/10.3390/life12040479] [PMID: 35454969]

[106] Catani MV, Rinaldi F, Tullio V, Gasperi V, Savini I. Comparative analysis of phenolic composition of six commercially available chamomile (Matricaria chamomillaL.) extracts: Potential biological implications. Int J Mol Sci 2021; 22(19): 10601.
[http://dx.doi.org/10.3390/ijms221910601] [PMID: 34638940]

[107] Piknová Ľ, Brežná B, Kuchta T. Detection of gluten-containing cereals in food by 5′-nuclease real-time polymerase chain reaction. J Food Nutr Res 2008; 47(3): 114-9.

[108] de Sousa JS. Enzymatic treatment of celiac disease. J Pediatr Gastroenterol Nutr 2004; 38(2): 229.
[PMID: 14734892]

[109] Auricchio R, Troncone R. Can celiac disease be prevented? Front Immunol 2021; 12: 672148.
[http://dx.doi.org/10.3389/fimmu.2021.672148] [PMID: 34054850]

[110] Baranenko D, Bespalov V, Nadtochii L, *et al.* Development of encapsulated extracts on the basis of meadowsweet (Filipendula ulmaria) in the composition of functional foods with oncoprotective properties. Agro Res 2019; 17(5): 1829-38.

[111] Edwards SE, da Costa Rocha I, Williamson EM, *et al.* Phytopharmacy: An evidence-based guide to herbal medicinal products Chicester. John Wiley & Sons 2015.
[http://dx.doi.org/10.1002/9781118543436]

[112] Marti T, Molberg Ø, Li Q, Gray GM, Khosla C, Sollid LM. Prolyl endopeptidase-mediated destruction of T cell epitopes in whole gluten: chemical and immunological characterization. J Pharmacol Exp Ther 2005; 312(1): 19-26.
[http://dx.doi.org/10.1124/jpet.104.073312] [PMID: 15358813]

[113] Matuz J, Bartók T, Mórocz-Salamon K, Bóna L. Structure and potential allergenic character of cereal proteins I. Protein content and amino acid composition. Cereal Res Commun 2000; 28(3): 263-70.
[http://dx.doi.org/10.1007/BF03543603]

[114] Stepniak D, Spaenij-Dekking L, Mitea C, *et al.* Highly efficient gluten degradation with a newly identified prolyl endoprotease: implications for celiac disease. Am J Physiol Gastrointest Liver Physiol 2006; 291(4): G621-9.
[http://dx.doi.org/10.1152/ajpgi.00034.2006] [PMID: 16690904]

[115] Pastorino G, Cornara L, Soares S, Rodrigues F, Oliveira MBPP. Liquorice (*Glycyrrhiza glabra*): A phytochemical and pharmacological review. Phytother Res 2018; 32(12): 2323-39.
[http://dx.doi.org/10.1002/ptr.6178] [PMID: 30117204]

[116] Karkanis A, Martins N, Petropoulos SA, Ferreira ICFR. Phytochemical composition, health effects, and crop management of liquorice (*Glycyrrhiza glabra* L.): A medicinal plant. Food Rev Int 2018; 34(2): 182-203.
[http://dx.doi.org/10.1080/87559129.2016.1261300]

[117] Gowthaman V, Sharma D, Biswas A, Deo C. Liquorice (glycyrrhiza glabra) herb as a poultry feed additive- A review. Letters In Animal Biology 2021; 1(2): 14-20.
[http://dx.doi.org/10.62310/liab.v1i2.68]

[118] Stenman SM, Venäläinen JI, Lindfors K, *et al.* Enzymatic detoxification of gluten by germinating wheat proteases: Implications for new treatment of celiac disease. Ann Med 2009; 41(5): 390-400.
[http://dx.doi.org/10.1080/07853890902878138] [PMID: 19353359]

[119] Tsai ML, Wu CT, Lin TF, Lin WC, Huang YC, Yang CH. Chemical composition and biological properties of essential oils of two mint species. Trop J Pharm Res 2013; 12(4): 577-82.
[http://dx.doi.org/10.4314/tjpr.v12i4.20]

[120] Zhao H, Ren S, Yang H, *et al.* Peppermint essential oil: its phytochemistry, biological activity, pharmacological effect and application. Biomed Pharmacother 2022; 154: 113559.
[http://dx.doi.org/10.1016/j.biopha.2022.113559] [PMID: 35994817]

[121] Bai JC, Fried M, Corazza GR, *et al.* World Gastroenterology Organisation global guidelines on celiac disease. J Clin Gastroenterol 2013; 47(2): 121-6.
[http://dx.doi.org/10.1097/MCG.0b013e31827a6f83] [PMID: 23314668]

[122] Howlett K, Galbo H, Lorentsen J, *et al.* Effect of adrenaline on glucose kinetics during exercise in adrenalectomised humans. J Physiol 1999; 519(3): 911-21.
[http://dx.doi.org/10.1111/j.1469-7793.1999.0911n.x] [PMID: 10457100]

[123] Kagnoff MF. Overview and pathogenesis of celiac disease. Gastroenterology 2005; 128(4) (Suppl. 1): S10-8.
[http://dx.doi.org/10.1053/j.gastro.2005.02.008] [PMID: 15825116]

[124] Khan RU, Fatima A, Naz S, Ragni M, Tarricone S, Tufarelli V. Perspective, opportunities and challenges in using fennel (*Foeniculum vulgare)* in poultry health and production as an eco-friendly alternative to antibiotics: a review. Antibiotics (Basel) 2022; 11(2): 278.
[http://dx.doi.org/10.3390/antibiotics11020278] [PMID: 35203880]

[125] Makharia GK. Current and emerging therapy for celiac disease. Front Med (Lausanne) 2014; 1: 6.
[http://dx.doi.org/10.3389/fmed.2014.00006] [PMID: 25705619]

[126] Pinier M, Fuhrmann G, Verdu E, *et al.* Prevention measures and exploratory pharmacological treatments of celiac disease. Off J Am Coll Gastroenterol 2014; 105: 2551-61.
[http://dx.doi.org/10.1038/ajg.2010.372]

[127] Setty M, Hormaza L, Guandalini S. Celiac Disease. Mol Diagn Ther 2008; 12(5): 289-98.
[http://dx.doi.org/10.1007/BF03256294] [PMID: 18803427]

[128] Braun L. Slippery elm. J Complement Med 2006; 5(1).

[129] Bonamico M, Thanasi E, Mariani P, *et al.* Duodenal bulb biopsies in celiac disease: a multicenter study. J Pediatr Gastroenterol Nutr 2008; 47(5): 618-22.
[http://dx.doi.org/10.1097/MPG.0b013e3181677d6e] [PMID: 18979585]

[130] Ciacci C, Maiuri L, Caporaso N, *et al.* Celiac disease: *In vitro* and *in vivo* safety and palatability of wheat-free sorghum food products. Clin Nutr 2007; 26(6): 799-805.
[http://dx.doi.org/10.1016/j.clnu.2007.05.006] [PMID: 17719701]

[131] Mota MAL, Landim JSP, Targino TSS, Silva SFR, Silva SL, Pereira MRP. Evaluation of the anti-inflammatory and analgesic effects of green tea (Camellia sinensis) in mice. Acta Cir Bras 2015; 30(4): 242-6.
[http://dx.doi.org/10.1590/S0102-865020150040000002] [PMID: 25923256]

[132] Dias R, Brás NF, Fernandes I, Pérez-Gregorio M, Mateus N, Freitas V. Molecular insights on the interaction and preventive potential of epigallocatechin-3-gallate in Celiac Disease. Int J Biol Macromol 2018; 112: 1029-37.
[http://dx.doi.org/10.1016/j.ijbiomac.2018.02.055] [PMID: 29447966]

[133] Zhang YZ, Li YY. Inflammatory bowel disease: Pathogenesis. World J Gastroenterol 2014; 20(1): 91-9.
[http://dx.doi.org/10.3748/wjg.v20.i1.91] [PMID: 24415861]

[134] Vezza T, Rodríguez-Nogales A, Algieri F, Utrilla M, Rodriguez-Cabezas M, Galvez J. Flavonoids in inflammatory bowel disease: a review. Nutrients 2016; 8(4): 211.
[http://dx.doi.org/10.3390/nu8040211] [PMID: 27070642]

[135] Van Buiten CB, Lambert JD, Elias RJ. Green tea polyphenols mitigate gliadin-mediated inflammation and permeability *in vitro*. Mol Nutr Food Res 2018; 62(12): 1700879.
[http://dx.doi.org/10.1002/mnfr.201700879] [PMID: 29704403]

[136] Van Buiten CB, Lambert JD, Sae-tan S, Elias RJ. Inhibition of gliadin digestion by green tea polyphenols and the potential implications for celiac disease. FASEB J 2017; 31(S1): 974-23.
[http://dx.doi.org/10.1096/fasebj.31.1_supplement.974.23]

[137] Saeidnia S, Manayi A, Vazirian M. Echinacea purpurea: Pharmacology, phytochemistry and analysis methods. Pharmacogn Rev 2015; 9(17): 63-72.
[http://dx.doi.org/10.4103/0973-7847.156353] [PMID: 26009695]

[138] Vimalanathan S, Arnason JT, Hudson JB. Anti-inflammatory activities of *Echinacea* extracts do not correlate with traditional marker components. Pharm Biol 2009; 47(5): 430-5.
[http://dx.doi.org/10.1080/13880200902800204]

[139] Abascal K, Yarnell E. Treatments for recurrent aphthous stomatitis. Altern Complement Ther 2010; 16(2): 100-6.
[http://dx.doi.org/10.1089/act.2010.16205]

[140] Hill LL, Foote JC, Erickson BD, Cerniglia CE, Denny GS. Echinacea purpurea supplementation stimulates select groups of human gastrointestinal tract microbiota. J Clin Pharm Ther 2006; 31(6): 599-604.
[http://dx.doi.org/10.1111/j.1365-2710.2006.00781.x] [PMID: 17176365]

[141] Sánchez E, Laparra JM, Sanz Y. Discerning the role of Bacteroides fragilis in celiac disease pathogenesis. Appl Environ Microbiol 2012; 78(18): 6507-15.
[http://dx.doi.org/10.1128/AEM.00563-12] [PMID: 22773639]

[142] Karim N. Impact of dietary measures in autoimmune diseases. J Bahria Uni Med Dental Coll 2012; 9(1): 01-2.

[143] Dwita L, Yati K, Gantini S. The anti-inflammatory activity of Nigella sativa balm sticks. Sci Pharm 2019; 87(1): 3.
[http://dx.doi.org/10.3390/scipharm87010003]

[144] Shende V, Hedaoo SA, Ansari MH, Bhomle P, Mahapatra DK. Re-highlighting the potential natural resources for treating or managing the ailments of gastrointestinal tract origin. Applied Pharmaceutical Practice and Nutraceuticals. Apple Academic Press 2021; pp. 105-20.
[http://dx.doi.org/10.1201/9781003054894-8]

[145] Anheyer D, Frawley J, Koch AK, *et al.* Herbal medicines for gastrointestinal disorders in children and adolescents: a systematic review. Pediatrics 2017; 139(6): e20170062.
[http://dx.doi.org/10.1542/peds.2017-0062] [PMID: 28562281]

CHAPTER 8

Beneficial Effects of Berry Fruits on Autoimmune Diseases

Yasin Ozdemir[1,*], Aysun Ozturk[1] and **Fatih Gokhan Erbas[2]**

[1] *Department of Food Technologies, Ataturk Horticultural Central Research Institution, Yalova 77100, Türkiye*

[2] *Department of Pomiculture, Ataturk Horticultural Central Research Institution Yalova 77100, Türkiye*

Abstract: The prevalence of autoimmune diseases in developed societies suggests the use of natural products for prevention and treatment. At the beginning of preventive approaches, the idea of regularly consuming herbal products that can have positive effects on autoimmune diseases and making them a part of the diet is common. Beneficial phytochemicals can be reached by consuming these herbal products directly and/or the products obtained from them. In addition, numerous studies have demonstrated that berries offer the potential to protect against autoimmune diseases if they are consumed regularly with their phytochemicals, especially phenols, anthocyanins, vitamins, and specific minor components. There are also studies on the effects of these phytochemicals on autoimmune diseases. It is stated that the regular consumption of berry fruits increases the quality of life, and the protective effect it provides is much easier and less costly than the treatment of autoimmune diseases. This chapter is aimed at revealing the potential of berry fruits to protect from autoimmune diseases, reduce the negative effects of the disease, and/or support treatment. Although studies on the beneficial effects of berries have increased in recent years, they are still behind other fruits.

Keywords: Autoimmune diseases, Anthocyanins, Berry fruits, Diet, Herbal products, Phytochemicals, Phenols, Quality of life.

INTRODUCTION

Well-known berries are strawberry, raspberry, blueberry, blackberry, gooseberry, redcurrant, currant, and cranberry. Boysenberry, bilberry, jostaberry, cloudberry, loganberry, and lingonberry are more rarely known berry fruits. Berry fruits represent an important fresh product variety in Europe in terms of production volume and economic profitability [1, 2].

---

[*] **Corresponding author Yasin Ozdemir:** Department of Food Technologies, Ataturk Horticultural Central Research Institution, Yalova 77100, Türkiye; Tel: +903322232781; E-mail: yasin.ozdemir@tarimorman.gov.tr

Cennet Ozay & Gokhan Zengin (Eds.)

Berry berries have a special taste and unique texture. In addition, berry fruits offer a very different experience than other fruits with their striking and bright colours, delicate textures, and different shapes. In this way, they win the appreciation of consumers. Berry fruits are a group of fruits that have attracted intense interest not only for their sensory qualities but also for the beneficial components they have [3].

Growing conditions such as climate, soil structure, irrigation, number of sunny days, variety, and maturity level directly affect the phytochemical content of berry fruits [4, 5]. Berries contain many phytochemicals, fibers, vitamins, and minerals. Berries also have a high concentration of polyphenols, so it is possible to use them for treating various diseases pharmacologically by acting on oxidative stress and inflammation [6]. In studies, it has been reported that berry fruits can be a source of functional components that can be used in the food and pharmaceutical industries due to their unique phytochemical composition [7, 8]. Studies on not only fruit but also berry seeds have shown that they have high health potential. For this reason, examining the functional properties of berry seeds and determining their effects on health have been among the topics of interest in recent years. In addition, studies report that berry seeds can have beneficial effects on autoimmune diseases. Studies on the by-products formed after the processing of berry fruits indicate that extracts that can be effective in the prevention of autoimmune diseases can be made with the tip in the raw material [9, 10]. Consumption of berries or berry products with high phytochemical content is expected to provide an advantage for protection from autoimmune diseases. It should not be forgotten that the variety, amount, and frequency of their consumption in the diet are very effective in the health benefits that will emerge [11, 12].

It is reported that unhealthy living conditions such as less physical activity during the day, unbalanced diet, stressful lifestyle, insufficient sleep, and air pollution weaken the immune system and weaken people's defence against diseases. It has been stated that this situation not only weakens the immune system but also causes problems with the immune system [13]. It is reported that autoimmune diseases also fall into this group. Autoimmune diseases are conditions in which the immune system mistakenly damages healthy cells in the body. Your immune system works to protect the body from diseases and infections. The immune system can distinguish between foreign cells and body cells and detect foreign cells as disease agents. But in case of an autoimmune disease, the immune system may perceive parts of your body, such as the joints or skin, as foreign and unfortunately begin to attack these healthy cells or tissues [14]. The reported number of autoimmune diseases is increasing every year. Some of those are celiac diseases, type 1 diabetes, psoriasis, rheumatoid arthritis, inflammatory bowel disease, multiple sclerosis, Guillain, chronic inflammatory demyelinating polyneuropathy, Graves' disease, Hashimoto's thyroiditis, myasthenia gravis, scleroderma, and vasculitis [15, 16].

In order to be protected from diseases in unhealthy living conditions, the search for plants offered by nature to people attracts the attention of scientists. With this point of view, it has been reported that pharmaceutical raw materials and food supplements have been developed, and successful results have been obtained with previous studies. This chapter's purpose is to assemble and analyze the current studies on the beneficial effects of berry fruits on autoimmune diseases. Also, it aims at providing a collective perspective for consumers and scientists.

EFFECT OF BERRIES ON AUTOIMMUNE DISEASES

Both autoimmune diseases and the characteristics of berry fruits are not widely known. Increasing studies on this subject may be beneficial for raising awareness. This section of the chapter provides a review of studies investigating the effects of some berries on autoimmune diseases.

Effect of Berries on Vasculitis

Berry consumption has been associated with a reduction in all-cause mortality [17]. Epidemiological studies and meta-analyses have reported the positive effect of polyphenols and polyphenol-rich foods on vascular function [18, 19]. Since all berry fruits are rich in polyphenols, it suggests that their regular consumption may be beneficial for the prevention of vascular diseases. It has also been reported that anthocyanins protect against cardiovascular and neurodegenerative diseases [20]. Berry berries are already characterised by their rich anthocyanin content. Therefore, it is accepted that both phenol and anthocyanin contents may be effective in preventing vascular diseases and have positive effects on vascular functions [19, 21]. It has been stated that protective effects may be seen on vascular function depending on the regular consumption of berry fruits in the diet, the frequency, amount, and type of consumption [19, 22].

A study investigating the effect of a single serving of blueberries (250 g) in elderly subjects ($\geq$ 60 years) evaluated the effects of bioactive substances on markers of oxidative stress, inflammation, and vascular function following blueberry ingestion. In the study, it was reported that blueberries slowed vascular dysfunction and the development of cardiovascular diseases and showed potential beneficial effects on vascular function [23]. Post-harvest processing, such as pressing, pasteurisation, and conventional and vacuum drying, can significantly affect the polyphenol (including anthocyanin) and vitamin content of berries, and therefore their bioactivities and effects on vasculitis risk factors are also influenced [24 - 26].

Effect of Berries on Multiple Sclerosis

Epidemiological studies associate regular, moderate intake of blueberries and/or anthocyanins with improved neuroprotection. These findings are supported by biomarker-based evidence from human clinical studies [27]. Polyphenols in the diet have been shown to reduce oxidative stress and the risk of neurological disorders such as multiple sclerosis and Alzheimer's disease. Aronia is well known for its strong antioxidant content [28]. Thus, the consumption of Aronia and similar high-antioxidant fruits can be beneficial against these diseases. Blueberry-supplemented feeding studies on different mouse models have reported the therapeutic effects of blueberry on multiple sclerosis [29]. *J. communis* berry extracts with different solvents (methanol, water, and ethyl acetate) displayed moderate to potent growth inhibitory activity against multiple sclerosis [30].

Effect of Berries on Inflammatory Bowel Disease

As a result of *in vitro*, *in vivo*, and clinical studies, it has been reported that polyphenols have the potential to alleviate inflammatory bowel disease. It has been reported that consuming fruits containing rich polyphenols, such as berries preserves the epithelial barrier function, regulates intestinal flora, inhibits oxidation damage, and thus reduces the negative effects of inflammatory bowel disease [31 - 33]. It was reported that diet has an important role in both the emergence of inflammatory bowel disease and reducing the negative effects experienced during this disease. However, it is difficult to draw definite conclusions due to the complex nature of the disease and its multifactorial effects in nutrition studies [34]. As a result of a study on rats, it was reported that rats that fed strawberries every day had reduced symptoms of inflammatory bowel disease compared to the control group, and consuming strawberries showed protective effects [35].

Black raspberry extract added to the diet of mice increased Akkermansia. The number of Akkermansia has been reported to be higher in healthy intestines and lower in intestines with inflammatory diseases or metabolic disorders [36]. In a study on mice, dietary blueberries and/or broccoli altered the gut microbiota and colon metabolism. However, it has been reported that more clinical research is needed to determine the positive effects of blueberry and/or broccoli consumption on colon health [37].

Complex polyphenols are metabolised into smaller phenolic compounds in the gut. In healthy subjects, phenolic compounds reaching the intestine generally increase the number of Bifidobacterium, Lactobacillus, and Akkermansia. This suggests that berry fruits or compounds have a prebiotic-like effect. Berry berries have been shown to relieve symptoms of intestinal inflammation through the modulation of pro-inflammatory cytokines [31, 38].

Effect of Berries on Psoriasis

Some herbal extracts have shown promising results in the treatment of psoriasis, especially when consumed with antipsoriatic drugs [39, 40]. Blackberry extract, some herbal extracts, and fish oil have been reported to have beneficial antipsoriatic properties [39, 41, 42]. Berry extract with gold nanoparticles was used as a material for curing psoriatic lesions after exposure to UVB radiation. Compared to the samples treated with berries extract alone, more successful results were obtained in the samples in which berry extract and gold nanoparticles were applied together [43].

The effect of berry extracts in silver nanoparticles on psoriasis patients was studied, and the cytotoxic effect of Ag nanoparticles was determined. Epicatechin and Albizia adianthifolia leaves have been used as a source of an –OH functional group on the nanoparticles, and cytotoxic effect was not reported [44].

Berries are a rich source of anthocyanin and cyanidin. The research was performed on psoriasis patients by using gold nanoparticles with anthocyanin cyanidin 3-O-glucoside and cyanidin 3-O-sambubioside in moisturizing creams. Their inhibition effects on psoriatic inflammation were reported [43]. There is increasing evidence of the benefits of flavonoids for preventing and treating many skin disorders, including psoriasis [45]. Chrysanthemin a specific phenol present in blackcurrant and raspberries inhibits UVB irradiation-induced damage and inflammation in an animal study [46]. Berries are high in antioxidants, flavonoids, fibre, and some nutrients, which may support your skin's ability to fight inflammation related to psoriasis [47].

Effect of Berries on Rheumatoid Arthritis

Fruits, such as berries and pomegranates are rich sources of a variety of dietary bioactive compounds, especially polyphenolic flavonoids that have been associated with antioxidant, anti-inflammatory, and analgesic effects. Emerging research demonstrates the protective role of fruits and their polyphenols in pre-clinical, clinical, and epidemiological studies of osteoarthritis and rheumatoid arthritis. In this context, commonly available fruits, such as blueberries, raspberries, strawberries, and pomegranates have shown promising results in reducing pain and inflammation in experimental models, and in human clinical studies of arthritis [48 - 50].

Berry berries have many phytochemicals. Since they are a rich source of polyphenols and flavonoids associated with antioxidant, anti-inflammatory, and analgesic effects, their effects on arthritis have been investigated [51, 52]. Studies have shown that regularly consumed fruits and their phenols play a protective role in preclinical, clinical, and epidemiological studies on osteoarthritis and rheumatoid arthritis. The effects of fruits such as blueberries, raspberries, pomegranates, and strawberries on arthritis have been studied in animal studies and human arthritis clinical studies and reported promising results in reducing pain and inflammation [48, 49].

Decreases in disease activity scores and joint pain of rheumatoid arthritis in adults were found to be lower in the groups that consumed pomegranate extracts (eight weeks, 250 mg day−1) compared to those that did not consume the extracts [53]. Quercetin (one of the important phenols in berry fruits) consumption (eight weeks, 500 mg day−1) decreased the disease activity scores, joint pain, and stiffness in rheumatoid arthritis of adults [50]. Consumption of pomegranate juice for six weeks showed a different beneficial effect on knee osteoarthritis in adults [54].

Consumption of strawberry beverages during 26 weeks decreased matrix metalloproteinases and total knee pain in adults with knee osteoarthritis [49]. Consumption of *J. communis* berry extracts was reported to inhibit moderate to potent growth against bacterial triggers of rheumatoid arthritis [30]. Orally consumed pomegranate juice (4, 10, and 20 mL kg^{-1}) for 2 weeks decreased chondrocyte damage and inflammation in synovial fluid was determined in the rodent model of mono-iodoacetate-induced osteoarthritis [55].

In the rodent model of collagen-induced arthritis, raspberry fruit extract (15 mg crude extract per kg) every 24 h for 12 days inhibited the paw eodema, decreased the histological damage score and articular destruction, and improved the clinical features of arthritis [56]. Blueberry fruit extract decreased histological damage, decreased Cox-2 and iNOS improved the clinical features of arthritis in the rodent model of collagen-induced arthritis [51]. Hesperidin, which is a berry and citrus Phenolic Compound, inhibited fibroblast-like synoviocyte proliferation and DNA methyltransferase-1 expression and decreased the inflammation arthritis of rodents [57]. Fruit extracts of silver berry (*E. angustifolia*) decreased the oedema and inflammation of rodents that had collagen-induced arthritis [58]. Pomegranate fruit extract decreased histological damage score and cytokines in the synovial fluid of the rabbit model of surgically-induced osteoarthritis [52].

Effect of Berries on Type 1 Diabetes

Berry fruits contain many effective components, especially anthocyanins and proanthocyanidins. In this way, it has been reported that it can suppress the increase in blood sugar levels and contribute to the improvement of diabetes and other metabolic disorders [59]. Although clinical studies on the anti-diabetic effects of berries and especially their polyphenols are limited, epidemiological data have reported the beneficial effects of consumption of berry fruit or berry anthocyanins on the development and/or management of type 1 diabetes [60].

Blackberry, a traditional and complementary medicine in India, is accepted as a medicine that helps in controll diabetes [61]. It has been reported that the presence of berries in the diet reduces the severity or slows down the progression of diabetes and many other diseases that may occur due to ageing. As a result of their findings, it has been reported that phytochemicals in berry fruits exhibit antiglycative activity [62]. The fruit, seeds, and even juice of jamunu play an important role in the treatment of diabetes. It has been reported that the fruit, seed, or fruit juice of Blackberries may be beneficial in the treatment of diabetes [61].

Consumption of berry fruits has been noted to have an effect similar to that of diabetes medications. In a study on diabetic mice, it was reported that the ethanolic extract of aronia fruit may be beneficial in the treatment of type 1 diabetes [63]. Oral administration of alcoholic extracts of blackberry seed to diabetic patients has been found to reduce blood sugar and glucose levels [61]. Some foods or drugs that inhibit alpha-amylase and alpha-glucosidase activity limit glucose absorption. It has been reported that the increase in blood sugar almost completely stopped in mice after consuming Aronia berry extract for 6 weeks [63]. In another study, it was reported that anthocyanins increase the function and insulin sensitivity of adipocytes [64]. A study confirmed the anti-diabetic activity of Aronia berry, and it can be expected to increase utilisation according to the results [65, 66]. Another study found that berry fruits with a relatively lower glycemic index may have higher positive effects on diabetes [67].

Consuming blueberries can help improve insulin sensitivity in overweight men and women [68]. Blueberry anthocyanins have been shown to reduce insulin sensitivity and hyperglycemia. The diet supplemented with blueberry powder improves glucose tolerance in mice, normalises glucose metabolism, and has been reported to improve insulin sensitivity in humans [69, 70].

Mice consuming ellagic acid (extracted from red raspberries) for 12 weeks have been reported to improve diabetic status by increasing insulin levels and reducing fasting glucose [71]. Raspberry extract is one of the most effective fruits for inhibiting alpha-amylase. It has also been reported that proanthocyanidins are one of the important inhibitors of alpha-amylase activity [72, 73].

Anthocyanins and ellagic acid antioxidants have been reported to have beneficial effects in diabetic animals and humans [71, 74, 75]. Strawberry also reported an inhibiting effect on glucosidase and angiotensin-1-converting enzymes [76]. Some studies have reported that cranberries and cranberry products may be beneficial in relieving insulin-related disorders [77].

IMMUNOMODULATORY EFFECT OF BERRIES

It has been reported that blueberry can protect against autoimmune diseases because it has immunomodulatory, anti-inflammatory, and neuroprotective properties [78]. Blueberry-fed mice with experimental autoimmune encephalomyelitis have been reported to have significantly lower motor disability scores, as well as significantly more myelin preservation in the lumbar spinal cord, compared with the control group [78]. Chilean berry extract decreased the expression of proinflammatory cytokines (IL-1β and TNF-α) in a culture of mononuclear cells observed, which indicates the immunomodulatory activity against inflammation [79]. It has been reported that berry fruits show potential positive effects on the proper functioning of the immune system. However, more clinical studies are required to fully understand the immunomodulation mechanisms provided by berry fruits [80, 81].

CONCLUDING REMARKS

Berry fruits have various categories of phytochemicals, especially phenolic compounds (phenolic acids, flavonoids, anthocyanins, flavonols, tannins, procyanidins, phenolic acid esters, *etc.*), which ensure different health-beneficial properties. These rich sources of phytochemicals also explain the protective effects of berries against autoimmune diseases. Berry fruits or their products also have the potential to reduce the severity and inflammation of autoimmune diseases. Studies on the beneficial effects of berry fruits have an important place in the regulation of the intestinal system and the strengthening and proper functioning of the immune system. It is known that autoimmune diseases are closely related to intestinal health and the immune system. For this reason, it is thought that berry fruits have new potential for autoimmune system diseases, both directly against specific autoimmune diseases and by contributing to the regulation of the intestine and immune system. From this perspective, future studies will better understand the possibilities of using berry fruits and their specific components in the prevention and treatment of autoimmune diseases.

Although it has beneficial effects on many diseases, such as autoimmune diseases, berry fruits and products are consumed less than other fruits. The short shelf life of berry fruits is seen as a barrier to widespread consumption, since they are relatively expensive, spoil quickly, and have delicate textures. Making berry fruits more accessible with new agricultural practises and developing different berry products in the food industry will offer new opportunities to consumers.

The health effects attributed to fruits are closely related to the bioaccessibility of their phytochemicals. The low bioavailability of phytochemicals, especially phenols, in berry fruit limits their beneficial effects on health. Changes in the content and bioaccessibility of these active ingredients should be taken into account during the processing of food products, especially extracts to be produced from berry fruits.

Although there are thousands of studies on the beneficial effects of berry fruits, such as the prevention and treatment of different diseases, it is seen that the number of studies on the effects of berry fruits on autoimmune diseases is less. On the other hand, no studies have been found on the effects of berry fruit on some autoimmune diseases such as Guillain -Barre syndrome, chronic inflammatory demyelinating polyneuropathy, Graves' disease, Hashimoto's thyroiditis, myasthenia gravis, and scleroderma. It is thought that these diseases are much rarer than common diseases such as cancer or cardiovascular diseases, and the effects of berry fruits on these diseases are relatively more difficult to determine, making studies on this subject more difficult. On the other hand, it should not be overlooked that these issues are untouched. In addition, determining that berry fruits or the products obtained from them are effective against these diseases will provide both high health benefits and high blood potential.

In this study, literature on the effects of berry fruits, products, or active substances on relatively more common autoimmune diseases has been discussed. These autoimmune diseases in which the beneficial effects of berry fruits or products have been determined are vasculitis, multiple sclerosis, inflammatory bowel disease, psoriasis, rheumatoid arthritis, and type 1 diabetes. It has been reported that some active substances in berry fruits are beneficial for these diseases. It may inspire new studies on obtaining and purifying these active substances from fruit or by-products.

In research on determining the contents and beneficial effects of berry fruits, information on the variety or cultivar name, maturity status, and growing conditions and places should be given together with the berry's name. In this way, it will be possible to make more objective evaluations. To study the beneficial effects of berry fruits in stages, it is important to express the material concretely and to give the content information first. Subsequently, reporting of bioavailability and beneficial effects may lead to more beneficial and comparable results.

The desire of consumers to be protected from diseases by feeding natural foods is increasing day by day. From this point of view, it is expected that the consumption of berry fruits will increase in the coming years. Agricultural practises that will increase the yield and quality in berry agriculture without moving away from naturalness will be beneficial for both consumers and farmers.

REFERENCES

[1]   Macori G, Gilardi G, Bellio A, *et al.* Microbiological parameters in the primary production of berries: A pilot study. Foods 2018; 7(7): 105.
[http://dx.doi.org/10.3390/foods7070105] [PMID: 29976895]

[2]   Kljajić N, Vuković P, Arsić S. Production and foreign trade exchange of raspberries: Case study of Serbia. Western Balkan Journal of Agricultural Economics and Rural Development 2023; 5(1): 91-105.
[http://dx.doi.org/10.5937/WBJAE2301091K]

[3]   Skrovankova S, Sumczynski D, Mlcek J, Jurikova T, Sochor J. Bioactive compounds and antioxidant activity in different types of berries. Int J Mol Sci 2015; 16(10): 24673-706.
[http://dx.doi.org/10.3390/ijms161024673] [PMID: 26501271]

[4]   Taghavi T, Siddiqui RK, Rutto L. The effect of preharvest factors on fruit and nutritional quality in strawberry. Strawberry - Pre- and Post-Harvest Management Techniques for Higher Fruit Quality 2019.
[http://dx.doi.org/10.5772/intechopen.84619]

[5]   Teker T. A study of kaolin effects on grapevine physiology and its ability to protect grape clusters from sunburn damage. Sci Hortic (Amsterdam) 2023; 311: 111824.
[http://dx.doi.org/10.1016/j.scienta.2022.111824]

[6]   Golovinskaia O, Wang CK. Review of functional and pharmacological activities of berries. Molecules 2021; 26(13): 3904.
[http://dx.doi.org/10.3390/molecules26133904] [PMID: 34202412]

[7]   Ilić T, Dodevska M, Marčetić M, Božić D, Kodranov I, Vidović B. Chemical characterization, antioxidant and antimicrobial properties of goji berries cultivated in Serbia. Foods 2020; 9(11): 1614.
[http://dx.doi.org/10.3390/foods9111614] [PMID: 33172053]

[8]   Jan B, Parveen R, Zahiruddin S, Khan MU, Mohapatra S, Ahmad S. Nutritional constituents of mulberry and their potential applications in food and pharmaceuticals: A review. Saudi J Biol Sci 2021; 28(7): 3909-21.
[http://dx.doi.org/10.1016/j.sjbs.2021.03.056] [PMID: 34220247]

[9]   Jurendić T, Ščetar M. Aronia melanocarpa products and by-products for Health and Nutrition: A Review. Antioxidants 2021; 10(7): 1052.
[http://dx.doi.org/10.3390/antiox10071052] [PMID: 34209985]

[10]   Ćirić I, Sredojević M, Dabić Zagorac D, Fotirić-Akšić M, Meland M, Natić M. Bioactive phytochemicals from berries seed oil processing by-products. Reference Series in Phytochemistry 2021; pp. 1-23.
[http://dx.doi.org/10.1007/978-3-030-63961-7_19-1]

[11]   Tran PHL, Tran TTD. Blueberry supplementation in neuronal health and protective technologies for efficient delivery of Blueberry Anthocyanins. Biomolecules 2021; 11(1): 102.

[http://dx.doi.org/10.3390/biom11010102] [PMID: 33466731]

[12]   Benedetti G, Zabini F, Tagliavento L, Meneguzzo F, Calderone V, Testai L. An overview of the health benefits, extraction methods and improving the properties of pomegranate. Antioxidants 2023; 12(7): 1351.
[http://dx.doi.org/10.3390/antiox12071351] [PMID: 37507891]

[13]   Meletis CD, Wilkes K. Immune Competence and Minimizing Susceptibility to COVID-19 and Other Immune System Threats. Altern Ther Health Med 2020; 26(S2): 94-9.
[PMID: 33245701]

[14]   Jeong H, Lee B, Han SJ, Sohn DH. Glucose metabolic reprogramming in autoimmune diseases. Anim Cells Syst 2023; 27(1): 149-58.
[http://dx.doi.org/10.1080/19768354.2023.2234986] [PMID: 37465289]

[15]   Porpora MG, Scaramuzzino S, Sangiuliano C, *et al.* High prevalence of autoimmune diseases in women with endometriosis: a case-control study. Gynecol Endocrinol 2020; 36(4): 356-9.
[http://dx.doi.org/10.1080/09513590.2019.1655727] [PMID: 31476950]

[16]   Lerner A, Jeremias P, Matthias T. The world incidence and prevalence of autoimmune diseases is increasing. International Journal of Celiac Disease 2016; 3(4): 151-5.
[http://dx.doi.org/10.12691/ijcd-3-4-8]

[17]   Aune D, Giovannucci E, Boffetta P, *et al.* Fruit and vegetable intake and the risk of cardiovascular disease, total cancer and all-cause mortality—a systematic review and dose-response meta-analysis of prospective studies. Int J Epidemiol 2017; 46(3): 1029-56.
[http://dx.doi.org/10.1093/ije/dyw319] [PMID: 28338764]

[18]   Istas G, Wood E, Le Sayec M, *et al.* Effects of aronia berry (poly)phenols on vascular function and gut microbiota: a double-blind randomized controlled trial in adult men. Am J Clin Nutr 2019; 110(2): 316-29.
[http://dx.doi.org/10.1093/ajcn/nqz075] [PMID: 31152545]

[19]   Martini D, Marino M, Angelino D, *et al.* Role of berries in vascular function: a systematic review of human intervention studies. Nutr Rev 2019; 78(3): nuz053.
[http://dx.doi.org/10.1093/nutrit/nuz053] [PMID: 31365093]

[20]   Mattioli R, Francioso A, Mosca L, Silva P. Anthocyanins: A comprehensive review of their chemical properties and health effects on cardiovascular and Neurodegenerative Diseases. Molecules 2020; 25(17): 3809.
[http://dx.doi.org/10.3390/molecules25173809] [PMID: 32825684]

[21]   Ahles S, Joris PJ, Plat J. Effects of Berry Anthocyanins on cognitive performance, vascular function and cardiometabolic risk markers: A systematic review of randomized placebo-controlled intervention studies in humans. Int J Mol Sci 2021; 22(12): 6482.
[http://dx.doi.org/10.3390/ijms22126482] [PMID: 34204250]

[22]   Xu L, Tian Z, Chen H, Zhao Y, Yang Y. Anthocyanins, anthocyanin-rich berries, and cardiovascular risks: Systematic Review and meta-analysis of 44 randomized controlled trials and 15 prospective cohort studies. Front Nutr 2021; 8: 747884.
[http://dx.doi.org/10.3389/fnut.2021.747884] [PMID: 34977111]

[23]   Del Bo' C, Tucci M, Martini D, *et al.* Acute effect of blueberry intake on vascular function in older subjects: Study protocol for a randomized, controlled, crossover trial. PLoS One 2022; 17(12): e0275132.
[http://dx.doi.org/10.1371/journal.pone.0275132] [PMID: 36454906]

[24]   Srivastava A, Akoh CC, Yi W, Fischer J, Krewer G. Effect of storage conditions on the biological activity of phenolic compounds of blueberry extract packed in glass bottles. J Agric Food Chem 2007; 55(7): 2705-13.
[http://dx.doi.org/10.1021/jf062914w] [PMID: 17348670]

[25]   Hartmann A, Patz CD, Andlauer W, Dietrich H, Ludwig M. Influence of processing on quality parameters of strawberries. J Agric Food Chem 2008; 56(20): 9484-9.
[http://dx.doi.org/10.1021/jf801555q] [PMID: 18821768]

[26]   Wojdyło A, Figiel A, Oszmiański J. Effect of drying methods with the application of vacuum microwaves on the bioactive compounds, color, and antioxidant activity of strawberry fruits. J Agric Food Chem 2009; 57(4): 1337-43.
[http://dx.doi.org/10.1021/jf802507j] [PMID: 19170638]

[27]   Kalt W, Cassidy A, Howard LR, *et al.* Recent research on the health benefits of blueberries and their anthocyanins. Adv Nutr 2020; 11(2): 224-36.
[http://dx.doi.org/10.1093/advances/nmz065] [PMID: 31329250]

[28]   Sultana R. Aronia melanocarpa:a review of potential antioxidants on neuroprotection and cognitive performance. JOURNAL OF DRUG VIGILANCE AND ALTERNATIVE THERAPIES 2021; 1(3): 92-100.
[http://dx.doi.org/10.52816/JDVAT.2021.1301]

[29]   Seeram NP. Emerging research supporting the positive effects of berries on human health and disease prevention. J Agric Food Chem 2012; 60(23): 5685-6.
[http://dx.doi.org/10.1021/jf203455z] [PMID: 22066828]

[30]   Fernandez A, Edwin Cock I. The therapeutic properties of *Juniperus communis* L.: Antioxidant capacity, bacterial growth inhibition, anticancer activity and toxicity. Pharmacogn J 2016; 8(3): 273-80.
[http://dx.doi.org/10.5530/pj.2016.3.17]

[31]   Zhong W, Gong J, Su Q, *et al.* Dietary polyphenols ameliorate inflammatory bowel diseases: advances and future perspectives to maximize their nutraceutical applications. Phytochem Rev 2023..
[http://dx.doi.org/10.1007/s11101-023-09866-z]

[32]   Nakase H, Uchino M, Shinzaki S, *et al.* Evidence-based clinical practice guidelines for inflammatory bowel disease 2020. J Gastroenterol 2021; 56(6): 489-526.
[http://dx.doi.org/10.1007/s00535-021-01784-1] [PMID: 33885977]

[33]   Liu S, Zhao W, Lan P, Mou X. The microbiome in inflammatory bowel diseases: from pathogenesis to therapy. Protein Cell 2021; 12(5): 331-45.
[http://dx.doi.org/10.1007/s13238-020-00745-3] [PMID: 32601832]

[34]   Haskey N, Gibson D. An examination of diet for the maintenance of remission in inflammatory bowel disease. Nutrients 2017; 9(3): 259.
[http://dx.doi.org/10.3390/nu9030259] [PMID: 28287412]

[35]   Chassaing B, Aitken JD, Malleshappa M, Vijay-Kumar M. Dextran sulfate sodium (DSS)-induced colitis in mice. Curr Protoc Immunol 2014; 104(1): 25.1-, 14.
[http://dx.doi.org/10.1002/0471142735.im1525s104] [PMID: 24510619]

[36]   Pan P, Lam V, Salzman N, *et al.* Black raspberries and their anthocyanin and fiber fractions alter the composition and diversity of gut microbiota in F-344 rats. Nutr Cancer 2017; 69(6): 943-51.
[http://dx.doi.org/10.1080/01635581.2017.1340491] [PMID: 28718724]

[37]   Paturi G, Mandimika T, Butts CA, *et al.* Influence of dietary blueberry and broccoli on cecal microbiota activity and colon morphology in mdr1a−/− mice, a model of inflammatory bowel diseases. Nutrition 2012; 28(3): 324-30.
[http://dx.doi.org/10.1016/j.nut.2011.07.018] [PMID: 22113065]

[38]   Lavefve L, Howard LR, Carbonero F. Berry polyphenols metabolism and impact on human gut microbiota and health. Food Funct 2020; 11(1): 45-65.
[http://dx.doi.org/10.1039/C9FO01634A] [PMID: 31808762]

[39]   Murphy EC, Schaffter SW, Friedman AJ. Nanotechnology for psoriasis therapy. Curr Dermatol Rep 2019; 8(1): 14-25.

[http://dx.doi.org/10.1007/s13671-019-0248-y]

[40] Bakshi H, Nagpal M, Singh M, Dhingra GA, Aggarwal G. Treatment of psoriasis: A comprehensive review of entire therapies. Curr Drug Saf 2020; 15(2): 82-104.
[http://dx.doi.org/10.2174/22123911MTAziOTU84] [PMID: 31994468]

[41] Crisan D, Scharffetter-Kochanek K, Crisan M, *et al.* Topical silver and gold nanoparticles complexed with *Cornus mas* suppress inflammation in human psoriasis plaques by inhibiting NF-κB activity. Exp Dermatol 2018; 27(10): 1166-9.
[http://dx.doi.org/10.1111/exd.13707] [PMID: 29906306]

[42] Chen X, Hong S, Sun X, *et al.* Efficacy of fish oil and its components in the management of psoriasis: a systematic review of 18 randomized controlled trials. Nutr Rev 2020; 78(10): 827-40.
[http://dx.doi.org/10.1093/nutrit/nuz098] [PMID: 31995220]

[43] Crisan M, David L, Moldovan B, *et al.* New nanomaterials for the improvement of psoriatic lesions. J Mater Chem B Mater Biol Med 2013; 1(25): 3152-8.
[http://dx.doi.org/10.1039/c3tb20476f] [PMID: 32260915]

[44] David L, Moldovan B, Vulcu A, *et al.* Green synthesis, characterization and anti-inflammatory activity of silver nanoparticles using European black elderberry fruits extract. Colloids Surf B Biointerfaces 2014; 122: 767-77.
[http://dx.doi.org/10.1016/j.colsurfb.2014.08.018] [PMID: 25174985]

[45] Gębka N, Adamczyk J, Gębka-Kępińska B, Mizgała-Izworska E. The role of flavonoids in prevention and treatment of selected skin diseases. Journal of Pre-Clinical and Clinical Research 2022; 16(3): 99-107.
[http://dx.doi.org/10.26444/jpccr/152551]

[46] Pratheeshkumar P, Son YO, Wang X, *et al.* Cyanidin-3-glucoside inhibits UVB-induced oxidative damage and inflammation by regulating MAP kinase and NF-κB signaling pathways in SKH-1 hairless mice skin. Toxicol Appl Pharmacol 2014; 280(1): 127-37.
[http://dx.doi.org/10.1016/j.taap.2014.06.028] [PMID: 25062774]

[47] Čižmárová B, Hubková B, Tomečková V, Birková A. Flavonoids as promising natural compounds in the prevention and treatment of selected skin diseases. Int J Mol Sci 2023; 24(7): 6324.
[http://dx.doi.org/10.3390/ijms24076324] [PMID: 37047297]

[48] Basu A, Schell J, Scofield RH. Dietary fruits and arthritis. Food Funct 2018; 9(1): 70-7.
[http://dx.doi.org/10.1039/C7FO01435J] [PMID: 29227497]

[49] Schell J, Scofield R, Barrett J, *et al.* Strawberries improve pain and inflammation in obese adults with radiographic evidence of knee osteoarthritis. Nutrients 2017; 9(9): 949.
[http://dx.doi.org/10.3390/nu9090949] [PMID: 28846633]

[50] Javadi F, Ahmadzadeh A, Eghtesadi S, *et al.* The effect of quercetin on inflammatory factors and clinical symptoms in women with rheumatoid arthritis: A double-blind, randomized controlled trial. J Am Coll Nutr 2017; 36(1): 9-15.
[http://dx.doi.org/10.1080/07315724.2016.1140093] [PMID: 27710596]

[51] Figueira ME, Oliveira M, Direito R, *et al.* Protective effects of a blueberry extract in acute inflammation and collagen-induced arthritis in the rat. Biomed Pharmacother 2016; 83: 1191-202.
[http://dx.doi.org/10.1016/j.biopha.2016.08.040] [PMID: 27551767]

[52] Akhtar N, Khan NM, Ashruf OS, Haqqi TM. Inhibition of cartilage degradation and suppression of PGE_2 and MMPs expression by pomegranate fruit extract in a model of posttraumatic osteoarthritis. Nutrition 2017; 33: 1-13.
[http://dx.doi.org/10.1016/j.nut.2016.08.004] [PMID: 27908544]

[53] Ghavipour M, Sotoudeh G, Tavakoli E, Mowla K, Hasanzadeh J, Mazloom Z. Pomegranate extract alleviates disease activity and some blood biomarkers of inflammation and oxidative stress in Rheumatoid Arthritis patients. Eur J Clin Nutr 2017; 71(1): 92-6.

[http://dx.doi.org/10.1038/ejcn.2016.151] [PMID: 27577177]

[54] Ghoochani N, Karandish M, Mowla K, Haghighizadeh MH, Jalali MT. The effect of pomegranate juice on clinical signs, matrix metalloproteinases and antioxidant status in patients with knee osteoarthritis. J Sci Food Agric 2016; 96(13): 4377-81.
[http://dx.doi.org/10.1002/jsfa.7647] [PMID: 26804926]

[55] Hadipour-Jahromy M, Mozaffari-Kermani R. Chondroprotective effects of pomegranate juice on monoiodoacetate☐induced osteoarthritis of the knee joint of mice. Phytother Res 2010; 24(2): 182-5.
[http://dx.doi.org/10.1002/ptr.2880] [PMID: 19504467]

[56] Figueira ME, Câmara MB, Direito R, *et al.* Chemical characterization of a red raspberry fruit extract and evaluation of its pharmacological effects in experimental models of acute inflammation and collagen-induced arthritis. Food Funct 2014; 5(12): 3241-51.
[http://dx.doi.org/10.1039/C4FO00376D] [PMID: 25322288]

[57] Liu Y, Sun Z, Xu D, *et al.* Hesperidin derivative-11 inhibits fibroblast-like synoviocytes proliferation by activating Secreted frizzled-related protein 2 in adjuvant arthritis rats. Eur J Pharmacol 2017; 794: 173-83.
[http://dx.doi.org/10.1016/j.ejphar.2016.10.004] [PMID: 27720921]

[58] Motevalian M, Shiri M, Shiri S, Shiri Z, Shiri H. Anti-inflammatory activity of *Elaeagnus angustifolia* fruit extract on rat paw edema. J Basic Clin Physiol Pharmacol 2017; 28(4): 377-81.
[http://dx.doi.org/10.1515/jbcpp-2015-0154] [PMID: 28358712]

[59] Kellogg J, Wang J, Flint C, *et al.* Alaskan wild berry resources and human health under the cloud of climate change. J Agric Food Chem 2010; 58(7): 3884-900.
[http://dx.doi.org/10.1021/jf902693r] [PMID: 20025229]

[60] Edirisinghe I, Burton-Freeman B. Anti-diabetic actions of Berry polyphenols – Review on proposed mechanisms of action. J Berry Res 2016; 6(2): 237-50.
[http://dx.doi.org/10.3233/JBR-160137]

[61] Bhowmik D, Gopinath H, Kumar BP, Duraivel S, Aravind G, Kumar KP. Sampath. Traditional and Medicinal Uses of Indian Black Berry. J Pharmacogn Phytochem 2013; 1(5): 36-41.

[62] Thangthaeng N, Poulose SM, Miller MG, Shukitt-Hale B. Preserving brain function in aging: The anti-glycative potential of Berry Fruit. Neuromolecular Med 2016; 18(3): 465-73.
[http://dx.doi.org/10.1007/s12017-016-8400-3] [PMID: 27166828]

[63] Jeon YD, Kang SH, Moon KH, *et al.* The effect of Aronia Berry on type 1 diabetes *in vivo* and *in vitro*. J Med Food 2018; 21(3): 244-53.
[http://dx.doi.org/10.1089/jmf.2017.3939] [PMID: 29470134]

[64] Tsuda T. Regulation of adipocyte function by anthocyanins; possibility of preventing the metabolic syndrome. J Agric Food Chem 2008; 56(3): 642-6.
[http://dx.doi.org/10.1021/jf073113b] [PMID: 18211021]

[65] Jenkins DJA, Srichaikul K, Kendall CWC, *et al.* The relation of low glycaemic index fruit consumption to glycaemic control and risk factors for coronary heart disease in type 2 diabetes. Diabetologia 2011; 54(2): 271-9.
[http://dx.doi.org/10.1007/s00125-010-1927-1] [PMID: 20978741]

[66] Du H, Li L, Bennett D, *et al.* Fresh fruit consumption in relation to incident diabetes and diabetic vascular complications: A 7-y prospective study of 0.5 million Chinese adults. PLoS Med 2017; 14(4): e1002279.
[http://dx.doi.org/10.1371/journal.pmed.1002279] [PMID: 28399126]

[67] Bondonno NP, Davey RJ, Murray K, *et al.* Associations between fruit intake and risk of diabetes in the ausdiab cohort. The Journal of Clinical Endocrinology &amp. J Clin Endocrinol Metab 2021; 106(10): e4097-108.
[http://dx.doi.org/10.1210/clinem/dgab335] [PMID: 34076673]

[68]   Stull AJ, Cash KC, Johnson WD, Champagne CM, Cefalu WT. Bioactives in blueberries improve insulin sensitivity in obese, insulin-resistant men and women. J Nutr 2010; 140(10): 1764-8.
[http://dx.doi.org/10.3945/jn.110.125336] [PMID: 20724487]

[69]   Takikawa M, Inoue S, Horio F, Tsuda T. Dietary anthocyanin-rich bilberry extract ameliorates hyperglycemia and insulin sensitivity *via* activation of AMP-activated protein kinase in diabetic mice. J Nutr 2010; 140(3): 527-33.
[http://dx.doi.org/10.3945/jn.109.118216] [PMID: 20089785]

[70]   Elks CM, Terrebonne JD, Ingram DK, Stephens JM. Blueberries improve glucose tolerance without altering body composition in obese postmenopausal mice. Obesity (Silver Spring) 2015; 23(3): 573-80.
[http://dx.doi.org/10.1002/oby.20926] [PMID: 25611327]

[71]   Chao C, Mong M, Chan K, Yin M. Anti-glycative and anti-inflammatory effects of caffeic acid and ellagic acid in kidney of diabetic mice. Mol Nutr Food Res 2010; 54(3): 388-95.
[http://dx.doi.org/10.1002/mnfr.200900087] [PMID: 19885845]

[72]   McDougall GJ, Shpiro F, Dobson P, Smith P, Blake A, Stewart D. Different polyphenolic components of soft fruits inhibit α-amylase and α-glucosidase. J Agric Food Chem 2005; 53(7): 2760-6.
[http://dx.doi.org/10.1021/jf0489926] [PMID: 15796622]

[73]   Grussu D, Stewart D, McDougall GJ. Berry polyphenols inhibit α-amylase *in vitro*: identifying active components in rowanberry and raspberry. J Agric Food Chem 2011; 59(6): 2324-31.
[http://dx.doi.org/10.1021/jf1045359] [PMID: 21329358]

[74]   Panchal SK, Ward L, Brown L. Ellagic acid attenuates high-carbohydrate, high-fat diet-induced metabolic syndrome in rats. Eur J Nutr 2013; 52(2): 559-68.
[http://dx.doi.org/10.1007/s00394-012-0358-9] [PMID: 22538930]

[75]   Calvano A, Izuora K, Oh EC, Ebersole JL, Lyons TJ, Basu A. Dietary berries, insulin resistance and type 2 diabetes: an overview of human feeding trials. Food Funct 2019; 10(10): 6227-43.
[http://dx.doi.org/10.1039/C9FO01426H] [PMID: 31591634]

[76]   da Silva Pinto M, de Carvalho JE, Lajolo FM, Genovese MI, Shetty K. Evaluation of antiproliferative, anti-type 2 diabetes, and antihypertension potentials of ellagitannins from strawberries (Fragaria × ananassa Duch.) using *in vitro* models. J Med Food 2010; 13(5): 1027-35.
[http://dx.doi.org/10.1089/jmf.2009.0257] [PMID: 20626254]

[77]   Paquette M, Medina Larqué AS, Weisnagel SJ, *et al.* Strawberry and cranberry polyphenols improve insulin sensitivity in insulin-resistant, non-diabetic adults: a parallel, double-blind, controlled and randomised clinical trial. Br J Nutr 2017; 117(4): 519-31.
[http://dx.doi.org/10.1017/S0007114517000393] [PMID: 28290272]

[78]   Xin J, Feinstein DL, Hejna MJ, Lorens SA, McGuire SO. Beneficial effects of blueberries in experimental autoimmune encephalomyelitis. J Agric Food Chem 2012; 60(23): 5743-8.
[http://dx.doi.org/10.1021/jf203611t] [PMID: 22243431]

[79]   Guerrero Muñoz E, Alarcón Lozano M. Berries Chilenos (Aristotelia chilensis y Berberis microphylla) inhiben la producción de citoquinas proinflamatorias en células mononucleares humanas. Escuela de Tecnología Médica 2015.

[80]   Dong A, Yu J, Chen X, Wang LS. Potential of dietary supplementation with berries to enhance immunity in humans. J Food Bioact 2021; 16: 19-24.
[http://dx.doi.org/10.31665/JFB.2021.16289]

[81]   Correa-Betanzo J, Padmanabhan P, Corredig M, Subramanian J, Paliyath G. Complex formation of blueberry (Vaccinium angustifolium) anthocyanins during freeze-drying and its influence on their biological activity. J Agric Food Chem 2015; 63(11): 2935-46.
[http://dx.doi.org/10.1021/acs.jafc.5b00016] [PMID: 25727778]

CHAPTER 9

The Role of Herbal Therapy in the Treatment of Graves' Disease and Hashimoto Thyroiditis

Mehmet Tolga Kafadar[1,*] and **Baran Demir**[1]

[1] *Department of General Surgery, Faculty of Medicine, Dicle University, Diyarbakır 21280, Türkiye*

Abstract: Currently, Hashimoto's thyroiditis (HT) and Graves' disease (GD) are the foremost conditions that people think of when discussing autoimmune thyroid disorders. While radioactive iodine (RAI) treatment, anti-thyroid drugs, and surgical resection are currently at the forefront for GD; thyroid replacement therapy is used for HT. Many studies are being performed to develop new treatment methods for Graves and Hashimoto thyroiditis patients who do not respond to traditional treatments. While herbal treatments are being tried for GD, studies are being carried out on changing nutritional habits or additional food supplements for HT. While there are currently many studies on traditional Chinese medicine in the literature for GD, nutrients for HT are considered complementary treatments using their anti-inflammatory and antioxidant properties. In patients with HT, the need for levothyroxine increases, especially due to possible interactions of gliadin with thyroid antigens, the presence of lactose components in levothyroxine preparations, and damage to the intestinal villi in those with lactose intolerance. Therefore, the course of the disease may be better in HT patients with additional dietary recommendations.

Keywords: Autoimmune thyroid diseases, Chinese medicine, Hashimoto's thyroiditis, Graves' disease, Herbal therapy, Hyperthyroidism, Hypothyroidism, Thyroglobulin, Thyrotoxicosis.

INTRODUCTION

The prevalence of autoimmune diseases (AIDs) is gradually increasing worldwide. Autoimmune diseases are seen in approximately 5% of the general population in developed countries and their cause is multifactorial and is not fully known. The first diseases that come to mind when it comes to autoimmune thyroid diseases (ATD) are Graves' Disease (GD) and Hashimoto thyroiditis (HT). Clinically, HT usually manifests with hypothyroidism and GD with thyrotoxicosis [1].

---

* **Corresponding author Mehmet Tolga Kafadar:** Department of General Surgery, Faculty of Medicine, Dicle University, Diyarbakır 21280, Türkiye; Tel: +90 4122488001; E-mail: drtolgakafadar@hotmail.com

Cennet Ozay & Gokhan Zengin (Eds.)

Graves' disease (GD) is an autoimmune disease defined by diffuse thyroid enlargement of the thyroid gland and elevated blood thyroid hormone levels. Patients suffer from symptoms of thyrotoxicosis including excessive sweating, irritability, palpitations, weakness, fatigue, heat intolerance, and insomnia. Anti-thyroid drugs are currently used as the first step in treatment against GD. Thyroidectomy or ablation with radioactive iodine (RAI) causes permanent hypothyroidism and necessitates life-long thyroid hormone replacement therapy [7].

Also called chronic lymphocytic thyroiditis, Hashimoto thyroiditis (HT) is currently regarded as the most frequent AID. HT is characterized by the existence of circulating autoantibodies against thyroglobulin (TG), thyroid peroxidase (TPO) and lymphocytes infiltrating the thyroid tissue. Although hyperthyroidism and euthyroidism phases are observed in HT, most patients eventually develop hypothyroidism. Early diagnosis and intervention are particularly important as high thyroid autoantibody levels cause lower quality of life in euthyroid HT patients. It involves the substitution of thyroid hormones to address hypothyroidism associated with HT [2]. This chapter aims to evaluate the effects of herbs and herbal metabolites on the management of Hashimoto's thyroiditis and Graves' disease.

AUTOIMMUNE THYROID DISEASES

Worldwide, there is a gradual increase in the prevalence of autoimmune diseases. The etiology of autoimmune diseases is multifaceted and remains incompletely understood. However, it is thought that T-lymphocytes escaping from central and peripheral tolerance mechanisms trigger autoimmunity. The organ most affected by these diseases is the thyroid gland. The first diseases that come to mind when it comes to autoimmune thyroid diseases (ATD) are Hashimoto thyroiditis (HT) and Graves' Disease (GD). Clinically, HT usually manifests with hypothyroidism, and GD with thyrotoxicosis. These disorders can emerge in genetically susceptible individuals with the addition of environmental factors [1]. Other autoimmune diseases such as vitiligo, rheumatoid arthritis, myasthenia gravis, coeliac disease, and primary adrenal insufficiency may accompany ATDs [2].

Although HT is most commonly seen between 45 and 65 years of age, it may also be seen in children. Its prevalence in adults is reported to be 5%. The prevalence of autoimmune thyroid diseases in school-age children is reportedly 2.5% [2].

The Pathophysiology of Graves' Disease

Graves' disease (GD) is an autoimmune disease characterized by diffuse enlargement of the thyroid gland and elevated blood thyroid hormone levels. It is most commonly seen in women of 20-40 years of age. Patients suffer from symptoms of thyrotoxicosis including excessive sweating, irritability, palpitations, weakness, fatigue, heat intolerance, and insomnia. Blood TSH level is low, T3 and/or T4 levels are elevated. In addition, increased vascularization and parenchymal heterogeneity of the thyroid gland, and the presence of TSH Receptor Antibody (TRAB) are sufficient to make the diagnosis [3].

In GD, there is an abnormal activation of the immune system and a loss of immune tolerance against TSHR [4]. In addition, hydrophilic muco-polysaccharides proinflammatory cytokines released as a result of the effect of TRAB on TSHR on the surface of fibroblasts cause local edema, congestion, and exophthalmos in the eye [5].

Recent research has indicated that the insulin-like growth factor-1 receptor (IGF-1R) plays a crucial role as both a significant factor and autoantigen in the development of Graves' ophthalmopathy (GO) [6, 7] (Fig. **1**).

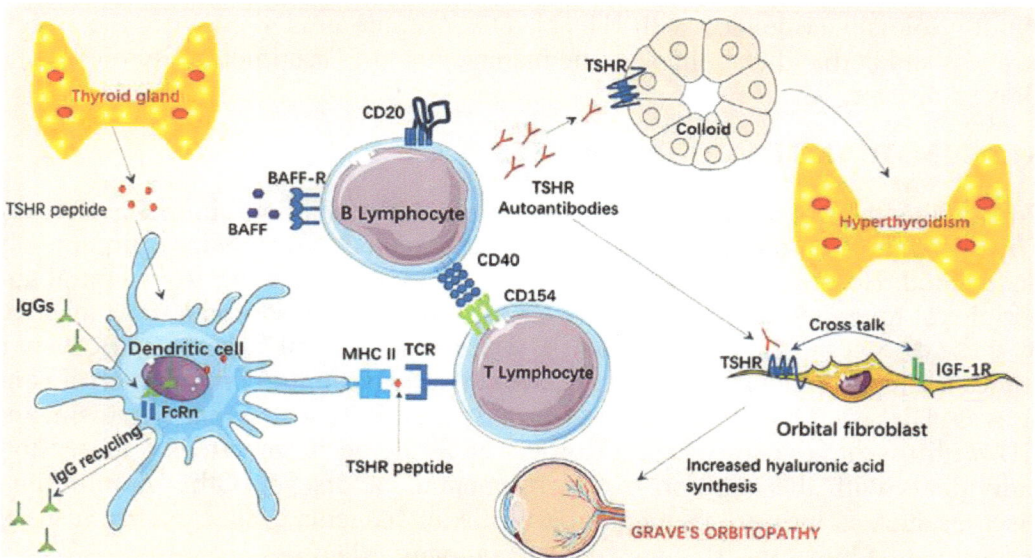

Fig. (1). Pathogenesis of Graves Hyperthyroidism and Orbitopathy [7].

Large amounts of TRAB are released from B lymphocytes as a result of humoral immune response activation. TRAB, which is released from B lymphocytes, is divided into two groups, namely inductor TRAB and inhibitor TRAB [8]. Circulating TRAB acts like a TSH agonist and binds to TSHR to stimulate thyroid cells to proliferate and get hypertrophied. As a result, the expression of the thyroglobulin, thyroid peroxidase, and sodium-ion cotransporter genes is promoted. Consequently, thyroid hormone production is increased and hyperthyroidism occurs [4].

Moreover, the B cell activating factor (BAFF), belonging to the TNF cytokine family, assumes a crucial function in the activation, differentiation, and survival of B lymphocytes. Elevated circulating levels of BAFF have been observed in individuals with various AIDs, including Graves' disease. In this context, there is a demonstrated correlation between higher levels of thyroid hormones and TRAB with the serum BAFF level [9]. The interaction between BAFF and its receptor on the surface of B lymphocytes serves as the second signal to initiate an adaptive humoral immune response.

TRAB is positive in 90% of Graves's patients and pathognomic for GD. It is believed that stimulating TRAB is responsible for hyperthyroidism in GD [10]. TRAB is useful in predicting treatment response to antithyroid therapy and recurrence after the treatment of GD. In patients with high antibody levels, stopping the drug will lead to recurrence. Anti-TPO is positive in 75% of Graves patients [11]. In genetically susceptible individuals, GD is triggered by infections, psychological stress, pregnancy, drugs, and sex-associated factors. In GD, the total T3/total T4 ratio is usually above 20. GD is a disease characterized by remissions and relapses.

In half of Graves's patients, the clinical symptoms may be accompanied by ocular symptoms. Dermopathy and acropathy can also be found in addition to oculopathy. It is known that CXCL10, which is released from thyrocytes, fibroblasts, and preadipocytes by the effect of IFN-γ, contributes to the pathogenesis of oculopathy in GD. There are studies indicating that blood CXCL10 levels are higher in patients with active Graves or relapses. It has been observed that blood CXCL10 levels dropped after those patients were treated with thyroidectomy or radioactive iodine [12].

THE TRADITIONAL TREATMENT OF GRAVES' DISEASE

Currently, anti-thyroid drugs represent the initial treatment approach for Graves' disease (GD). Thyroidectomy or ablation with radioactive iodine (RAI) causes permanent hypothyroidism and necessitates life-long thyroid hormone replacement therapy. In patients with active GD, high-dose intravenous corticosteroids or immunoglobulins may be administered to alleviate inflammation and reduce orbital congestion. Orbital decompression surgery and post-globular radiotherapy are alternative options for managing Graves' ophthalmopathy (GO). However, the widespread utilization of these treatments is constrained by their associated side effects [13].

There are currently three classical treatment methods for Graves hyperthyroidism: anti-thyroid drugs (ATD), total thyroidectomy (TX), and RAI therapy. Anti-thyroid drugs are used as the first-line treatment [14]. Propylthiouracil (PTU) and Methimazole (MMI) are the two drugs used for this purpose. MMI inhibits iodination, a process catalyzed by thyroid peroxidase [15]. MMI is considered the standard ATD having an acceptable, low side effect profile, longest half-life, and highest efficacy [16].

Nevertheless, the effectiveness of antithyroid drug therapy in GD is constrained. A more radical therapy involving RAI or TX can be selected in patients with sustained TRAB elevation or hyperthyroidism at the 18th month of medical therapy or those with a recurrence after the completion of therapy. Radioactive iodine treatment should be avoided in patients with Graves' disease who have active Graves' ophthalmopathy or a history of smoking [17].

Available GD therapies have many adverse effects. In a study, 2,430 newly diagnosed Graves patients were sampled from 13 endocrinology clinics in Sweden; the remission rates for ATD, RAI, and surgery were reported as 45.3% (351/774), 81.5% (324/264), and 96.3% (52/54), respectively [18]. In the same study, it was reported that the remission rate was even lower when ATD was re-administered to patients with GD recurrence after remission had been achieved with ATD (29.4%). Recurrences after treatment are one of the main problems in the management of GD; a large goiter size has been linked to an increased recurrence risk in a significant manner. In patients for whom ATD was selected as the first-line therapy, the chances of averting ablation were merely 50.3% and the likelihood of having a long-term normal thyroid function was only 40% [18]. In addition, several studies have suggested that the risk of hypothyroidism after RAI therapy is much higher than the risk after ATD. Furthermore, it has been reported that GO is exacerbated by increased TRAB after RAI therapy. In a study, the incidence of GO was reported to be 15% for RAI and 2% for MMI [19]. It was reported that oral steroid prophylaxis for GO is effective and safe after RAI therapy [20]. There is a life-long need for thyroxine replacement therapy after surgical treatment; calcium-phosphate imbalance due to a low PTH level may also be seen [21].

In order to predict the likelihood of recurrence at the start of treatment of hyperthyroidism in GD, GREAT (Graves' Recurrent Events after Treatment) score and the Clinical Severity Score (CSS) have been developed [22].

The clinical demand for novel treatment regimens of Graves' disease has led to the development of many novel treatment ideas including biologics, low-molecule peptides, immunomodulators, and teprotumumab. Since the elements of

Traditional Chinese Medicine (TCM) possess unique therapeutic effects and mechanisms of action, they attract the increasing attention of modern medicine. Nutraceuticals belong to TCM, defined as food or food parts that provide medical or health benefits, including the prevention or treatment of different pathological conditions and thyroid diseases. Nutraceuticals have a place within complementary medicines, positioned in a field between food, food supplements, and pharmaceuticals. The market of some nutraceuticals such as thyroid supplements has been increasing in recent years [23].

The Role of Herbal Therapy in the Treatment of Graves' Disease

Diosgenin

Diosgenin is a natural steroidal saponin found in large quantities in *Dioscorea bulbifera* [24]. It has been shown that diosgenin successfully controls hyperthyroidism and goiter in mice with Graves' disease while it has a little effect on thyroxine expression and thyroid tissue in mice with normal thyroid tissue. It has also been observed that high-dose diosgenin treatment had an extremely low and statistically non-significant effect on intact thyroid tissue. Therefore, it is believed that diosgenin selectively affects hypertrophied thyroid tissue rather than normal thyroid tissue and has a quite low likelihood of causing hypothyroidism. It is thought that the target of diosgenin is not TRAB expression but thyroid cell proliferation [24].

Beyond thyroid receptor antibodies, numerous growth factors play a role in cell proliferation in Graves' disease. Among these, IGF-1 is regarded as the most significant factor [25]. Diosgenin inhibits thyroid cell proliferation of IGF-1 origin *in vitro* by reducing the expressions of IGF-1, cyclin D, NF-κB, and proliferating cell nuclear antigen [26]. Studies have shown that diosgenin could concurrently prevent the overexpression of proteins associated with proliferation in mice's thyroid glands, which suggests that diosgenin is a potential new drug candidate for the treatment of Graves' disease [25].

Resveratrol

Resveratrol, the bioactive phytochemical of the plant *Reynoutria japonica*, a stilbenoid produced by plants in response to injury, is associated with elevated levels of Cu/Zn superoxide dismutase and glyoxal oxidase [27]. Research indicates that orbital fibroblasts exhibit heightened sensitivity to oxidative stress, establishing a connection between oxidative stress and the pathogenesis of Graves' ophthalmopathy. It has been demonstrated that resveratrol reduces oxidative stress and increases the nuclear and transcriptional activity of Factor 2 (NRF2), thereby increasing the ability to bind to antioxidant genes (ARE) [28]. In another study, it was shown that resveratrol reduces the production of reactive oxygen species (ROS) and human heme oxygenase 1 (HO^{-1}) caused by oxidative stress and inhibits lipogenesis and lipid droplet accumulation [29]. Resveratrol enhances the nuclear translocation of NRF2, stimulates the activation of the NRF2-ARE pathway, and induces the expression of the antioxidant gene ARE in cultured orbital fibroblasts. In summary, resveratrol demonstrates the potential to alleviate symptoms associated with oxidative stress by activating the NRF2-ARE pathway. Moreover, it can inhibit the adipogenesis of orbital fibroblasts *in vivo* by reducing ROS production.

Icariin

Icariin, the bioactive compound of the plant *Epimedium brevicornum* (Berberidaceae), inhibits the differentiation of preadipocytes into adipocytes by suppressing autophagy; it mediates these events by blocking the activation of the protein kinase/rapamycin mechanical target (AMPK/mTOR) pathway activated by 5'-adenosine phosphate [30]. Moreover, *E. brevicornum* has the potential to diminish the accumulation of orbital adipose cells during the inactive phase of Graves' ophthalmopathy, contributing to its therapeutic effect. This effect may be elucidated by heightened expressions of death receptor (Fas)/death receptor ligand and apoptosis [31].

Celastrol

Celastrol, the bioactive triterpenoid ingredient of the plant *Celastrus orbiculatus* (Celastraceae), is a promising drug for treating diverse inflammatory diseases and AIDs [7]. Cytokines play a pivotal role in the development of Graves' ophthalmopathy and are crucial for both the initiation and sustenance of inflammation. Studies have reported elevated mRNA expression of IL-1β in the orbital tissues of Graves' ophthalmopathy patients, indicating that IL-1β plays a role in mediating inflammatory responses [32]. It was shown that Celastrol significantly inhibits IL-1β and thus inhibits the production of orbital fibroblast cytokines IL-6, IL-8, intercellular adhesion molecule (ICAM-1), and cyclooxygenase (COX-2) of IL-1β origin [33, 34]. It is also recognized that COX-2 is the key to the inflammatory response of GO patients, and COX-2 expression is positively associated with increasing severity of orbital diseases [34]. IL-1β promotes orbital fibroblasts through the activation of the NF-κB pathway in patients with GO-producing high levels of COX-2. Celastrol inhibits the production of the cytokines IL-6, IL 8, ICAM-1, and COX-2 in orbital fibroblasts induced by IL-1β, which suppresses inflammation and prevents GO from progressing further [35].

Gypenosides

These are the active pharmacological saponin components in *Gynostemma pentaphyllum* and possess various biological activities. It has been observed that Gypenosides can regulate immune cell activation and cytokine expression and have the potential to suppress the inflammatory reaction associated with various diseases [36, 37]. Gypenosides possess both anti-inflammatory and antioxidant activities. These activities are made possible by signal transducer and transcription activator STAT1 and STAT3 signal pathways. By inhibiting the expression of the STAT-1 pathway, they inhibit the production of chemokine 10 (IP 10)/CXC-chemokine ligand 10 (CXCL10) of (IFN)-y origin in the orbital fibroblasts of the GO patients; in this way, they can prevent orbital inflammation [38]. STAT3 signal pathway plays an anti-inflammatory, antioxidant, and immunomodulatory role in chronic respiratory tract diseases, breast cancer, and hepatic inflammation [39, 40]. Inflammation of the orbital tissues and oxidative stress injury are the major pathogenetic mechanisms of GO (Li and others, 2016; Rotondo Dottore and others, 2017). Therefore, the signal pathways targeted by Gynostevenosides in the treatment of GO include STAT1 and STAT3 [41].

Astragaloside IV

Astragaloside IV, an active component of *Astragalus mongholicus,* exhibits antioxidant and anti-inflammatory activities and shows therapeutic potential in various ischemic and inflammatory diseases [42]. IL-1β upregulates the mRNA expression of inflammatory cytokines such as IL-6, IL-8, TNF-α, and monocyte chemotactic protein-1 in cultured orbital fibroblasts. Treatment with AS-IV significantly decreased IL-1β-induced production of inflammatory cytokines *in vitro*. *In vivo*, it demonstrated a reduction in orbital inflammation, fat accumulation, collagen deposition, and macrophage infiltration in GO. The protective impact of AS-IV on GO has also been associated with a decrease in autophagy activity in both orbital fibroblasts and orbital tissues [42].

Ingredients from Prunella vulgaris

Spica Prunellae (SP), derived from *Prunella vulgaris* is a traditional antipyretic botanic remedy extensively distributed in Northeast Asia [43]. SP is widely used for thyroid disorders such as goiter and subacute thyroiditis [41]. It is regarded as an important component in many herbal formulations in GO treatment [44]. According to the Joint Center gene pathway network, rutin, ursolic acid and quercetin entered interaction with the main active ingredients and many targets showing important roles in the anti-GO system [43].

Quercetin is a flavonoid phytoestrogen exhibiting antioxidant and anti-inflammatory properties and limiting proliferation in orbital fibroblasts. It has been reported that ursolic acid and rutin promote apoptosis and regulate the immune system in cell and animal models [43]. PI3K-Akt signal pathway plays an important role in both immune inflammation and proliferation, apoptosis; this process may be an effective target for SP [45]. With respect to immune inflammation, it has been confirmed that the pro-inflammatory cytokines COX-2, IL-6, and TNFa play a role in the pathogenesis of GO. Previous studies have shown that COX-2 is reduced with decreasing GO clinical activity scores and is now regarded as critical for the anti-inflammatory process in patients with GO [34, 46]. COX-2 takes part in the biosynthesis of prostaglandins that play a key role in inflammation. IL-6 is related to the pathogenesis of autoimmune disorders and it has been reported that the AKT/NF-κB signal pathway contributes to IL-6 production in the retro bulbar space during GO activity [47]. Similarly, it has been demonstrated that the AKT/NF- κB signal pathway mediates inflammation and higher serum TNF levels in GO. It has been currently reported that some TNF inhibitors like SP achieved promising results in GO patients regardless of rare side effects [48]. Recent research has indicated that orbital fibroblasts overexpress TSHR and activate the PI3K-Akt pathway, boosting the expression and proliferation of inflammatory genes. Additionally, the PI3K-Akt signal pathway contributes to the progression of GO by participating in the proliferation of the pre-orbital adipose cells. Caspase 3 (CASP3) activation is one of the final steps of the apoptosis and SP activates CASP3 to exert a proapoptotic activity in GO [49].

Triptolide

Triptolide, extracted from *Tripterygium wilfordii*, has been observed to induce T cell apoptosis, reduce IL-2 synthesis, and inhibit NF-κB expression and T cell proliferation [50, 51]. Triptolide IFN-y-induced RF activation reduces the expressions of HLA-DR, ICAM-1, and CD40 in GO. It has been shown that thanks to these effects, it inhibits cellular proliferation and hyaluronic acid (HA) synthesis and mitigates exophthalmos, diplopia, and clinical signs of periorbital edema and congestion [52].

Bupleurum Saponins from Bupleurum falcatum

Bupleurum falcatum (Bupleuri radix with strong antioxidant effects), has been shown to have favorable effects on hyperthyroidism symptoms induced by levothyroxine (LT4) [53].

In addition to all these herbs, the effects of compounds such as *Prunella vulgaris* L. (Lamiaceae; Prunellae spica fruit), *Bupleurum falcatum* L. (Apiaceae; Bupleuri radix), *Fritillaria thunbergia* Miq (Liliaceae; Fritillaria thunbergia bulb), and

Paeonia lactiflora Pall (Paeoniaceae; Paeonia species flowers and stems), *etc.* on autoimmune diseases and Graves' disease will be examined in later stages.

THE PATHOPHYSIOLOGY AND TRADITIONAL TREATMENT OF HASHIMOTO DISEASE

Also called chronic lymphocytic thyroiditis, Hashimoto thyroiditis (HT) is currently considered the most common autoimmune disease. HT is characterized by the existence of circulating autoantibodies against thyroid peroxidase (TPO), thyroglobulin (TG) and lymphocytes infiltrating the thyroid tissue. Although hyperthyroid, euthyroid states are seen in HT, many patients eventually develop a hypothyroid state [54]. In a cross-sectional study performed in China, the positivity rates of the anti-TPO antibodies (TPOAb) and anti-Tg antibodies (TgAb) in adults were found to be 10.19% and 9.70%, respectively [55]. Recent studies have suggested that TgAb and TPOAb can increase the risk of both thyroid cancer and thyroid nodules [56, 57]. Higher levels of thyroid autoantibodies not only cause hypothyroidism, but they also have an important effect on the progression of HT disease. There are studies indicating that higher thyroid autoantibody levels in euthyroid HT patients may lead to a lower quality of life score and vestibular dysfunction [58, 59]. Therefore, early diagnosis and intervention are particularly important. The treatment involves thyroid hormone replacement for HT-related hypothyroidism. The main pharmacotherapeutic agent is levothyroxine [57].

The Effect of Nutrition on the Treatment of Hashimoto's Disease

Diet can be a supplementary treatment for Hashimoto's disease by affecting thyroid function and anti-inflammatory features. Although it is not clear yet which diet strategy would be most beneficial, a large number of studies have been conducted on this subject. While genetic factors are responsible for 70-80% of the risk, environmental factors are responsible for the remaining 20-30%. Thus, the elimination of environmental factors and the nutritional effect is believed to be effective in treating HT and improving its course. So, more research is needed on the nutritional factors, which have a protective role in HT.

As far as we know, reviews and meta-analyses published so far have focused on the importance of selected nutrients that is selenium, vitamin D, iodine, gluten, zinc, iron, and guatrogens, in HT [60 - 62]. Some of these nutritional factors such as selenium and vitamin D have been proven to be related to HT pathogenesis [60, 63]. It has been shown that selenium supplementation significantly decreases autoantibody levels [64]; however, the clinical efficacy of selenium supplements is yet controversial. Moreover, available clinical evidence regarding the effect of dietary factors on HT is still insufficient and inconclusive.

Gluten Diet

Elimination of gluten from the diet is the treatment of several diseases including Coeliac disease, Duhring disease, wheat allergy, or non-coeliac gluten sensitivity (NCGS) [65]. Coeliac disease is more common in individuals with Hashimoto's disease [66]. This may lead to a higher levothyroxine requirement for treatment due to a lower levothyroxine absorption capacity of the gastrointestinal system [67]. Although there are studies indicating that eliminating gluten from the diet causes reductions in antibody titers, the prevailing opinion is that eliminating gluten from the diet does not provide sufficient clinical benefit unless there is a medical indication [68, 69].

Lactose Diet

There are studies indicating that a vast majority of patients with HT taking LT+ have lactose intolerance [70, 71]. Lactose is a common component of levothyroxine formulations and may cause impaired LT4 efficacy in sensitive individuals [72]. Lactose intolerance is associated with intestinal villus injury that results in bacterial overgrowth, malabsorption, and higher LT4 dose requirements. Although there are several studies recommending a search for lactose intolerance in case of high levothyroxine dose requirements or resistance to treatment and difficulty in controlling TSH [71, 73], Marabotto *et al.* [74] reported that they did not observe any difference between the cumulative LT4 dose requirements of Hashimoto patients with and without lactose intolerance. Available studies have reported that the lactose diet, like the gluten diet, provides adequate clinical benefit in HT.

Nigella sativa

There are studies reporting that *N. Sativa* treatment provided significant decreases in TSH level, weight, BMI, and waist circumference in HT patients treated with levothyroxine. In this study, an increase in T3 level was also observed. However, Anti-TPO, T4, nesfatin-1, and vascular endothelial growth factor 8VEGF) levels were not altered. In a meta-analysis by Song *et al.* [75], obesity was found to be correlated to Hashimoto's disease. A significant correlation was found between high anti-TPO levels and obesity; however, no relationship was found between a positive anti-TGA result and obesity. According to three meta-analyses, other studies have demonstrated that selenium supplementation led to a decrease in antibody titers, although the quality of evidence is low [76 - 78].

CONCLUSION

In conclusion, there is insufficient literature data as to which nutritional/dietary interventions contribute to success in the management of metabolic parameters and body weight in Hashimoto patients. It is difficult to establish the role of nutritional intervention over the stated parameters in Hashimoto's disease due to several factors. First of all, the number of available studies is low and the interventions are diversified. Furthermore, there is a possibility that patient-related and non-patient related factors may have manipulated the results. Secondly, the disease is not a homogenous condition and the variability between patients is large. Studies have not addressed the basic source of critical nutrients such as iodine, selenium, and iron, and these may show differences between countries and individuals. Hence, there is a great need for further research to clearly determine what type of nutritional intervention would be most beneficial for patients with Hashimoto's thyroiditis.

REFERENCES

[1]   Onbaşı K. Autoimmunity and thyroid. Turkiye Klinikleri J Immun Allergy-Special Topics 2018; 11(1): 16-21.

[2]   Pyzik A, Grywalska E, Matyjaszek-Matuszek B, Roliński J. Immune disorders in Hashimoto's thyroiditis: what do we know so far? J Immunol Res 2015; 2015: 1-8.
        [http://dx.doi.org/10.1155/2015/979167] [PMID: 26000316]

[3]   Canpolat GA, Erdoğan MF. Graves hastalığı ve tedavi stratejileri. Türkiye Klinikleri J Endocrin-Special Topics 2014; 7(3): 41-7.

[4]   Smith TJ, Hegedüs L. Graves' Disease. N Engl J Med 2016; 375(16): 1552-65.
        [http://dx.doi.org/10.1056/NEJMra1510030] [PMID: 27797318]

[5]   Armengol MP, Juan M, Lucas-Martín A, *et al.* Thyroid autoimmune disease: demonstration of thyroid antigen-specific B cells and recombination-activating gene expression in chemokine-containing active intrathyroidal germinal centers. Am J Pathol 2001; 159(3): 861-73.
        [http://dx.doi.org/10.1016/S0002-9440(10)61762-2] [PMID: 11549579]

[6]   Wang Y, Smith TJ. Current concepts in the molecular pathogenesis of thyroid-associated ophthalmopathy. Invest Ophthalmol Vis Sci 2014; 55(3): 1735-48.
        [http://dx.doi.org/10.1167/iovs.14-14002] [PMID: 24651704]

[7]   He Q, Dong H, Gong M, *et al.* New Therapeutic Horizon of Graves' Hyperthyroidism: Treatment Regimens Based on Immunology and Ingredients From Traditional Chinese Medicine. Front Pharmacol 2022; 13: 862831.
        [http://dx.doi.org/10.3389/fphar.2022.862831] [PMID: 35462920]

[8]   Diana T, Wüster C, Kanitz M, Kahaly GJ. Highly variable sensitivity of five binding and two bio-assays for TSH-receptor antibodies. J Endocrinol Invest 2016; 39(10): 1159-65.
        [http://dx.doi.org/10.1007/s40618-016-0478-9] [PMID: 27197966]

[9]   Lin JD, Wang YH, Fang WF, *et al.* Serum BAFF and thyroid autoantibodies in autoimmune thyroid disease. Clin Chim Acta 2016; 462: 96-102.
        [http://dx.doi.org/10.1016/j.cca.2016.09.004] [PMID: 27616625]

[10]   Antonelli A, Ferrari SM, Corrado A, Di Domenicantonio A, Fallahi P. Autoimmune thyroid disorders. Autoimmun Rev 2015; 14(2): 174-80.

[http://dx.doi.org/10.1016/j.autrev.2014.10.016] [PMID: 25461470]

[11]   Öztürk CB, Özgen G. Otoimmün tiroid hastalıkları. Türkiye Klinikleri J Endocrin-Special Topics 2010; 3(2): 18-23.

[12]   Antonelli A, Fallahi P, Elia G, *et al.* Graves' disease: Clinical manifestations, immune pathogenesis (cytokines and chemokines) and therapy. Best Pract Res Clin Endocrinol Metab 2020; 34(1): 101388.
[http://dx.doi.org/10.1016/j.beem.2020.101388] [PMID: 32059832]

[13]   He Z, Tian Y, Zhang X, *et al.* Anti-tumour and immunomodulating activities of diosgenin, a naturally occurring steroidal saponin. Nat Prod Res 2012; 26(23): 2243-6.
[http://dx.doi.org/10.1080/14786419.2011.648192] [PMID: 22235932]

[14]   Bartalena L. Diagnosis and management of Graves disease: a global overview. Nat Rev Endocrinol 2013; 9(12): 724-34.
[http://dx.doi.org/10.1038/nrendo.2013.193] [PMID: 24126481]

[15]   Taurog A, Riesco G, Larsen PR. Formation of 3,3'-diiodothyronine and 3',5',3-triiodothyronine (reverse T3) in thyroid glands of rats and in enzymatically iodinated thyroglobulin. Endocrinology 1976; 99(1): 281-90.
[http://dx.doi.org/10.1210/endo-99-1-281] [PMID: 939197]

[16]   Cooper DS. Antithyroid drugs in the management of patients with Graves' disease: an evidence-based approach to therapeutic controversies. J Clin Endocrinol Metab 2003; 88(8): 3474-81.
[http://dx.doi.org/10.1210/jc.2003-030185] [PMID: 12915620]

[17]   Kahaly GJ. Management of Graves thyroidal and extrathyroidal disease. An Update. J Clin Endocrinol Metab 2020; 105(12): 3704-20.
[http://dx.doi.org/10.1210/clinem/dgaa646] [PMID: 32929476]

[18]   Starling S. Long-term treatment outcomes for Graves disease. Nat Rev Endocrinol 2019; 15(11): 628.
[http://dx.doi.org/10.1038/s41574-019-0268-5] [PMID: 31548694]

[19]   El Kawkgi OM, Ross DS, Stan MN. Comparison of long-term antithyroid drugs versus radioactive iodine or surgery for Graves' disease: A review of the literature. Clin Endocrinol (Oxf) 2021; 95(1): 3-12.
[http://dx.doi.org/10.1111/cen.14374] [PMID: 33283314]

[20]   Rosetti S, Tanda ML, Veronesi G, *et al.* Oral steroid prophylaxis for Graves' orbitopathy after radioactive iodine treatment for Graves' disease is not only effective, but also safe. J Endocrinol Invest 2020; 43(3): 381-3.
[http://dx.doi.org/10.1007/s40618-019-01126-2] [PMID: 31587179]

[21]   Jørgensen CU, Homøe P, Dahl M, Hitz MF. Postoperative chronic hypoparathyroidism and quality of life after total thyroidectomy. JBMR Plus 2021; 5(4): e10479.
[http://dx.doi.org/10.1002/jbm4.10479] [PMID: 33869995]

[22]   Masiello E, Veronesi G, Gallo D, *et al.* Antithyroid drug treatment for Graves' disease: baseline predictive models of relapse after treatment for a patient-tailored management. J Endocrinol Invest 2018; 41(12): 1425-32.
[http://dx.doi.org/10.1007/s40618-018-0918-9] [PMID: 29946800]

[23]   Benvenga S, Ferrari SM, Elia G, *et al.* Nutraceuticals in thyroidology: A review of *in vitro* and *in vivo* animal studies. Nutrients 2020; 12(5): 1337.
[http://dx.doi.org/10.3390/nu12051337] [PMID: 32397091]

[24]   Cai H, Wang Z, Zhang H, *et al.* Diosgenin relieves goiter *via* the inhibition of thyrocyte proliferation in a mouse model of Graves' disease. Acta Pharmacol Sin 2014; 35(1): 65-73.
[http://dx.doi.org/10.1038/aps.2013.133] [PMID: 24241350]

[25]   Völzke H, Friedrich N, Schipf S, *et al.* Association between serum insulin-like growth factor-I levels and thyroid disorders in a population-based study. J Clin Endocrinol Metab 2007; 92(10): 4039-45.
[http://dx.doi.org/10.1210/jc.2007-0816] [PMID: 17666480]

[26]   Ren M, Zhong X, Ma C, *et al.* Insulin-like growth factor-1 promotes cell cycle progression *via* upregulation of cyclin D1 expression through the phosphatidylinositol 3-kinase/nuclear factor-κB signaling pathway in FRTL thyroid cells. Acta Pharmacol Sin 2009; 30(1): 113-9.
[http://dx.doi.org/10.1038/aps.2008.8] [PMID: 19060913]

[27]   Lucini L, Baccolo G, Rouphael Y, Colla G, Bavaresco L, Trevisan M. Chitosan treatment elicited defence mechanisms, pentacyclic triterpenoids and stilbene accumulation in grape (Vitis vinifera L.) bunches. Phytochemistry 2018; 156: 1-8.
[http://dx.doi.org/10.1016/j.phytochem.2018.08.011] [PMID: 30149150]

[28]   Gong W, Li J, Chen Z, *et al.* Polydatin promotes Nrf2-ARE anti-oxidative pathway through activating CKIP-1 to resist HG-induced up-regulation of FN and ICAM-1 in GMCs and diabetic mice kidneys. Free Radic Biol Med 2017; 106: 393-405.
[http://dx.doi.org/10.1016/j.freeradbiomed.2017.03.003] [PMID: 28286065]

[29]   Kim CY, Lee HJ, Chae MK, Byun JW, Lee EJ, Yoon JS. Therapeutic effect of resveratrol on oxidative stress in Graves' orbitopathy orbital fibroblasts. Invest Ophthalmol Vis Sci 2015; 56(11): 6352-61.
[http://dx.doi.org/10.1167/iovs.15-16870] [PMID: 26436888]

[30]   Li H, Yuan Y, Zhang Y, Zhang X, Gao L, Xu R. Icariin inhibits AMPK-dependent autophagy and adipogenesis in adipocytes *in vitro* and in a model of Graves' orbitopathy *in vivo*. Front Physiol 2017; 8: 45.
[http://dx.doi.org/10.3389/fphys.2017.00045] [PMID: 28243204]

[31]   Zhang R, Tan J, Wang R, *et al.* Analysis of risk factors of rapid thyroidal radioiodine-131 turnover in Graves' disease patients. Sci Rep 2017; 7(1): 8301.
[http://dx.doi.org/10.1038/s41598-017-08475-z] [PMID: 28811561]

[32]   Wakelkamp IMMJ, Bakker O, Baldeschi L, Wiersinga WM, Prummel MF. TSH-R expression and cytokine profile in orbital tissue of active *vs.* inactive Graves' ophthalmopathy patients. Clin Endocrinol (Oxf) 2003; 58(3): 280-7.
[http://dx.doi.org/10.1046/j.1365-2265.2003.01708.x] [PMID: 12608932]

[33]   Chen LF, Greene WC. Shaping the nuclear action of NF-κB. Nat Rev Mol Cell Biol 2004; 5(5): 392-401.
[http://dx.doi.org/10.1038/nrm1368] [PMID: 15122352]

[34]   Konuk EBY, Konuk O, Misirlioglu M, Menevse A, Unal M. Expression of cyclooxygenase-2 in orbital fibroadipose connective tissues of Graves' ophthalmopathy patients. Eur J Endocrinol 2006; 155(5): 681-5.
[http://dx.doi.org/10.1530/eje.1.02280] [PMID: 17062883]

[35]   Li H, Yuan Y, Zhang Y, *et al.* Celastrol inhibits IL-1β-induced inflammation in orbital fibroblasts through the suppression of NF-κB activity. Mol Med Rep 2016; 14(3): 2799-806.
[http://dx.doi.org/10.3892/mmr.2016.5570] [PMID: 27484716]

[36]   Wang X, Yang L, Yang L, *et al.* Gypenoside IX suppresses P38 MAPK/Akt/NFκB signaling pathway activation and inflammatory responses in astrocytes stimulated by proinflammatory mediators. Inflammation 2017; 40(6): 2137-50.
[http://dx.doi.org/10.1007/s10753-017-0654-x] [PMID: 28822019]

[37]   Wang F, Dang Y, Wang J, Zhou T, Zhu Y. Gypenosides attenuate lipopolysaccharide-induced optic neuritis in rats. Acta Histochem 2018; 120(4): 340-6.
[http://dx.doi.org/10.1016/j.acthis.2018.03.003] [PMID: 29559175]

[38]   Pu W, Bai R, Zhou K, *et al.* Baicalein attenuates pancreatic inflammatory injury through regulating MAPK, STAT 3 and NF-κB activation. Int Immunopharmacol 2019; 72: 204-10.
[http://dx.doi.org/10.1016/j.intimp.2019.04.018] [PMID: 30999210]

[39]   Alhusaini A, Faddaa L, Ali HM, Hassan I, El Orabi NF, Bassiouni Y. Amelioration of the protein expression of Cox2, NFκB, and STAT-3 by some antioxidants in the liver of sodium fluoride-

intoxicated rats. Dose Response 2018; 16(3)
[http://dx.doi.org/10.1177/1559325818800153]

[40]   Natarajan K, Meganathan V, Mitchell C, Boggaram V. Organic dust induces inflammatory gene
        expression in lung epithelial cells *via* ROS-dependent STAT-3 activation. Am J Physiol Lung Cell
        Mol Physiol 2019; 317(1): L127-40.
        [http://dx.doi.org/10.1152/ajplung.00448.2018] [PMID: 31042082]

[41]   Li K, Li H, Xu W, *et al.* Research on the potential mechanism of gypenosides on treating thyroid-
        associated ophthalmopathy based on network pharmacology. Med Sci Monit 2019; 25: 4923-32.
        [http://dx.doi.org/10.12659/MSM.917299] [PMID: 31268042]

[42]   Li H, Zhang Y, Min J, Gao L, Zhang R, Yang Y. Astragaloside IV attenuates orbital inflammation in
        Graves' orbitopathy through suppression of autophagy. Inflamm Res 2018; 67(2): 117-27.
        [http://dx.doi.org/10.1007/s00011-017-1100-0] [PMID: 29127443]

[43]   Zhang Y, Li X, Guo C, Dong J, Liao L. Mechanisms of Spica Prunellae against thyroid-associated
        Ophthalmopathy based on network pharmacology and molecular docking. BMC Complementary
        Medicine and Therapies 2020; 20(1): 229.
        [http://dx.doi.org/10.1186/s12906-020-03022-2] [PMID: 32689994]

[44]   Yang K, Guo KQ, Wu HY. [Clinical effect of Prunellae Oral Liquid on goiter with different thyroid
        function]. Chung Kuo Chung Hsi I Chieh Ho Tsa Chih 2007; 27(1): 37-9.
        [PMID: 17302062]

[45]   Bahn RS. Graves' Ophthalmopathy. N Engl J Med 2010; 362(8): 726-38.
        [http://dx.doi.org/10.1056/NEJMra0905750] [PMID: 20181974]

[46]   Vondrichova T, de Capretz A, Parikh H, *et al.* COX-2 and SCD, markers of inflammation and
        adipogenesis, are related to disease activity in Graves' ophthalmopathy. Thyroid 2007; 17(6): 511-7.
        [http://dx.doi.org/10.1089/thy.2007.0028] [PMID: 17614770]

[47]   Gillespie EF, Raychaudhuri N, Papageorgiou KI, *et al.* Interleukin-6 production in CD40-engaged
        fibrocytes in thyroid-associated ophthalmopathy: involvement of Akt and NF-κB. Invest Ophthalmol
        Vis Sci 2012; 53(12): 7746-53.
        [http://dx.doi.org/10.1167/iovs.12-9861] [PMID: 23092922]

[48]   Kapadia MK, Rubin PAD. The emerging use of TNF-alpha inhibitors in orbital inflammatory disease.
        Int Ophthalmol Clin 2006; 46(2): 165-81.
        [http://dx.doi.org/10.1097/00004397-200604620-00014] [PMID: 16770161]

[49]   Zhu J, Zhang W, Zhang Y, Wang Y, Liu M, Liu Y. Effects of *Spica prunellae* on caspase-3-associated
        proliferation and apoptosis in human lung cancer cells *in vitro*. J Cancer Res Ther 2018; 14(4): 760-3.
        [http://dx.doi.org/10.4103/jcrt.JCRT_1289_16] [PMID: 29970649]

[50]   Li H, Liu ZH, Dai CS, Liu D, Li LS. Triptolide inhibits proinflammatory factor-induced over-
        expression of class II MHC and B7 molecules in renal tubular epithelial cells. Acta Pharmacol Sin
        2002; 23(9): 775-81.
        [PMID: 12230943]

[51]   Qiu D, Kao PN. Immunosuppressive and anti-inflammatory mechanisms of triptolide, the principal
        active diterpenoid from the Chinese medicinal herb Tripterygium wilfordii Hook. f. Drugs R D 2003;
        4(1): 1-18.
        [http://dx.doi.org/10.2165/00126839-200304010-00001] [PMID: 12568630]

[52]   Yan S, Wang Y. Inhibitory effects of Triptolide on interferon-γ-induced human leucocyte antigen-DR,
        intercellular adhesion molecule-1, CD40 expression on retro-ocular fibroblasts derived from patients
        with Graves' ophthalmopathy. Clin Exp Ophthalmol 2006; 34(3): 265-71.
        [http://dx.doi.org/10.1111/j.1442-9071.2006.01190.x] [PMID: 16671908]

[53]   Kim SM, Kim SC, Chung IK, Cheon WH, Ku SK. Antioxidant and protective effects of bupleurum
        falcatum on the L-thyroxine-induced hyperthyroidism in rats. Evid Based Complement Alternat Med

2012; 2012: 1-12.
[http://dx.doi.org/10.1155/2012/578497] [PMID: 22888365]

[54]   Caturegli P, De Remigis A, Rose NR. Hashimoto thyroiditis: Clinical and diagnostic criteria. Autoimmun Rev 2014; 13(4-5): 391-7.
[http://dx.doi.org/10.1016/j.autrev.2014.01.007] [PMID: 24434360]

[55]   Li Y, Teng D, Ba J, *et al.* Efficacy and safety of long-term universal salt iodization on thyroid disorders: Epidemiological evidence from 31 provinces of mainland China. Thyroid 2020; 30(4): 568-79.
[http://dx.doi.org/10.1089/thy.2019.0067] [PMID: 32075540]

[56]   Wu X, Lun Y, Jiang H, *et al.* Coexistence of thyroglobulin antibodies and thyroid peroxidase antibodies correlates with elevated thyroid-stimulating hormone level and advanced tumor stage of papillary thyroid cancer. Endocrine 2014; 46(3): 554-60.
[http://dx.doi.org/10.1007/s12020-013-0121-x] [PMID: 24338678]

[57]   Xu W, Huo L, Chen Z, *et al.* The Relationship of TPOAb and TGAb with risk of thyroid nodules: A large epidemiological study. Int J Environ Res Public Health 2017; 14(7): 723.
[http://dx.doi.org/10.3390/ijerph14070723] [PMID: 28678169]

[58]   Bektas Uysal H, Ayhan M. Autoimmunity affects health-related quality of life in patients with Hashimoto's thyroiditis. Kaohsiung J Med Sci 2016; 32(8): 427-33.
[http://dx.doi.org/10.1016/j.kjms.2016.06.006] [PMID: 27523457]

[59]   Chiarella G, Russo D, Monzani F, *et al.* Hashimoto Thyroiditis and Vestibular Dysfunction. Endocr Pract 2017; 23(7): 863-8.
[http://dx.doi.org/10.4158/EP161635.RA] [PMID: 28534686]

[60]   Danailova Y, Velikova T, Nikolaev G, *et al.* Nutritional Management of Thyroiditis of Hashimoto. Int J Mol Sci 2022; 23(9): 5144.
[http://dx.doi.org/10.3390/ijms23095144] [PMID: 35563541]

[61]   Ihnatowicz P, Drywień M, Wątor P, Wojsiat J. The importance of nutritional factors and dietary management of Hashimoto's thyroiditis. Ann Agric Environ Med 2020; 27(2): 184-93.
[http://dx.doi.org/10.26444/aaem/112331] [PMID: 32588591]

[62]   Szczuko M, Syrenicz A, Szymkowiak K, *et al.* Justification of the gluten-free diet in the course of Hashimoto's disease. Nutrients 2022; 14(9): 1727.
[http://dx.doi.org/10.3390/nu14091727] [PMID: 35565695]

[63]   Groenewegen KL, Mooij CF, van Trotsenburg ASP. Persisting symptoms in patients with Hashimoto's disease despite normal thyroid hormone levels: Does thyroid autoimmunity play a role? A systematic review. J Transl Autoimmun 2021; 4: 100101.
[http://dx.doi.org/10.1016/j.jtauto.2021.100101] [PMID: 34027377]

[64]   Hu S, Rayman MP. Multiple nutritional factors and the risk of Hashimoto's thyroiditis. Thyroid 2017; 27(5): 597-610.
[http://dx.doi.org/10.1089/thy.2016.0635] [PMID: 28290237]

[65]   Al-Toma A, Volta U, Auricchio R, *et al.* European Society for the Study of Coeliac Disease (ESsCD) guideline for coeliac disease and other gluten-related disorders. United European Gastroenterol J 2019; 7(5): 583-613.
[http://dx.doi.org/10.1177/2050640619844125] [PMID: 31210940]

[66]   Dore MP, Fanciulli G, Rouatbi M, Mereu S, Pes GM. Autoimmune thyroid disorders are more prevalent in patients with celiac disease: A retrospective case-control study. J Clin Med 2022; 11(20): 6027.
[http://dx.doi.org/10.3390/jcm11206027] [PMID: 36294348]

[67]   Virili C, Bassotti G, Santaguida MG, *et al.* Atypical celiac disease as cause of increased need for thyroxine: a systematic study. J Clin Endocrinol Metab 2012; 97(3): E419-22.

[http://dx.doi.org/10.1210/jc.2011-1851] [PMID: 22238404]

[68] Malandrini S, Trimboli P, Guzzaloni G, Virili C, Lucchini B. What about tsh and anti-thyroid antibodies in patients with autoimmune thyroiditis and celiac disease using a gluten-free diet? A systematic review. Nutrients 2022; 14(8): 1681.
[http://dx.doi.org/10.3390/nu14081681] [PMID: 35458242]

[69] Szostak-Wegierek D, Bednarczuk T. The validity of gluten-free diet in Hashimoto's thyroiditis: Statement of the expert committee of the section of medical dietetics of the Polish Society for Parenteral, Enteral Nutrition and Metabolism (POLSPEN). Adv Clin Nutr 2018; 47: 33-47.

[70] Krysiak R, Szkróbka W, Okopień B. The effect of gluten-free diet on thyroid autoimmunity in drug-naïve women with Hashimoto's thyroiditis: A pilot study. Exp Clin Endocrinol Diabetes 2019; 127(7): 417-22.
[http://dx.doi.org/10.1055/a-0653-7108] [PMID: 30060266]

[71] Asik M, Gunes F, Binnetoglu E, et al. Decrease in TSH levels after lactose restriction in Hashimoto's thyroiditis patients with lactose intolerance. Endocrine 2014; 46(2): 279-84.
[http://dx.doi.org/10.1007/s12020-013-0065-1] [PMID: 24078411]

[72] Ruchała M, Szczepanek-Parulska E, Zybek A. The influence of lactose intolerance and other gastro-intestinal tract disorders on L-thyroxine absorption. Endokrynol Pol 2012; 63(4): 318-23.
[PMID: 22933169]

[73] Cellini M, Santaguida MG, Gatto I, et al. Systematic appraisal of lactose intolerance as cause of increased need for oral thyroxine. J Clin Endocrinol Metab 2014; 99(8): E1454-8.
[http://dx.doi.org/10.1210/jc.2014-1217] [PMID: 24796930]

[74] Marabotto E, Ferone D, Sheijani AD, et al. Prevalence of lactose intolerance in patients with Hashimoto thyroiditis and impact on LT4 replacement dose. Nutrients 2022; 14(15): 3017.
[http://dx.doi.org/10.3390/nu14153017] [PMID: 35893871]

[75] Song R, Wang B, Yao Q, Li Q, Jia X, Zhang J. The impact of obesity on thyroid autoimmunity and dysfunction: A systematic review and meta-analysis. Front Immunol 2019; 10: 2349.
[http://dx.doi.org/10.3389/fimmu.2019.02349] [PMID: 31681268]

[76] Toulis KA, Anastasilakis AD, Tzellos TG, Goulis DG, Kouvelas D. Selenium supplementation in the treatment of Hashimoto's thyroiditis: a systematic review and a meta-analysis. Thyroid 2010; 20(10): 1163-73.
[http://dx.doi.org/10.1089/thy.2009.0351] [PMID: 20883174]

[77] Wichman J, Winther KH, Bonnema SJ, Hegedüs L. Selenium supplementation significantly reduces thyroid autoantibody levels in patients with chronic autoimmune thyroiditis: A systematic review and meta-analysis. Thyroid 2016; 26(12): 1681-92.
[http://dx.doi.org/10.1089/thy.2016.0256] [PMID: 27702392]

[78] Winther KH, Wichman JEM, Bonnema SJ, Hegedüs L. Insufficient documentation for clinical efficacy of selenium supplementation in chronic autoimmune thyroiditis, based on a systematic review and meta-analysis. Endocrine 2017; 55(2): 376-85.
[http://dx.doi.org/10.1007/s12020-016-1098-z] [PMID: 27683225]

SUBJECT INDEX

A

Acid(s) 26, 65, 92, 94, 146, 148, 149, 150
  amino 26
  chebulinic 92
  cinnamic 65
  docosahexaenoic 146
  Folic 94
  lipoic 148, 149, 150
Action 30, 31, 172
  anti-inflammatory 31
  coating 172
  immunosuppressive 30
Activation 11, 31, 33, 53
  inflammasome 31
  macrophage 33
  of cytokine-producing cells 11
  tyrosine kinase 53
Activities 26, 27, 29, 33, 37, 59, 61, 72, 90, 92, 93, 113, 114, 115, 116, 143, 148, 191, 207
  anti-inflammatory 26, 27, 72, 93, 113, 115, 207
  antibacterial 114
  anticancer 92
  anticholinesterase 148
  antiglycative 191
  antioxidant enzymes 59
  autoimmune 90
  catalase 61
  cytokine 29
  inflammatory 33, 37
  myeloperoxidase 116
  oligodendrocyte 143
Adipocytes 191, 206
Adipogenesis 206
Air pollution 7, 86, 108, 186
Alzheimer's disease 140, 188
AMPK activation and regulation 70
Anaerobic bacteria 161
Analgesic 12, 92, 138, 141, 142
  anti-diarrheal 141

Analgesic properties 169
Angiogenesis 27, 93
Anthelmintic agent 173
Anti-bacterial effects 113
Anti-diabetic effects 191
Anti-hemorrhoidal agent 168
Anti-inflammatory 13, 14, 26, 30, 32, 37, 68, 71, 85, 90, 101, 113, 114, 115, 137, 140, 141, 142, 144, 146, 148, 168, 170, 173
  agent 32, 142, 170
  drugs 101
  effects 26, 68, 90, 113, 114, 115, 141, 148, 168, 173
  properties 13, 14, 30, 37, 71, 85, 101, 137, 140, 144, 146
  effect 115
Anti-microbial effects 138
Anti-neuroinflammatory effects 139
Anti-ulcerogenic properties 170
Antiallergenic effects 171
Antibacterial effect 166
Antibodies 12, 13, 24, 30, 52, 53, 111
  antinuclear 24
Anticancer effects 147
Antidiabetic 48, 55, 56, 57, 58, 59, 60, 61, 62, 64, 65, 66, 73, 116
  agents 48
  effect 55, 56, 57, 58, 59, 60, 61, 62, 64, 65, 66, 73
  properties 116
Antimicrobial 10, 92, 114, 159, 171, 174
  activities 114
  effect 114
  peptides 10
  properties 171
Antioxidant 13, 14, 67, 68, 70, 71, 72, 91, 92, 114, 115, 128, 142, 143, 144, 146, 148, 159, 189, 200, 205, 206, 207
  enzymes 72
  genes 205, 206
  natural 148
  properties 67, 91, 128, 143, 146, 200

T

U

www.ingramcontent.com/pod-product-compliance
Lightning Source LLC
Chambersburg PA
CBHW050832220326
41598CB00006B/359